From Competence to Excellence in Gastroenterology

THE STOMACH

A. B. R. Thomson

www.giandhepatology.com

athoms47@uwo.ca

FROM COMPETENCE TO EXCELLENCE
The Stomach

© A.B.R. Thomson

From Competence to Excellence in Gastroenterology

THE STOMACH

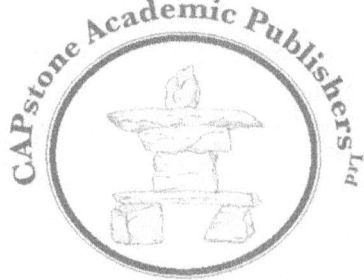

CAPstone (Canadian Academic Publishers Ltd) is a not-for-profit company dedicated to the use of the power of education for the betterment of all persons everywhere.

"For the Democratization of Knowledge"

© A.B.R. Thomson

ARE YOU PREPARING FOR EXAMS IN GENERAL INTERNAL MEDICINE OR IN GASTROENTEROLOGY AND HEPATOLOGY?

See the full range of examination preparation and review publications from CAPstone on Amazon.com

For no cost viewing, please consult: www.giandhepatology.com

Gastroenterology and Hepatology

First Principles of Gastroenterology and Hepatology in Adults and Children – Volume I - Gastroenterology, 7th edition (ISBN: 978-1494345624).

First Principles of Gastroenterology and Hepatology in Adults and Children - Volume II - Hepatology and Paediatrics, 7th edition (ISBN: 978-1494345501).

GI Practice Review, 2nd edition (ISBN: 978-1475219951).

Endoscopy and Diagnostic Imaging Part I (ISBN: 978-1477400579).

Endoscopy and Diagnostic Imaging Part II (ISBN: 978-1477400654).

Scientific Basis for Clinical Practice in Gastroenterology and Hepatology (ISBN: 978-1475226645).

Guideline–Based Therapy in Gastroenterology and Hepatology.

General Internal Medicine

Achieving Excellence in the OSCE. Part I. Cardiology to Nephrology (ISBN: 978-1475283037).

Achieving Excellence in the OSCE. Part II. Neurology to Rheumatology (ISBN: 978-1475276978).

Bits and Bytes for Rounds in Internal Medicine (ISBN: 978-1478295365).

Mastering the Boards and Clinical Examinations. Part I. Cardiology, Endocrinology, Gastroenterology, Hepatology and Nephrology (ISBN: 978-1461024842).

Mastering the Boards and Clinical Examinations. Part II. Neurology to Rheumatology (ISBN: 978-1478392736)

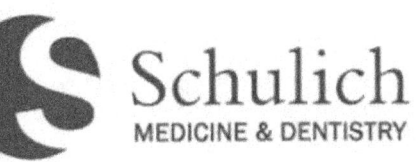 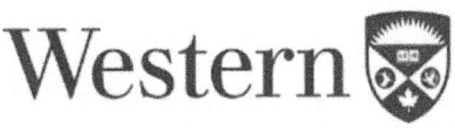

THE WESTERN WAY

FROM COMPETENCE TO EXCELLENCE
The Stomach

© A.B.R. Thomson

DISCLAIMER

The primary purpose of this publication is education. The author, editor and publisher acknowledge that the development of new material opens to way for possible errors – what is correct today might not be the standard of care tomorrow. Readers are advised to ensure that the doses of drugs which they use are in compliance with their country's product information, and that the use of any therapeutic agent, be it a pharmaceutical or a technology, should be guided by local guidelines. There is often a wide diversity of professional opinion, and guidelines from one country are not always congruent with another.

The authors, editor and publisher do not guarantee the safety, reliability, accuracy, completeness or usefulness of this material.

They disclaimer any and all liability for damage and claims that may result from the use of information, publications, technologies, products, and for series provided in this publication.

We have made every attempt to trace the holders of copyright for material reproduced in this book. If by some oversight we have omitted a copyright holder, please contact us.

Thank you

A. B. R. Thomson

FROM COMPETENCE TO EXCELLENCE
The Stomach

© A.B.R. Thomson

TABLE OF CONTENTS

Disclaimer	vi
GI Practice Review and The CANMED Objectives	xi
Acknowledgements	xv
Dedication	xvii

STOMACH	**1**
Gastric Anatomy	3
General Comments	6
Gastric Function	11
Immunohistochemistry (Immunostains) for Diagnosis of Gastric Pathology	11
Special Stains for Diagnosis of Gastric Pathologies	12
Immunostaining of Gastric Tumors	13
Gastric Acid Secretion	14
Redundant and overlapping pathways for acid secretion and inhibition	14
Fasting – Basal Gastric Acid Secretion	24
Turning "ON" Acid Secretion - Stimulated Gastric Acid Secretion	26
Neurocrine ("direct") pathway	26
Phases of Gastric Acid Secretion	27
Gastric Hydrochloric Acid Secretion at the Parietal Cell (Cellular) Level	29
Acid Rebound	33
Pharmaceutical Control of Acid Secretion	33
Hypergastrinemia: Gastrin and Disorders of Acid Secretion	35
Gastric Pepsinogen and Pepsin	39
Dyspepsia	43
Dyspepsia and Pregnancy	50
H. pylori Infection and Peptic Ulcer Disease (PUD)	51
Helicobactor pylori–Negative Peptic Ulcer Disease	67
Helicobactor pylori–Positive Peptic Ulcer Disease	68
Zollinger–Ellison Syndrome (ZES)	71
Acute Non–Variceal Upper GI Bleeding (NVUGIB; UGIB)	80
"Visible Vessel"	89
Recurrent and Persistent Ulcer Bleeding	100
Upper GI Bleeding from Possible Esophageal or Gastric Varices	104
Obscure GI Bleeding	107
Non–Steroidal Anti–Inflammatory Drugs (NSAIDs)	112

FROM COMPETENCE TO EXCELLENCE
The Stomach

© A.B.R. Thomson

Bariatric Surgery	124
Post–Operative Stomach	128
Obesity	136
Gastric Emptying and gastroparesis	140
Antral Filling and Pyloric Pump	164
Causes of Gastric Scarring and Slowed Gastric Emptying	169
Diabetes and Gastroparesis	170
Nausea and Vomiting	172
Post-operative Nausea and Vomiting	173
Vascular Lesions	182
Gastric Varices (GV)	182
Portal Hypertension Gastropathy (PHG)	185
Gastric Dieulafoy Lesion	190
Gastric Antral Vascular Ectasia (GAVE; Watermelon Stomach)	191
Acute Gastritis and Gastropathies	195
Environmental Multifocal Atrophic Gastritis (EMAG)	203
Autoimmune Metaplastic Atrophic Gastritis, Diffuse Corporal Atrophic Gastritis (AMAG and DCAG) or Type A Gastritis	203
Phlegmonous Gastritis	204
Collagenous Gastritis	210
NSAID–Induced Mucosal Damage	217
Carditis	220
Gastric Epithelial Dysplasia (GED)	221
Allergic Gastroenteropathy	224
Disseminated Eosinophilic Collagen Disease	224
Hypereosinophilic Syndrome (HES)	225
Active Chronic Antral Gastritis With Lymphoid Hyperplasia	225
Diffuse Antral Gastritis	226
Acute Erosive and Hemorrhagic Gastritis	227
Chronic Gastritis	231
Chronic Atrophic Gastritis of Body	233
Diffuse Corporal Atrophic Gastritis	234
Enterogastric Reflux Gastritis	235
Helicobacter Pylori (*H. pylori*)–Associated Gastritis	239
Autoimmune Gastritis (Autoimmune Metaplastic Atrophic Gastritis)	246
Gastritis Cystica Polyposa	251
Infectious Gastritis	252
Candidiasis	252
Cytomegalovirus (CMV)	255
Mycobacterial Gastritis	259

Suppurative (Phlegmonous) Gastritis	259
Granulomatous Gastritis	260
Lymphocytic Gastritis	264
Gastropathies causing Thickening of Gastric Folds	269
Ménétrier's Disease (MD)	271
Congestive Gastropathy	277
Hypertrophic Gastropathy (from Zollinger–Ellison syndrome)	277
Gastric Mucosal Calcinosis (GMC; Aluminocalcinosis)	280
Gastric Neoplasm	**281**
Gastric Polyps	281
Hyperplastic Fundic Polyp (HFuP)	283
Hyperplastic Foveolar polyp (HFoP)	283
Tumor–Like Lesion	283
Benign Gastric Ulcer	291
Fundic Gland Polyps	298
Gastric Neuroendocrine Tumors (NET)	305
Gastric Adenomas	313
Pyloric Gland Adenomas	317
Polyposis Syndromes	318
Gastritis Cytica Polyposa	319
Hyperplastic polyps (HP)	320
Gastric Foveolar Adenoma	324
Gastric Adenocarcinoma	326
Early Gastric Cancer (EGC)	357
Gastric Lymphoma	363
Gastric MALT Lymphoma	367
Gastric Diffuse Large B–Cell Lymphoma (DLBCL)	369
Burkitt Lymphoma	371
Gastric Stump Carcinoma	373
Stromal Tumors and Tissue Eosinophils	**376**
Inflammatory Fibroid Polyps (IFP)	378
Eosinophilic Gastritis	382
Allergic Gastroenteropathy	390
Disseminated Eosinophilic Collagen Disease	390
Hypereosinophilic Syndrome (HES)	390
Gastrointestinal Stromal Tumors (GIST)	391
Sunitinib	402
Sorafenib	403
Leiomyoma	404

FROM COMPETENCE TO EXCELLENCE
The Stomach

© A.B.R. Thomson

Heterotopia and Metaplasia	406
Pancreatic Heterotopia (Pancreatic Ectopia or Rest)	407
Paneth Cell Metaplasia	410
Thickened Basement Membrane	411
Apparent Fibrosis of Lamina Propria	411
Gastric Amyloid	412
Miscellaneous Gastric Conditions	418
Foamy Macrophages	420
Gastric Xanthomas	420
Signet-Ring Cell Carcinoma	427
Abbreviations	428
Suggested Reading	434
Index	440

Available at no cost online at www.giandhepatology.com

Photomicrographs available in colour at www.giandhepatology.com

FROM COMPETENCE TO EXCELLENCE
The Stomach

© A.B.R. Thomson

GI PRACTICE REVIEW AND THE CANMED OBJECTIVES

Medical expert
The discussion of complex cases provides the participants with an opportunity to comment on additional focused history and physical examination. They would provide a complete and organized assessment. Participants are encouraged to identify key features, and they develop an approach to problem-solving.

The case discussions, as well as the discussion of cases around a diagnostic imaging, pathological or endoscopic base provides the means for the candidate to establish an appropriate management plan based on the best available evidence to clinical practice. Throughout, an attempt is made to develop strategies for diagnosis and development of clinical reasoning skills.

Communicator
The participants demonstrate their ability to communicate their knowledge, clinical findings, and management plan in a respectful, concise and interactive manner. When the participants play the role of examiners, they demonstrate their ability to listen actively and effectively, to ask questions in an open–ended manner, and to provide constructive, helpful feedback in a professional and non-intimidating manner.

Collaborator
The participants use the "you have a green consult card" technique of answering questions as fast as they are able, and then to interact with another health professional participant to move forward the discussion and problem solving. This helps the participants to build upon what they have already learned about the importance of collegial interaction.

Manager
The participants are provided with assignments in advance of the three day GI Practice Review. There is much work for them to complete before as well as afterwards, so they learn to manage their time effectively, and to complete the assigned tasks proficiently and on time. They learn to work in teams to achieve answers from small group participation, and then to share this with other small group participants through effective delegation of work. Some of the material they must access demands that they use information technology effectively to access information that will help to facilitate the delineation of adequately broad differential diagnoses, as well as rational and cost effective management plans.

Health advocate
In the answering of the questions and case discussions, the participants are required to consider the risks, benefits, and costs and impacts of investigations and therapeutic alliances upon the patient and their loved ones.

Scholar
By committing to the pre- and post-study requirements, plus the intense three day active learning GI Practice Review with colleagues is a demonstration of commitment to personal education. Through the interactive nature of the discussions and the use of the "green consult card", they reinforce their previous learning of the importance of collaborating and helping one another to learn.

Professional
The participants are coached how to interact verbally in a professional setting, being straightforward, clear and helpful. They learn to be honest when they cannot answer questions, make a diagnosis, or advance a management plan. They learn how to deal with aggressive or demotivated colleagues, how to deal with knowledge deficits, how to speculate on a missing knowledge byte by using first principals and deductive reasoning. In a safe and supportive setting they learn to seek and accept advice, to acknowledge awareness of personal limitations, and to give and take 360^0 feedback.

Knowledge
The basic science aspects of gastroenterology are considered in adequate detail to understand the mechanisms of disease, and the basis of investigations and treatment. In this way, the participants respect the importance of an adequate foundation in basic sciences, the basics of the design of clinical research studies to provide an evidence-based approach, the designing of clinical research studies to provide an evidence-based approach, the relevance of their management plans being patient-focused, and the need to add "compassionate" to the Three C's of Medical Practice: competent, caring and compassionate.

"They may forget what you said, but they will never forget how you made them feel."

Carl W. Buechner, on teaching.

"With competence, care for the patient. With compassion, care about the person."

Alan B. R. Thomson, On Being a Physician.

PROLOGUE

Like any good story, there is no real beginning or ending, just an in-between glimpse of the passing of time, a peek into a reality of people's minds, thoughts, feelings, and beliefs. The truth as I know it has a personal perspective which drifts into the soul of creation. When does life begin, when does an idea become conceived, when do we see love or touch reality? A caring, supportive, safe, and stimulating environment creates the holding blanket, waiting for the energy and passion of those who dream, invent, create – disrupt the accepted, challenge the conventional, ask the questions with forbidden answers. Be a child of the 60's. Just as each of us is a speck of dust in the greater humanity, the metamorphosis of the idea is but a single sparkle in the limitlessness of the Divine Intelligence. We are the ideas, and they are us. No one of us is truly the only parent of the idea, for in each of us is bestowed the intertwined circle of the external beginning and the end....

...during a visit to the Division of Gastroenterology at the University of Ottawa several years ago, the trainees remarked how useful it would be to have more than two hours of learning exchange, a highly interactive tutorial with concepts, problem solving, collegial discussion, the fun and joys of discovery and successes. Ms. Jane Upshall of BYK Canada (Atlanta, Nycomed), who had sponsored two of these visiting Professorships, encouraged the possibility of the development of a longer program. Her successor, Lynne Vachon, supported the initial three day educational event for the trainees enrolled in the GI training program at the University of Ottawa. With her entrepreneurial foresight, wisdom, and enthusiasm, the idea began. Lynne's commitment to an event which benefited many of the future clinicians, who will care for ourselves and our loved ones, took hold. Then, thanks to the GI program directors in Ottawa and the University of Western Ontario, Nav Saloojee and Jamie Gregor, more trainees were exposed, future GI fellows talked with other trainees, and a grass roots initiative began. Had it not been for Nav and Jamie's willingness to take a risk on something new, had they not believed in me, then there would have been no further outreach. Thank you, Lynne, Nav, and Jamie. You were there at the beginning. I needed you.

By 2008, all but one GI program in the country gave their trainees time off work to participate in the three day event, GI Practice Review (GI-PR). The course is 90% unsponsored, and is gratis to the participants, (except for the cost of their enthusiastic participation!) I am happy to give back to the subspecialty that gave me so much for 33 years. I hope GI-PR is helpful to all trainees. I know that from these future leaders there will arise those who will continue to dedicate and donate their time, energy, and ability to the betterment of those who contribute to the continued improvement of our medical profession. The clinicians, the teachers, the researchers.

In the short span of ten years, more than 400 GI residents, coming from all the 14 training programs in Canada, have participated in the small group sessions in the GI practice review. I thank the training program directors who have supported GI-PR. Special appreciation as well to their many staff physicians who worked without their trainees for the three days of each program.

The idea for the electronic and hard copy summary of the "list of facts" came from the trainees who wished for an aide memoir. But the GI-PR is about more than lists and facts - it is about problem formulation, case discussions, review of endoscopy, histopathology, motility, diagnostic imaging. It is about having fun working together to learn. The subterfuge to gain interest in the basic sciences is the use of clinical scenarios to show the way to the importance of first principles. While the lists are here, the experience is in the performance.

The child will grow, the images will expand, the learning of all aspects of our craft will develop and flourish amongst persons of good will. Examinations will become second nature, as each clinical encounter, each person, each patient, becomes our test, the determination of clinical competence, of caring, of compassion. May these three C's become part of each of our life's narrative. And from this start comes Capstone Academic Publishing, an innovation for the highest quality and value in educational material, made available at cost, speaking in tongues, in the languages of many cultures, with the dialect of the true North strong and free, so that knowledge will be free at last.

Outstanding medical practice and true dedication to those from whom we receive both a privilege and pleasure of care, comes from much more than the GI-PR can give you, much more than Q & As, descriptions of diagnostic imaging or endoscopy stills or videos, histopathology or motility. True, we need all of these to jump over a very high bar. But to be a truly outstanding physician, you need to care for and care about people, and you must respect the dignity and rights of all others. You must strike a balance between love and justice, and you place your family and friends at the top of your wish-list of lifetime achievements.

For the skeptics who ask "What do you want from me?" I simply say "You are the future; I trust that in time you too will help young people to be the best they can be."

May good luck, good health, modesty, peace, and understanding be with you always. Through medicine, all persons of the world may come to share caring, respect, dignity, and justice.

Sincerely,

Alan Thomson

Emeritus Distinguished University Professor, U of A

Adjunct Professor, Western University, London, Canada

ACKNOWLEDGEMENTS

Patience and patients go hand in hand. So also does the interlocking of young and old, love and justice, equality and fairness. No author can have thoughts transformed into words, no teacher can make ideas become behavior and wisdom and art, without those special people who turn our minds to the practical - of getting the job done!

Thank you, Naiyana, for translating those scribbles (called my handwriting), into the still magical legibility of the electronic age. Sarah, thank you for your hard work and creativity.

My most sincere and heartfelt thanks go to the excellent persons at JP Consulting, and CapStone Academic Publishers. Jessica, you are brilliant, efficient, dedicated, and caring. Thank you most sincerely.

When Rebecca, Maxwell, Megan, Henry, Felix, Toby, Grady, and Jasper, ask about their Grandad, I will depend on James and Anne, Matthew and Allison, Jessica and Matt, and Benjamin to be understanding, generous, kind and forgiving. For what I was trying to say and to do was to make my professional life focused on the four C's and an "H"; competence, caring, compassion, and composure, as well as humour - and to make my very private personal life dedicated to family - to you all.

FROM COMPETENCE TO EXCELLENCE
The Stomach

© A.B.R. Thomson

DEDICATION

Dedicated to Jeannette Rita Cécile Mineault

My life began when I met you:

Your wit, your charm, your laughter,

Your love for children, your caring, your common sense.

As always, all ways, thank you for saying I do.

_ _ _ _ _ _ _ _ _ _

For the parents who gave us life

For the children and gradchildren who give us hope

For the teachers who gave us knowledge

For the partners who give us confidence, encouragement and meaning

FROM COMPETENCE TO EXCELLENCE
The Stomach

© A.B.R. Thomson

STOMACH

PRACTICE REVIEW
GASTROENTEROLOGY

© *A.B.R. Thomson*

FROM COMPETENCE TO EXCELLENCE
The Stomach

© *A.B.R. Thomson*

GASTRIC ANATOMY

Useful background: Gastric Anatomy
- Surface of the stomach is lined by mucous surface cells (MSC)
- Surface epithelium is invaginated to form gastric pits (foveolae)
- There is 1 gastric pit to 4 – 5 gastric glands

- Types of gastric glands
  - Cardiac glands
    - Branched and tortuous
    - Cell types
      - Mucous
      - Endocrine
      - Undifferentiated
  - Parietal glands (oxyntic or fundic) glands
    - Straight and tubular
    - Parts
      - Isthmus cells
        - Mucous
      - Neck cells
        - Mucous
        - Parietal
      - Base cells
        - Chief
        - Mucous
        - Parietal
    - Cell types
      - Chief (zymogen)
      - Mucous neck
      - Endocrine
      - Undifferentiated

- Pyloric (antral) glands
  - Coiled
  - Basilar cytoplasm
  - Cell types
    - Mucous
    - Endocrine

Comparison of enterochromaffin cells (EC) *vs* enterochromaffin–like (ECL) cells

	EC	ECL
Stain with silver		
– With reducing agent	–	+
– Without reducing agent	+	–
Contents		
– Serotonin	+	–
– Histamine	–	+
– Gastrin, somatostatin	–	+

> Diagnostic imaging

CT scan of the stomach, small and large bowels

- Position
- Distention
- Wall thickening
- Fold thickness
- Mesentery
- Enhancement

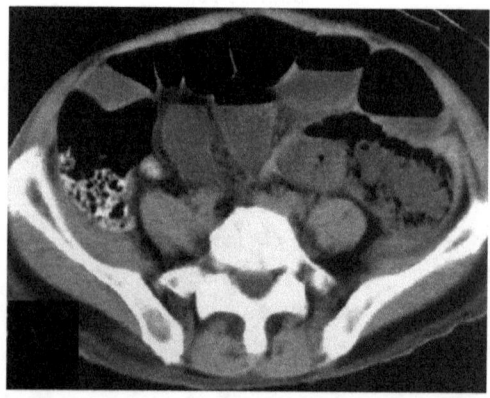

➤ Endoscopy

- What are the histological counterparts of the 5 layers of the GI tract wall seen on endoscopic ultrasound (EUS)?

	Histology	Colors	EUS layers
o Epithelial layers			
- Superficial	Mucosa	W white (hyperechoic)	1
- Deep	M. mucosa	B black (hypoechoic)	2
	Submucosal	W white	3
	M. propria	B black	4
	Serosa	W white	5

- Name the most common GI tumors in each GI stomach layers seen on EUS.

EUS layers	Tumors
2	o GIST
	o ECL
3	o Lipoma
	o ECL
4	o GIST
	o Glomus
	o Schwannoma

FROM COMPETENCE TO EXCELLENCE
The Stomach

© A.B.R. Thomson

> Histopathology

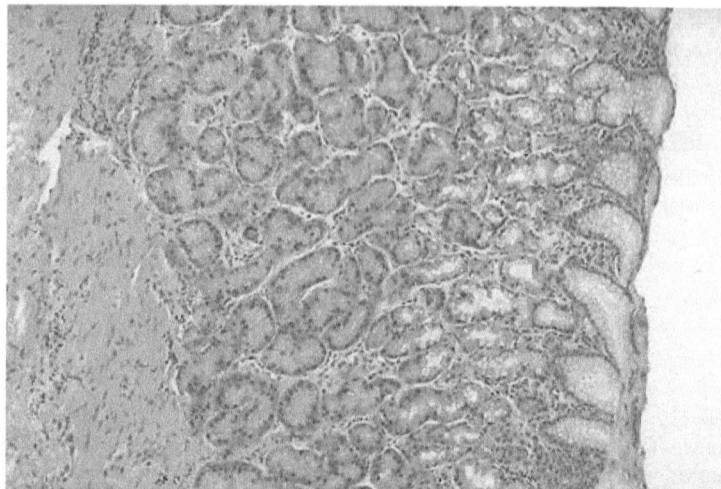

Normal appearance of the gastric fundal mucosa with short pits lined by pale columnar mucus cells into the long glands containing bright pink parietal cells that secrete hydrochloric acid.

http://library.med.utah.edu/WebPath/GIHTML/GI186.html

General Comments
- Foveolar cell hyperplasia represents a reaction to an injurious event, i.e. inflammation
- Pyloric cells with stacks of mucin → "pseudogoblet cells"
- Granulation tissue represents a response to injury
- Epithelial–like cells forming granuloma
- Non–necrotizing granuloma → think sarcoidosis
- Use polarized light to see if the refraction suggests a foreign body causing granulomatous reaction
- No globlet cells
- Lymphocytes → lymphoid aggregates → germinal centers → H. pylori chronic gastritis

- Positive toluidine blue, immunostain, silver (Warthin–Starry) stain, giemsa stain → *H. pylori*
- Distinguishing between type I and II intestinal metaplasia, based on the different types of mucin, has no predictive value; thus, is of little clinical use

➢ Goblet cells (look like stacked test tubes)
  o Mucin in columnar cells of duodenum – suggests gastric metaplasia
  o *H. pylori* can adhere to gastric metaplasia in duodenum (normally *H. pylori* does not adhere to duodenal mucosa, unless there is associated gastric metaplasia)
  o Immunostaining makes *H. pylori* look brown
  o Immunostaining gives greater sensitivity and specificity for diagnosis of *H. pylori*
  o *Helicobacter* species other than *H. pylori* can cause metaplasia
  o Stomach
    - Mucin (clear light pink)
    - Intracellular
    - Keratin (darker pink) intracellular
    - Extracellular, diffuse
      ▪ Amyloid in stroma, blood vessels
      ▪ Congo red stain, in amyloid becomes apple–green with birefringence
  o Corkscrew appearance in stomach
    - Think reactive gastropathy
    - Wisps of smooth muscle
  o Glands in stomach – secrete acid, mucin
  o Red stained cells, think parietal cells
  o Purple and blue cells, think chief cells
- Wharton – Starry stain for *H. pylori*
- Signet ring cells
  o Signet ring morphology in biopsies from gastric cardia may occur with Barrett epithelium, or in adenocarcinoma of the esophagus
  o Positive mucin stain; mucin pushes the nucleus to side of cell
  o Perinuclear halo from the Golgi

- Normal body and fundus
    - Foveolar compartment contains foveolae and gastric pits (1) covered by a layer of insoluble mucin
    - Pits are lined by columnar cells with abundant pale, eosinophilic cytoplasm containing mucin
    - Straight, parallel, evenly spaced tubular glands extend from the bases of the pits (2)
    - Mucous neck cells are concentrated near the neck, parietal cells in the midportion and chief cells in the base of the glands
    - Occasional inflammatory cells in the lamina propria (3)
    - A dilated lymphatic channel (4) is above the muscularis mucosae

- Normal foveolar compartment
    - Foveolar cell cytoplasm is abundant and clear or eosinophilic, and the nuclei are small, round, regular, and basally oriented
    - Cells in the proliferative zone (junction) of the foveolae and glands have less cytoplasm, and nuclei appear more basophilic
    - Absent mitotic figures
    - Capillary network located directly beneath the surface of the epithelium contains occasional circulating neutrophils
    - Cellular components in the lamina propria include stromal cells and (5) rare plasma cells

- Normal Antrum
    - Foveolar and glandular ratio is about 1:1
    - Glandular compartment consists of coiled, irregularly spaced, mucin–secreting glands
    - Plasma cells, lymphocytes, and eosinophils are more frequent in the antrum than in the body*
    - Foveolar hyperplasia in reactive gastropathy
    - In addition to foveolar hyperplasia, the lamina propria is edematous.
    - Dilated capillaries and venules
    - No inflammatory exudate
    - Foveolar hyperplasia in active chronic gastritis
    - Inflammation expands in the lamina propria

- Neutrophils infiltrate the epithelium
- Foveolae are tortuous, while epithelial cells show reactive and regenerative changes

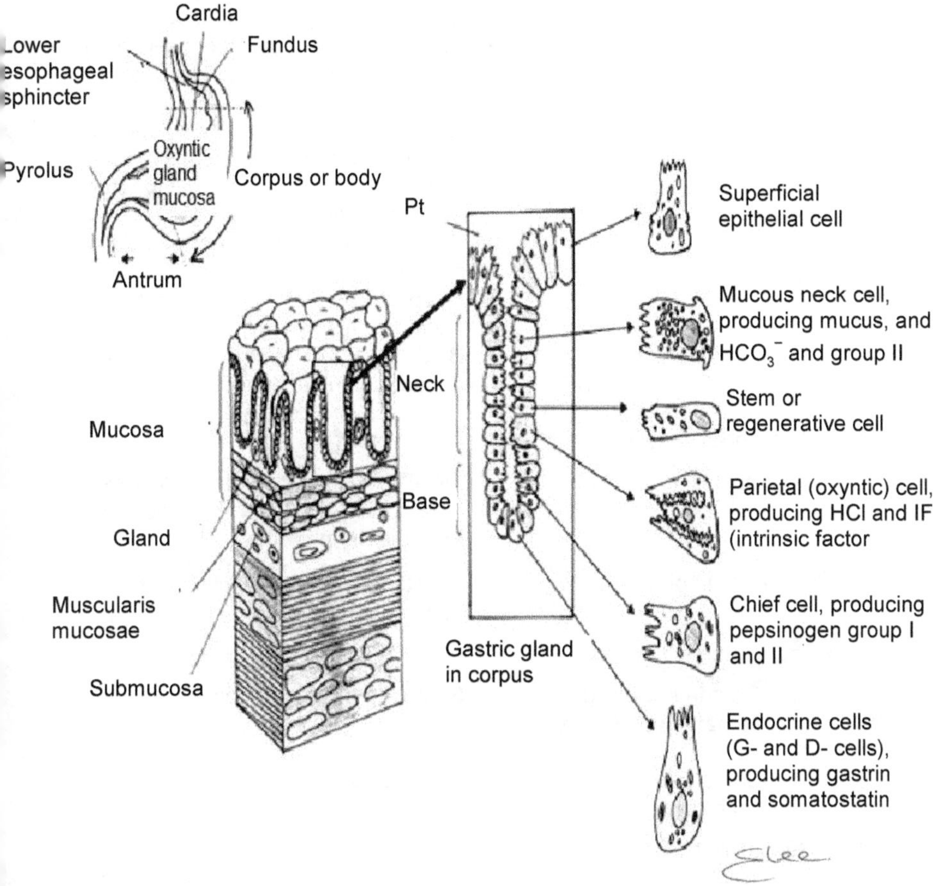

Adapted from: Boron–Walter, F. and Boulpaepemile, L. 2009. *Medical Physiology*. 2nd Edition, Figure 42-1, page 896.

- Name the cells of the stomach and their corresponding functions.

Cells	Functions
o Parietal (oxyntic) cells	
– Hydrochloric acid	• Provide optional pH for pepsin and gastric lipase (please see below) • Assist in duodenal inorganic iron absorption (reduction of food Fe^{3+} to Fe^{2+}) • Negative feedback of gastrin release (when intragastric acidity falls [↑ pH], serum gastrin concentration rises) • Stimulation of pancreatic HCO_3^- secretion • Suppression of the growth of microorganisms ingested in food
– Intrinsic factor	• Binding of vitamin B_{12} for subsequent ileal absorption
o Chief (peptic) cells	
– Pepsins	• Initial hydrolysis of dietary proteins • Liberation of vitamin B_{12} and Fe^{3+} from dietary proteins
o Superficial epithelial cells	• Maintain barrier function of the gastric membrane
o Endocrine cells	
– Gastrin secreting somatostatin G–cells	• Stimulate acid secretion
– Somatostatin secreting D–cells	• Inhibit acid secretion
o Mucous neck cells	
– Mucin and HCO_3^-	• Protection against noxious agents, including hydrochloric acid and pepsins

*In addition to assisting digestion and absorption of dietary proteins, hydrolysis of certain dietary proteins may render them harmless in individuals, who may be allergic to these proteins (i.e. pepsin may prevent the risk of developing certain food allergies)

> **SO YOU WANT TO BE A GASTROENTEROLOGIST!**
>
> The surfaces of the stomach and intestines possess several defense mechanisms, including trefoil factors.
>
> - What are the physiological effects of trefoil factors?
>   - Sources
>   - pS2
>   - Gastric mucus neck cells
>   - Spasmolysin
>   - Gastric antrum and pancreas
>   - Intestinal trefoil factor
>   - Goblet cells in the small intestines and colon
>   - Composition
>   - Cloverleaf shape
>   - 6 cysteine residues and 3 disulfide bonds
>   - Actions
>   - Secrete mucus in the mucosal surface
>   - Growth-promoting properties

Gastric Function

- Reservoir of food
- Synthesizing and secreting HCl and pepsinogen, as well as mucus and intrinsic factor
- Mixing of food with HCl and pepsinogen
- Control the release of partially digested food into the duodenum
- Assist in the control of appetite and food intake
- Gastric alcohol dehydrogenase metabolizes small amounts of ingested alcohol

In order to understand acid sensitive disease in the stomach, i.e. peptic ulcer disease causing gastric and duodenal ulcers, it is necessary to understand the initiation and termination of hydrochloric acid secretion at the organ and cellular levels.

IMMUNOHISTOCHEMISTRY (IMMUNOSTAINS) FOR THE DIAGNOSIS OF GASTRIC PATHOLOGY

IHC for infectious agent, i.e. *H. pylori*, CMV

Gastrin, chromogranin A, ECL hyperplasia

TGF–α	Ménétrier's disease
CD138	Amyloid precursors
K	Amyloid precursors
Λ	Amyloid precursors

Special Stains for the Diagnosis of Gastric Pathologies

Stains	Diagnosis
o Alizarin red	Calcium (gastric mucosal calcinosis)
o Chromogranin A	Pancreatic endocrine and islet cells
o Chymotrypsin	Pancreatic exocrine markers
o Congo red	Amyloid
o Genta stain	*H. pylori*
o Glucagon	Pancreatic endocrine and islet cells
o Insulin	Pancreatic endocrine and islet cells
o Lipase	Pancreatic exocrine markers
o Masson trichrome	Collagen
o Modified Giemsa	*H. pylori*
o Mucicarmine	Acidic mucin in goblet cells and signet ring cells
o Oil red	Lipid droplets
o Perioodic Acid Schiff (PAS) and Alcian blue (pH 2.5)	Mucin
o Potassium permanganate pretreatment and then Congo red	AA amyloid

Stains	Diagnosis
o Somatostatin	Pancreatic endocrine and islet cells
o Sudan black	Lipid droplets
o Sirius red, Sirius supra scarlet	Amyloid (red)
o Thioflavin T (fluorescent)	Amyloid
o Trypsin	Pancreatic exocrine markers
o Von Kossa	Calcium (gastric mucosal calcinosis)
o Warthin–Starry	*H. pylori*
o α–amylase	Pancreatic exocrine markers

Immunostaining of Gastric Tumors

IHC	Inflammatory fibroid polyp	Adenocarcinoma	NET
o CD34	+		
o Vimentin	+		
o Variable α–smooth muscle actin	+		
o Muscle specific actin	+		
o CD68	+		
o CEA		+	
o EMA		+	
o Variable CD7		+	
o Synaptophysin			+
o Chromogranin A			+
o Neuro–specific endolase			+

Abbreviation: NET, neuroendocrine tumor

GASTRIC ACID SECRETION

- What are the secretory cells of the stomach, and give one chemical, peptide or hormones that the cell secretes.
    - Goblet cells – mucus
    - Parietal cells – HCl, intrinsic factor
    - Chief cells – pepsinogen, gastric lipase
    - D–cells – somatostatin
    - G–cells – gastrin
    - Mast cells – histamine
    - Enterochromaffin–like cells – histamine

An understanding of the gastric parietal cell secretion of HCl and G–cell secretion of stimulatory gastrin, as well as D–cell secretion of inhibitory somatostatin, is important to understand the pathophysiology of UD, as well as the gastric effects of hypergastrinemia, including the ZES of the sporadic or MEN types.

Redundant and overlapping pathways for acid secretion and inhibition

- **Parietal cells**
    - Secretory vesicles are lined with membrane containing the H^+ / K^+ ATPase acid–secreting pump
    - With food stimulation, secretory vesicles traffic and incorporated into the luminal membrane of the parietal cells → forming secretory canaliculi
    - The pathway for K^+ to reach the H^+ / K^+ ATPase is in a short–circuited state during fasting
    - Upon stimulation, this pathway allows access of K^+ to the H^+ / K^+ ATPase exchange of H^+ for K^+ → HCl secretion
    - Parietal cell is stimulated by cephalic, gastric and intestinal components with activation occurring through the following:
        - ↑ Ca_i^{2+} (intracellular Ca^{2+})
        - ↑ cAMP → cAMP–dependent PK (protein kinase) cascade
    - When activation of the parietal cell ceases, or inhibition increases, the H^+ / K^+ ATPase in the parietal cell membrane moves back (reinternalization) into the cytoplasmic side of the cell
    - Reinternalization of the H^+ / K^+ ATPase occurs through the cytoplasmic tail of the β subunit of the enzyme

- **Acetylcholine**
  - Cephalic phase is responsible for about 30% of total stimulated acid secretion.
  - Gastric phase is responsible for about 60 – 65% of total stimulated acid secretion.
  1) Sites, smell, and tastes of food activate the dorsal motor nucleus (DMN) of the vagus nerve in the medulla
  - Distention of the gastric wall by food results to:
    - ↑ acid secretion by activating the vagal afferent and efferent pathways (vagovagal) and the ENS reflexes
  2) Parasympathetic preganglionic nerves release acetylecholine (Ach), gastrin–releasing peptide (GRP), and vasoactive intestinal peptide (VIP) neurons
  3) Ach binds to M3 receptors, which directly stimulates (+) parietal cells in the fundus (oxyntic mucosa), to secrete HCl
  - Hormonal ("indirect") pathway (release of gastrin from the G–cell, and its action on the CCK–2 receptor of the parietal cell, as well as the release of the gastrin–releasing peptide (GRP) from the vagus nerve, and the action of GRP on the G–cell
  - GRP from PPP or ENS neurons activated by luminal protein also stimulate gastrin secretion
  - Ach stimulates the antral G cells to release gastrin
  - Vagal Ach → D–cell secretion of SST
  - VIP neurons, activated by low grade gastrc distention, stimulate SST → inhibit gastrin secretion
  4) Ach and GRP stimulates (+) G–cells to release gastrin (G)
  - Distention of the stomach stimulates VIP neurons
    - ↑ SST
    - Gastrin
  - Further distention → ↑ Ach
    - Binds to M3 receptors in the parietal cells
      - ↑ gastrin
      - ↓ somatostatin (SST)
  - VIP stimulates (+) D–cells → release SST; Ach inhibits (-) D–cells → release SST
  6) Ach neurons stimulate gastrin secretion directly, as well as indirectly, by inhibiting SST secretion (thus, eliminating its restraint on gastrin–containing G–cells)

7) Gastrin binds to CCK-2 receptors in the BM of parietal cells to stimulate HCl secretion
8) Gastrin stimulates ECL cells to produce histamine
9) Histamine stimulates (+) parietal cells (↑ HCl) and inhibits (-) H3 receptors in the D-cells (↓ SST)

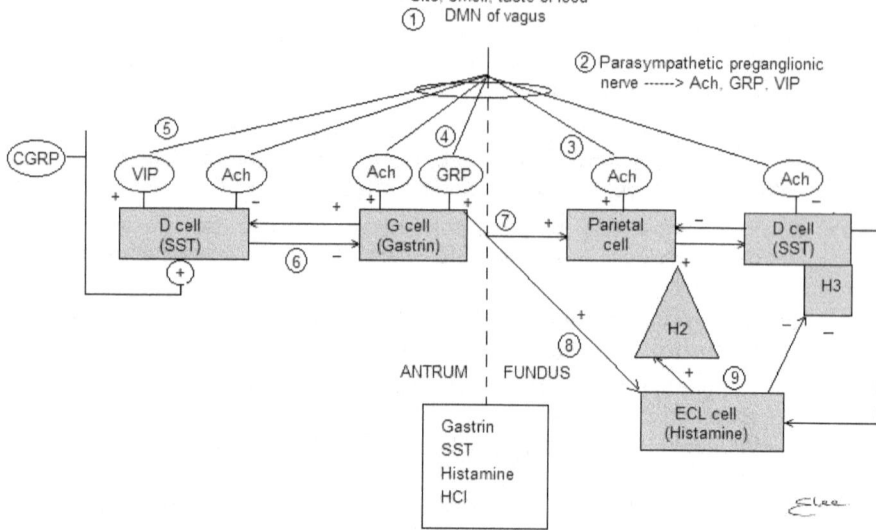

Abbreviations: Ach, acetylcholine; CGRP, calcitonin gene related peptide; ECL, enterochromafin-like cell; DMN, dorsal motor nucleus; GP, gastrin-releasing peptide; SST, somatostatin

- **Gastrin**
    - Gastrin is released from the G-cells in the gastric antrum due to:
        - Amino acids ([AA] protein and peptides) in the stomach
        - Distention of the stomach
    - Direct effect of AA → G-cells → ↑ gastrin
    - Indirect effects of AA
        - Activate Ach neurons
        - Activate GRP (gastrin related peptide) neurons → G cells → ↑ gastrin

- Gastrin binds to the following:
  - CCK–2 (CCK–B, or gastrin) receptors on
    - Parietal cells
    - ECL cells in body of stomach, adjacent to parietal cells
  - CCK–1 (CCK–A) receptors on D–cells, pancreas, gallbladder and the brain

Gastrin and their receptors (CCK–1 and CCK–2)

- Acute
  - Binds to CCK2 on
    - Parietal cells → ↑ secretion
    - Gastric ECL cells
  - ↑ synthesis of histamine in the ECL cells
  - ↑ release from the ECL cells of the following:
    - Histamine
    - Pituitary adenylate cyclase–activating polypeptide (PACAP)
    - Vasoactive intestinal peptides (VIP)
  - ↑ histamine binds to CCK1 receptors on the following
    - D cells → ↑ somatostatin (SST)
    - Gallbladder
    - Brain
    - ↑ somatostatin acts on G–cells → ↓ gastrin parietal cells → ↓ HCl
  - Paradoxical effects of gastrin
    - ↑ histamine release from ECL cells
      - ↑ HCl secretion
    - ↑ somatostatic release from D–cells
      - ↓ G release
      - ↓ HCl secretion
  - Major inhibitory mechanisms of somatostatin
    - ↓ gastrin–stimulated release of histamine from ECL cells
    - Antigens stimulate gastric mucosal mast cells → release of histamine

- Chronic
  - Causes hypertrophy of the parietal cells and ECL cells
- Hormonal ("indirect") Pathway

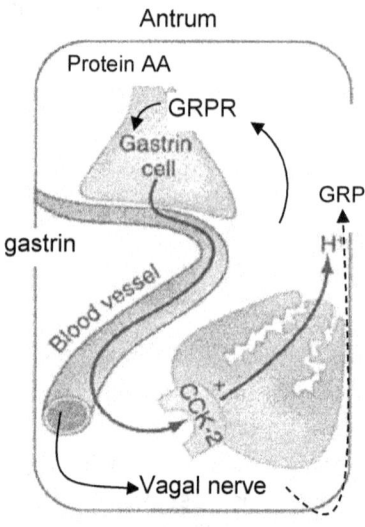

Hormonal

Abbreviations: CCK, cholecystokinin; GRPR, gastrin–releasing peptide receptor

- Products of protein digestion (i.e. peptides and amino acids)
  - Stimulate GRP (gastrin–releasing peptide) release from the vagal nerve endings
- GRP
  - Gastrin from the antral G–cells
  - Reduces the release of SST from the gastric body and antral D–cells
- Release of gastrin from the G–cells is mediated in the luminal and anti-luminal sides of the G–cell
- Gastrin, released from the antral G–cells, travels in the portal and to the systemic blood circulation to reach the parietal cells
- Gastrin binds to the CCK–2 receptor that directly activates CCK–2 receptors in the parietal cells → leading to the release of intracellular calcium (Ca^{2+}_i)
- This stimulates the post–translational modification of G–101 (101 amino acid containing gastrin) in the trans–Golgi apparatus of the endoplasmic reticulum (ER) of G–cells → resulting to G–17 and G–34

- - G–17 and G–34 are present as gastrin I (non–sulfated) and gastrin II (sulfated, respectively
  - In the plasma, G–17 is inherently more active, but is degraded faster than the less active but more slowly degraded G–34
  - Because of the differences in their inherent activity and rates of degradation in the plasma, G–17 and G–34 have similar potency, mole per mole
  - Parietal cell H^+ secretion is stimulated by way of CCK–B, Cq, PLC, IP3 and DAG
  - M3 and CCK–B receptors couple to a GTP–binding protein
  - GTP-binding protein receptor activates phospholipase C (PLC)

- **Histamine**
  - Ach and gastrin binding to the M3 and CCK–B receptors in the outer membrane of the enterochromafin–like cells (ECL) → release histamine from the ECL cells
  - Histamine released from oxyntic ECL cells diffuse to the parietal cells (paracrine effect), and ↑ release of GRP from peptidergic postganglionic
    - Parasympathetic (PPP) neurons
    - ENS neurons
  - Histamine released from the ECL and from the mast cells
    - Binds to histamine H2 receptor in the basolateral membrane (BM) of the parietal cell
  - Histamine coupled to Gls
    - Couples to Gls (another GTP–binding protein)
    - Activates adenyl cyclase (AC) to form cAMP
  - cAMP activates protein kinase A (PKA)
  - ↑ PKA → ↑ H^+ secretion

- **Somatostatin**
  o Acts by a paracrine pathway to ↓ gastrin release, which in turn ↓ acid secretion

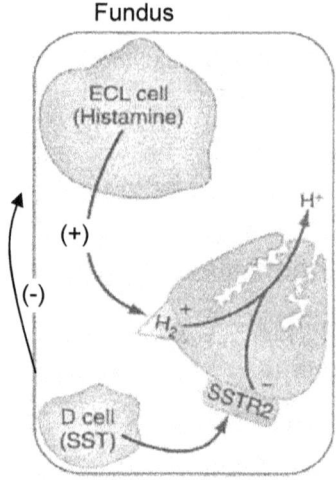

Adapted from: *Sleisenger and Fordtran's Gastrointestinal and Liver Disease*, Figure 49-1, page 818, 9th Edition, 2010.

  o H^+ in the stomach causes:
    - ↑ CGRP from extrinsic nerves → ↑ SST
  o H^+ has no effect on G–cells in the antrum
  o SST–28 is more abundant that SST–14
  o SST arises from the following:
    - D–cells in the gastric antrum and fundus
    - Duodenum
    - Islet cells of the pancreas
    - Neurons of the hypothalamus
  o SST inhibits the antral G–cell gastrin release → inhibits HCL secretion (protein → ↑ G, ↑ Ach, ↑ HCl, ↑ SST, ↓ G → ↓ HCl)
  o Alcohol, coffee, and peptones (partially digested protein) in the gastric lumen also stimulate the release of antral G–cell gastrin
  o SST binds to GI–coupled SSTR2
    - On basolateral membrane of the parietal cell → ↓ acid secretion (a redundant regulatory pathway)
    - On ECL cells and G–cells → tonically ↓ H^+ secretion

- This restraint is exerted
    - Directly in the parietal cell
    - Indirectly, by inhibiting histamine secretion from ECL cells and gastrin secretion from G–cells
- SST acts directly on ECL cells → ↓ histamine release, and thereby, to further ↓ acid secretion
- SST
    - ↓ antral gastrin release from antral G–cells
    - ↓ inhibits histamine release from ECL cells
- Histamine released from ECL cells act via H3 receptors on D–cells to inhibit SST secretion
- Acute infection with *Helicobacter pylori* also activates CGRP neurons → stimulate SST → inhibit gastrin secretion
- In duodenal ulcer patients, who are chronically infected with *H. pylori*, the organism or cytokines released from the inflammatory infiltrate inhibit SST → stimulate gastrin → secretion

Adapted from: *Sleisenger and Fordtran's Gastrointestinal and Liver Disease*. Figure 49-10, page 822, 9th Edition 2010.

- What are the factors responsible for the increase and/or decrease of the release of somatostatin from D–cells?

    - ↑ release (SST)
        - Gastric acidity (↑ H^+ → somatostatin → ↓ H^+ [feedback loop])
        - Minor distention of the stomach, acting through the VIP neurons
        - ↑ VIP activation
        - ↑ gastrin → ↑ somatostatin
            - ↓ ECL secretion of histamine
            - ↓ gastrin release

    - ↓ release
        - Major distention of the stomach
        - Ach

    - SST arises from D–cells in the gastric antrum and fundus, in the duodenum, in the islet cells of the pancreas, and by the neurons of the hypothalamus
        - SST is increased by luminal acid in the duodenum, but has no effects on the G–cells in the antrum
        - SST secretion is decreased by vagal Ach acting on the D–cell

- o SST binds to G1–coupled SSTR2 receptors in the parietal cells, as well as on the ECL cells and G–cells that tonically restrains acid secretion
- o This restraint is exerted directly on the parietal cell, as well as indirectly by inhibiting histamine secretion from ECL cells and gastrin secretion from G–cells
- o SST directly inhibits acid secretion by the parietal cells
  - SST and prostaglandin receptors for prostaglandin E2 (PGE2) couple to a GTP–binding protein in the BM of the parietal cell, (Gq, coupled with M3 receptor and CCKB receptor, Gs coupled by histamine–2 receptors, all in the cytosol of the parietal cell)
  - G1 inhibits the activity of Gs → reduces cAMP, PKA, and H^+–pumping by the canalicular membrane proton pump H^+, K^+–ATPase
  - PGE2 binds to EP3 (prostaglandin receptor) in the BM of parietal cell, PGE2–EP3 coupled to G1
  - Release of histamine from ECL cells
  - Binding of histamine to the H2 receptor of the parietal cell
  - Stimulation of acid secretion
  - Release of somatostatin from the D–cells
  - SST binds to the SSTR2 in the parietal cell → reducing acid secretion
  - SST reduces histamine release from the ECL cell
  - Neuroendocrine, hormonal, and paracrine pathways directly regulate parietal cell acid (H^+) secretion

- What peptides, other than somatostatin, inhibit acid secretion by ↓ ECL histamine release?

  - o Calcitonin gene–related peptide (CGRP)
  - o Peptide YY (PYY)
  - o Prostaglandins
  - o Galanin
  - o CCK–2 and CCK–2 receptors (G–protein–coupled receptors)
  - o Pertussis toxin–insensitive G–proteins
  - o Agonist stimulation of receptors

- **Prostaglandins**
  - Produced and stored in the gastric macrophages and capillary endothelial cells
  - ↓ acid secretion by inhibiting the following mechanisms:
    - ↓ gastrin–stimulated histamine release
    - ↓ histamine–stimulated parietal cell acid secretion
    - ↓ binding of histamine to H2 receptors
    - ↓ H⁺ secretion
    - ↓ SST release from D–cells

SO YOU WANT TO BE A GASTROENTEROLOGIST!

PYY is contained in the ECL cells in the terminal ileum and colon. Resection of the terminal colon (R. hemicolectomy) may be associated with increased gastric acid secretion, which sometimes results in diarrhea that responds to PPI–use.

- Explain the mechanism of surgically–induced increased acid secretion.
  - PYY inhibits gastrin–stimulated histamine release
  - This inhibition is lost with ileal resection and R. hemicolectomy

---

SO YOU WANT TO BE A GASTROENTEROLOGIST!

Histamine released from the ECL cells act on the H2–receptors in the basal membrane of the gastric body parietal cells → increasing HCl secretion.

- Explain the mechanism of action of H3 receptors altering gastric acid secretion.
  - Histamine stimulates H3 receptors to ↓ secretion of somatostatin from D–cells
    - ↓ somatostatin → ↓ inhibition of parietal cell acid inhibition (inhibits the inhibition, leading to stimulation)
    - ↑ HCl secretion

- **Other GI peptides**
  - Other peptides that inhibit acid secretion by ↓ ECL histamine release from ECL histamine release mechanism
    - Calcitonin gene-related peptide (CGRP)
    - Peptide YY (PYY)
    - Prostaglandins
    - Galanin
    - CCK-2 and CCK-2 receptors are G-protein-coupled receptors
    - Signaling by pertussis toxin-insensitive G-proteins
    - Agonist stimulation of receptors

➢ Distention
  - Initially, little distention
    - VIP neurons are activated to release somatostatin
    - Somatostatin inhibits antral G-cells
  - Then, more distention
    - Stimulation of the release of acetylcholine (Ach; cholinergic)
      - Directly stimulates M3 receptors in the parietal cell
      - ↑ gastrin
      - ↓ somatostatin

➢ AA in the stomach
  - Direct effects of AA → G cells → ↑ gastrin
  - Indirect effects of AA
    - Activate Ach neurons
    - Activate GRP neurons → G-cells → ↑ gastrin

Fasting Basal Gastric Acid Secretion
  - Gastric membrane permeability
    - Stomach produces large amount of acid (HCl), to start the digestion of food
    - Gastric membrane is designed to reduce back diffusion of acid into the wall of the stomach
    - Mucus is produced and released from the following:
      - Glands in the gastric antrum (a neutral glycoprotein)
      - Surface and neck cells containing both the neutral and acidic glycoproteins

- o Strong permeability or diffusion barrier for H^+ and Na^+ created by the following:
  - Tight junctions (TJs) between the gastric epithelial cells
  - Hydrophobicity of the lipid membranes of the cells
  - Secreted mucous and HCO_3^- from glands in the gastric antrum
  - Prostaglandins
  - Normal blood flow and capillary function
  - Normal cell proliferation
- o Alkaline microclimate adjacent to the gastric cellular membrane forms part of the unstirred water layer, which provides a pre–epithelial barrier to the back diffusion of HCl
- o Mucus is a viscous gel containing the following:
  - Water
  - Electrolytes
  - Phospholipids
  - Glycoproteins
- o Mucus is secreted as a result of Ach release from the vagus nerve
- o Vagus nerve is stimulated by irritation through:
  - Direct contact of food on the gastric mucosa
  - Indirect effects of chemicals, i.e. pickles and red peppers
- o Basal (interdigestive) gastric acid secretion
  - Basal acid output (BAO) is ~ 5 mEq/L
  - BAO is low in the morning and higher later in the day
  - BAO increases with the number of parietal cells, which increases in proportion to patient's body weight, and in response to chronic hypergastrinemia
  - Maximal stimulated acid secretion is also called the maximal acid output (MAO)
  - When gastric secretion is constantly stimulated, i.e. in patients with hypergastrinemia from Zollinger–Ellison Syndrome (ZES), the basal acid secretion is increased more than the stimulated secretion (BAO / MAO ~ 60%)

Turning "ON" Acid Secretion – Stimulated Gastric Acid Secretion

- Stimulated gastric HCl secretion
  - 3 pathways
    - Neurocrine (direct) pathway
    - Hormonal (indirect) pathway
    - Paracrine pathway
- Calcium
  - Phospholipase C (PLC) cleaves phosphatidyl inositol 4, 5–b1 phosphate (PIP2) in the BM of the parietal cell to inositol 1, 4, 5–triphosphate (IP3) and diacylglycerol (DAG)
  - IP3 releases Ca^{2+} stored in the endoplasmic reticulum of the cytosol of the parietal cell
  - M3 activates Ca^{2+} channel in the BM of the parietal cell, → further increase of the intracellular $Ca^{+2}[Ca^{+2}]i$
  - $Ca^{+2}{}_i$ is also increased from the Ca^{2+}–channels activating calmodulin-dependant protein kinase

Neurocrine ("direct") pathway
- Overlapping cephalic (CNS), gastric and intestinal phases, which enhance acid secretion
- Acetylcholine (Ach; neuronal stimulation), gastrin (hormonal) and histamine (paracrine) are the gastric stimulants
- Each of these have receptors (M3, CCK–B and histamine–2 receptors, respectively) on both, the parietal cells (direct pathway) and the enterochromafin cells, indirect pathway (ECL)

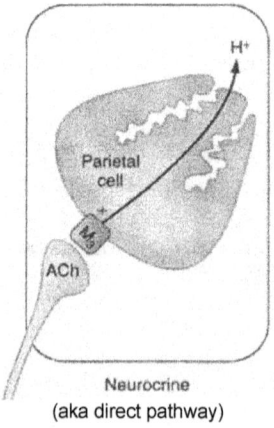

Parasympathetic preganglionic nerves

Neurocrine
(aka direct pathway)

Abbreviation: Ach, acetylcholine; M3, muscarinic receptor

Phases of Gastric Acid Secretion

➢ **Cephalic and Gastric Phases**

- Numerous peptide hormones produced by the GI tract involved in the regulation of gastric hydrochloric acid secretion

- Name the GI peptide hormones, their sources and action in the stomach.

Hormones	Sources	Actions
o Gastrin (G)	G–cells, antrum of stomach	↑ H^+ secretion
o Gastrin–releasing peptide (GRP)	Vagal nerve endings	↑ gastrin release
o Acetylcholine (Ach)	Vagal nerve endings	↑ HCL secretion
o Histamine	ECL cells; releases GRP from PPP and ENS neurons	↑ G from G–cells, ↓ SST from D–cells
o Secretin (S)	S–cells in small intestine	↑ HCO_3^- and fluid secretion by pancreatic ducts
o Somatostatin (SST)	D–cells of the stomach and duodenum, islet cells of pancreatic islets	↓ gastrin release
o Motilin	Endocrine cells in the upper GI tract	↑ smooth muscle contraction
o Peptide YY (PYY)	Endocrine cells in ileum and colon	↓ vagally mediated acid secretion

Printed with permission: Boron, Walter F. and Boulpaepemile, L. 2009. *Medical Physiology*. 2nd Edition, Table 41-1, page 889.

The Intestinal Phase

- Stimulation of Gastric and Acid Secretion
    - Protein digestion products (partially digested peptides and amino acids) stimulate duodenal G–cells to secrete gastrin, which stimulates the parietal cell
    - Protein digestion products act on an unknown intestinal endocrine cell to release an unknown hormone (named entero–oxyntin), which stimulates the gastric parietal cell to produce hydrochloric (HCl) acid
- Inhibition of Gastric Acid Secretion
    - In addition to the intestinal phase, which stimulates gastric acid secretion, there is an intestinal phase, which inhibits acid secretion
    - Loss of Gastric Stimulation
        - Loss of the stimulatory Ach, gastrin and histamine, as well as the emptying of the stomach and loss of gastric stimulatory signals, causes "inhibition" of the parietal cell acid secretion
- **Gastric Inhibitory Peptide** (GIP)
    - GIP is released from the K–cells in the duodenum and jejunum as the result of fat and glucose in the lumen
    - GIP reduces antral gastrin, and directly reduces acid secretion by the parietal cells
- **Secretin**
    - Fats, as well as acid in the duodenum, release secretion from S–cells in the small intestine
    - Gastric acid entering the duodenum initially causes an acidic environment in the lumen
    - As pH falls below 4.5, secretin is released from the duodenal S–cells
    - Secretin acts as an enterogastrone (inhibitor) in the intestinal phase of gastric acid secretion, inhibiting gastric parietal cell acid secretion
    - Secretion also stimulates pepsinogen secretion from the gastric chief cells
- **Prostaglandin E2** (PGE2)
    - PGE2
        - ↓ histamine from the ECL cells
        - ↓ gastrin release from the antral G–cells
- **Enterogastrones**

- In addition to SST, GIP, secretin and PGE2
  - Other enteric hormones (enterogastrones) inhibit gastric acid secretion
    - CCK
    - VIP
    - Gastric inhibiting peptide (GIP; better known as "glucose–dependent insulinotropic polypeptide")
    - Neurotensin (NT)
    - Peptide YY (PYY)

CLINICAL PHYSIOLOGICAL CHALLENGE – Turning Acid Secretion On and Off

- The stomach has a series of integrated control systems to mediate the secretion of HCl and pepsin to initiate the process of digestion of food.
- However, an excess of HCl and pepsin can damage the mucosa of the stomach and duodenum, causing ulceration with its associated problems of hemorrhage, obstruction and perforation.

• How stomach turns on and off hydrochloric (HCl) acid secretion?

- "Direct"

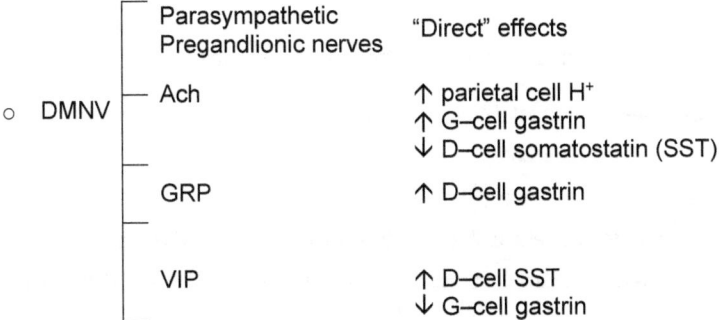

  - DMNV
    - Parasympathetic Pregandlionic nerves — "Direct" effects
    - Ach
      - ↑ parietal cell H^+
      - ↑ G–cell gastrin
      - ↓ D–cell somatostatin (SST)
    - GRP
      - ↑ D–cell gastrin
    - VIP
      - ↑ D–cell SST
      - ↓ G–cell gastrin

- "Indirect"
  - G–cell   Gastrin (G)   ↑ parietal cell H^+
  - D–cell   somatostatin (SST)   ↓ D–cell
  - ECL cell Histamine

Abbreviations: DMNV, dorsal motor nucleus of the vagus; CGRP, calcitonin gene–related peptide; SST, somatostatin

Gastric Hydrochloric Acid Secretion at the Parietal Cell (Cellular) **Level**

➤ Vocabulary of the components of parietal cell

Apical membrane	Cytosol	Basolateral membrane
H^+ / K^+ ATPase	Carbonic anhydrase (CA)	Na^+ / H^+ exchanger (NHE)
K^+ channel		Na^+ / K^+ ATPAse
Cl^- channel		K^+ channel
		Cl^- / HCO_3^- exchanger

➤ Requirements of the system
   o H^+ formed in the parietal cell is secreted across the apical membrane (AM)
   o Cl^- is needed to form HCl with H^+
   o Cl^- enters the parietal cell from the action in the basolateral membrane Cl^- / HCO_3^- exchanger
   o Cl^- leaves the cell through the AM Cl^- channel
   o The process is "energized" by the BM Na^+ / K^+ ATPase

See figure "Parietal Cell and H^+ Secretion"

QQQ4
- Explain the cellular acid secretion by the parietal cell.

   o Na^+ enters the parietal cell across the BM via any of the following:
      1) Na^+ / H^+ exchanger
      2) Na^+ / K^+ ATPase
   o K^+ enters the parietal cell across the BM by Na^+ / K^+ ATPase
      3) To avoid accumulation of K^+ in the parietal cell, K^+ may exit the parietal cell through the AM or BM K^+ channels
      4) CO_2 and water diffuse across the BM and into the cytosol of the parietal cell
      5) Carbonic anhydrase (CA) in the cytosol of the parietal cell forms H^+ plus HCO_3^- (from OH^- plus CO_2)
      6) Cl^- enters the parietal cell across the BM by the Cl^- / HCO_3^- exchanger
      7) The Cl^- needed to form HCl in the gastric lumen moves from the cytosol of the parietal cell across a Cl^- channel in the AM

PARIETAL CELL AND H⁺ SECRETION

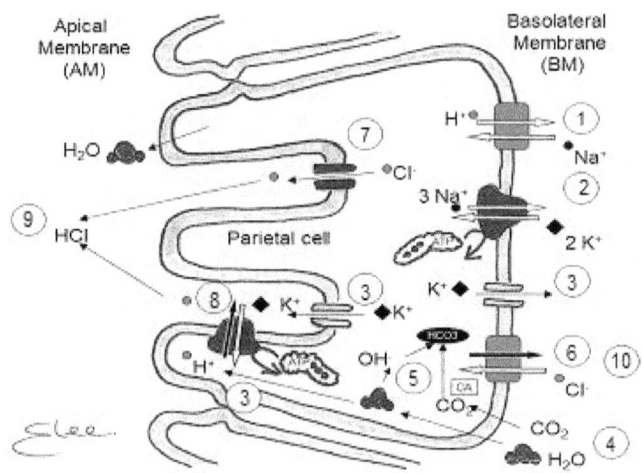

Adapted from: Boron, Walter F. and Boulpaepemile, L. 2009. *Medical Physiology*. 2nd Edition, Figure 42-4, page. 898.

8) Parietal cells in the gastric body have numerous tubulovesicles (TVs) containing inactive H^+ / K^+ ATPase ("the acid [or proton] pump")
   - Beta subunit of the H^+ / K^+ ATPase is the actual H^+ pump or catalytic unit
   - With stimulation of the parietal cell (neural, hormonal and paracrine factors), the activated PKA, PCA and Ca^{2+} activate H^+ / K^+ ATPase
   - Tubulovesicles (TVs) now contain activated H^+ / K^+ ATPase are inserted into the apical membrane (AM)
   - H^+ is actively secreted into the gastric lumen in exchange for K^+
   - H^+ in the cytosol of the parietal cell is removed by the proton pump from the AM, pumping H^+ into the external side of the AM

9) H^+ and Cl^- form HCl streaming through the overlying mucus and into the gastric lumen
   - Mucus layer reforms
     - Mucus layer prevents the back diffusion of HCl and pepsin towards the AM
   - Surface epithelial cells in the gastric body and antrum secrete HCO_3^-
   - HCO_3^- is trapped in the mucous or in unstirred water layer adjacent to the luminal side of the parietal cell AM

- This trapping of HCO_3^- in the mucus or in unstirred water layer form the alkaline microenvironment close to the AM
- This alkaline microclimate is protective to the luminal surface of the gastric cells, and thereby forms part of the diffusion or permeability barrier
- High concentration of H^+ in the gastric lumen does not readily diffuse through the mucus gel layer and in the alkaline microenvironment
- If any pepsin or acid manages to diffuse back into the mucous layer, pepsin becomes inactive because of the alkaline microclimate
- Back diffusion of acid from the gastric lumen into the cytosol of the parietal cell will also be partially neutralized

10 / 6) Cytosolic HCO_3^- formed from the CA effect on $CO_2 + H_2O$ exits across the BM by the Cl^- / HCO_3^- exchanger

Abbreviations: CCK, cholecystokinin; VIP, vasoactive intestinal peptide; PYY, peptide YY; ENS, enteric nervous system

---

CLINICAL PHYSIOLOGICAL CHALLENGE – Hypergastrinemia and Acid Hypersecretion

Case: A 35–year old man with dyspepsia and diarrhea have three ulcers in the second portion of the duodenum based on upper GI endoscopy. He did not take neither ASA nor NSAIDs, and his antral biopsies taken before acid lowering therapy were negative for *H. pylori*. A fasting serum gastrin concentration was 750 pg/ml. You suspect that he may be on gastric hypersecretory state.

Question:

- Explain the scientific basis of calcium infusion and secretin tests for Zollinger–Ellison Syndrome, and the rationale of measuring BAO and MAO to calculate the ratio BAO / MAO.

Abbreviations: BAO, basal acid output; MAO, maximal acid output

Acid Rebound

- Definition
  - An increase in acid secretion above the pretreatment values when an anti-secretory drug (i.e. PPI, H2RA) is suddenly discontinued
    - Magnitude of acid rebound usually ~ 15% may be sufficient to cause a post-treatment recurrence of symptoms

- Explain the pathophysiological mechanism(s) of acid rebound phenomenon occuring when an anti-secretory treatment is suddenly stopped.
  - Acid secretion inhibition → ↑ gastrin
    - Upregulation (hypertrophy or hyperplasia) of the following:
      - Parietal and G-cells (H^+ and gastrin)
      - Ach pathways
    - Down regulation of D-cells (somatostatin [SST])
  - Sudden stopping of PPIs
    - A given stimulus causes the following:
      - ↑ release of stimulatory gastrin and Ach
      - ↑ release of inhibitory SST

Pharmaceutical Control of Acid Secretion

Mechanism of Action of Proton Pump Inhibitors (PPIs)

1) PPIs are pro-drugs, coated to protect against damage by gastric HCl
2) PPI are rapidly absorbed in the upper small intestinal enterocytes and into the portal circulation where C_{max} of PPIs achieved in about 1 hour
3) PPIs reach the parietal cell from the portal and systemic bloodstreams and diffuse through the cytoplasm of the unstimulated, fasting and basal state parietal cell and accumulate in the acid environment of the secretory canaliculus
   - Proton pump (H^+ / K^+ ATPase) in the membrane of the canaliculi in the cytosol of the parietal cell is inactive during fasting, and does not bind to PPI or on its metabolites
4) With food intake, parietal cells are stimulated
   - In the stimulated state, canaliculi with inactive H^+ /K^+ ATPase ("inactive canaliculi") traffics to the AM of the parietal cell

5) In the stimulated active canaliculus, PPI becomes protonated and is trapped as a sulfenic acid, and then is degraded to sulfenamide (PPI–S)

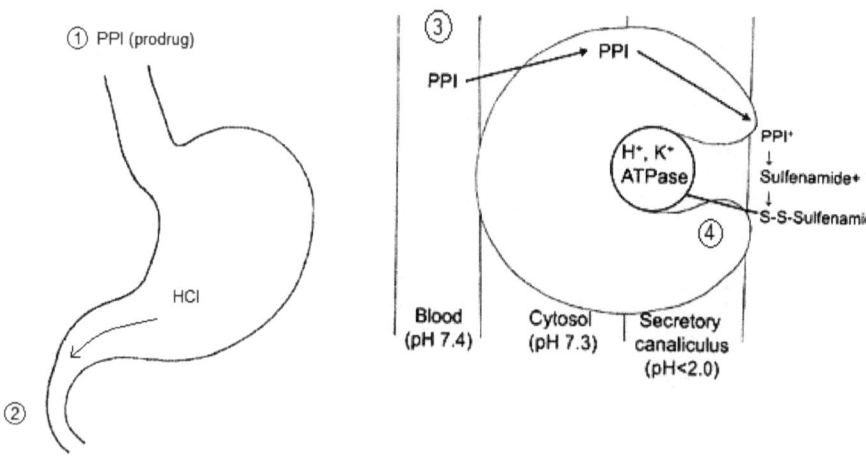

Adapted from: *Sleisenger and Fordtrans's Gastrointestinal and Liver Disease.* 10th ed. Philadelphia: Elsevier Saunders, 2016; Figure 50, page 849.

6) Canaliculi in the AM undergo a change in configuration with activation → exposure of their cysteine sites
   - Sulfenamide in PPI–S binds covalently to disulfide bonds in 1 or more cysteines of the H^+/K^+ ATPase
   - All PPIs bind to cysteine 813, omeprazole binds to cysteine 892, lansoprazole to cysteine 321, and pantoprazole to cysteine 822
7) PPI–S bound to canaliculi blocks H^+/K^+-ATPase (proton [H^+] pump) in the canaliculi of the AM and cause potent non–competitive secretion of HCl, regardless of method of stimulation (Ach, gastrin, histamine)

CLINICAL PHYSIOLOGICAL CHALLENGE – PK or PD of PPIs

Case: When an 18–year old man who has dyspepsia fails to respond to PPI od, he is reminded to take the medication half an hour before breakfast, and he now enjoys symptom–relief.

Question: Explain the pharmacokinetics and pharmacodynamics of PPIs, and why PPIs must be taken half an hour before the intake of food

- o Taking PPI half hour before meals provides the time necessary for PPI
  - To be absorbed across the jejunal enterocytes
  - To pass into the portal circulation
  - To diffuse across the basolateral (BM) of the parietal cell
  - To be metabolized to the PPI–sulfenamide (PPI—SS)
  - To be stimulated (for the canaliculi) to traffic to and inserted into the AM of the parietal cell, where the PPI–SS can bind to the exposed cysteine molecules in the H^+ / K^+ ATPase, and to markedly and non–competitively ↓↓ HCl secretion arising from all forms of stimulation
- o While the T1/2 of PPIs in the blood is about 1 hour, the irreversible binding of PPI to the H^+ / K^+ ATPase provides the biological half life (inhibition of H+ secretion of about 14 – 18 hours)
- o After 1 dose of PPI, only the H^+ / K^+ ATPase in the activated secretory canaliculi is inhibited, but some inactive canaliculi remains and more are formed
- o With each dosing of PPI, more of the canaliculi become inactivated
- o This explains why it takes several days of dosing with PPIs for a steady state of maximum acid inhibition to be achieved
- o With each dosing of PPI, more of the canaliculi become inactivated

Hypergastrinemia: Gastrin and Disorders of Acid Secretion
- o Serum gastrin level increases with food
- o Gastrin also increases when the antrum is distended (again, by food or diseases showing emptying of the stomach)
- o Gastrin is metabolized in the kidney (renal insufficiency → ↑ gastrin concentration in the serum)
- o There is negative feedback between gastrin level and acid secretion
- o When the parietal cell produces less acid, G–cells (gastrin–producing cells) lose the feedback inhibition from HCl
- o ↑ gastrin will be released → ↑↑ gastrin concentration
- o The serum gastric acid continues to increase, and acid levels in the stomach will also goes up and up because G–cell secretion from the tumor is not under the usual feedback control
- o Thus, to understand a disease due to hypersecretion of gastrin and acid, we need to understand the role of gastrin and acid, and the role of gastrin in the physiology of acid secretion
- Overview

- Where there is:
    - ↑ gastric H+, there is ↓ serum gastrin concentration
    - ↓ gastric H+, there is ↑ serum gastrin concentration
- Any condition reducing the number of parietal cells (i.e. gastric atrophy, atrophic gastritis) or function (i.e. PPI, H2RA, vagotomy) will lead to ↑ serum gastrin
- In chronic renal disease, there is ↓ breakdown and metabolism of gastrin → ↑ serum gastrin concentration
- In short bowel syndrome, loss of ileal inhibitors of the release of gastrin → ↑ serum gastrin → ↑ H+ secretion by the parietal cells
- When a person eats, the food (amino acids) and the stomach distention results in ↑ gastrin
- When there is a sporadic or MEN–1–associated gastrin–secreting tumor (gastrinoma), there is also ↑ serum gastrin

- The investigation of patient with confirmed fasting hypergastrinemia performed after a detailed history and physical examination.

➢ Laboratory tests
- Confirm fasting state from gastrin measurement
- Creatinine, calcium, PTH, chromogranin A (exclude renal failure)
- Schillings test, serum B_{12}
- Secretin infusion (increases paradoxically in ZES)
- TSN, urinary metanephrines
- Serum gastrin concentration
- Ca^{+2} infusion (G ↑↑)
- Basal and pentagastrin stimulated acid secretion (↑↑ BAO), BAO / MAO > 60% (ZES)
- Food–stimulated acid secretin (G–cell hyperplasia and hyperfunction)

- Endoscopy
  - EGD
    - Multiple ulcers in unusual sites
    - Biopsy of the antrum for G–cell number (to distinguish between G-cell hyperplasia [↑ G–cell number] vs G–cell hyperfunction, normal G-cell number); *H. pylori*
    - Thick gastric folds
  - EUS for possible tumor localization

- Diagnostic imaging
  - Abdominal ultrasound
  - CT of the head (pituitary fossa)
  - Octreotide scan
  - MBIG scan
  - CT scan of the abdomen
  - MRI of the abdomen
  - Parathyroid scan

Abbreviations: EUS, endoscopic ultrasound; ZES, Zollinger–Ellison syndrome

- Approach to hypergastrinemia
  - Is the patient fasting?
  - Have acid inhibitory medications been stopped?
  - Is renal function normal?
  - Is gastric acid being secreted? (i.e. in atrophic gastritis, there is no H^+ produced because of the atrophy of the parietal cells leading to ↑ serum gastrin concentration; but no acid peptic disease occurs because the ↑ gastrin cannot produce ↑ H^+ from the reduced number of parietal cells)
  - The presence of gastrinoma can be investigated by diagnostic imaging
    - To find the tumor (CT scan, EUS)
    - By laboratory testing, to determine the presence of the following:
      - ↑ acid secretion
      - ↑ serum gastrin concentration after an IV infusion of Ca^{2+}
      - ↓ serum gastrin concentration after an injection of secretin

> **CLINICAL CHALLENGE – Secretin Test for Gastrinoma**
>
> Case: A patient with aggressive peptic ulcer disease (PUD) complicated by hypercalcemia and diarrhea has fasting hypergastrinemia. A secretin infusion test is done to determine if the patient has biochemical evidences of gastrinoma.
>
> - Explain the increase in plasma concentration of gastrin after injection of secretin in patient with gastrinoma.

- Measurement of serum gastrin concentration
  - Calcium Infusion
    - Ca^{2+} infusion causes ↑ serum gastrin concentration in healthy individuals, but with same dose of $Ca2+$ infused, there is a higher increased in serum concentration if gastrinoma is present
  - Secretion Test for Gastrinoma
    - Normally, secretin causes ↑ gastrin and ↑ SST release
    - In healthy individuals, the following happens:
      - secretin → ↑ gastrin
      - ↑ SST → ↓ gastrin
    - In gastrinoma, the functional coupling of the release of gastrin and SST is lost, hence, the secretion of gastrin is unopposed by the injection of secretin, and the serum concentration of gastrin rises
    - Thus, the second approach to investigating whether hypergastrinemia is due to gastrinoma is to give the patient an injection of secretin
      - Observe the following after administration of secretin:
        - ↑ serum gastrin - suggestive of gastrinoma
        - ↓ serum gastrin - suggestive of no gastrinoma

- Measurement of basal and maximal acid output (BAO and MAO, respectively)
  - In response to injection of pentagastrin, in healthy individuals, there is ↑ BAO and ↑↑ MAO
  - In gastrinoma, there is ↑↑↑ BAO and ↑ MAO

- Why does the ratio BAO / MAO is higher with gastrinoma than in healthy individuals?

    o In gastrinoma, there is ↑ secretion of gastrin in both fed and fasting states, rather than just the ↑ gastrin secretion in response to food
    o This means that the acid secretion is stimulated all the time (↑↑ BAO, ↑ MAO), even when gastrinoma patient fasts
    o The ↑ BAO is greater than the ↑ MAO, so there is ↑ MAO and ↑ BAO / MAO (BAO / MAO > 60% suggestive of gastrinomas)

Gastric Pepsinogen and Pepsin

➢ Biochemistry
    o Pepsinogens are a group of proteolytic proenzymes, called zymogens
    o There are 3 isoforms of gastric pepsinogen
        - Group I pepsinogens
            ▪ Main pepsinogen
            ▪ Secreted from the gastric chief cells in the body of the stomach
        - Group II pepsinogens
            ▪ Secreted from the chief cells
            ▪ From mucous neck cells in the gastric cardia, body and antrum
        - Group III
            ▪ Pepsinogens
            ▪ Cathepsin E

➢ Physiology
    o Agonists of pepsinogen secretion from chief cells in the gastric body
        - Ach
        - Secretin
        - VIP
        - β_2–adrenergics
        - PGE2
        - Nitrogenous protein breakdown products (PBP) from food
            o ↑ secretion of gastrin from antral G–cells
            o CCK from I cells in the duodenum

- Affinity of CCK_A receptors is higher for CCK than for gastrin, whereas CCK_B receptors have greater affinity for gastrin than for CCK

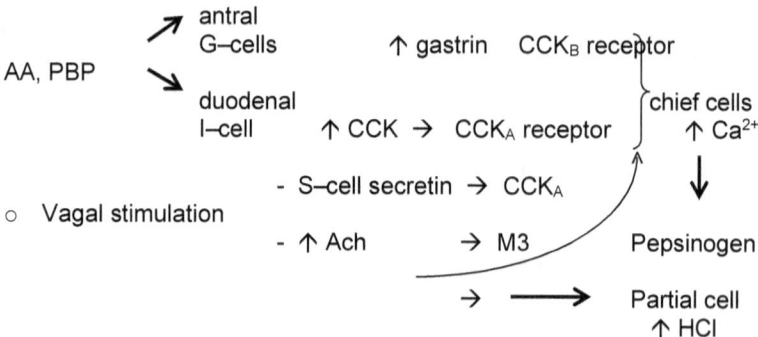

- There are receptors on the chief cells for secretin
  - M3 muscarinic receptor for Ach, and the CCK_A receptor for CCK
  - M3 or CKA stimulates chief cell pepsinogen secretion through an increased intracellular concentration of Ca^{+2}
- Pepsinogen secretory granules fuse with other secretory granules in the chief cells, and then fuse with the outer plasma membrane of the chief cells
- Both preformed and newly synthesized pepsinogen are secreted into the gastric lumen by compound exocytosis
- Pepsinogen secreted into the gastric lumen is an inactive enzyme precursor, which must be activated before it has proteolytic activity and can begin to digest protein

> Autoactivation of pepsinogen by pepsin
  - Most protein digestion occurs in the duodenum as the result of pancreatic trypsin
  - Gastric pepsin still plays an important role as an endopeptidase
  - Endopeptidase pepsin breaks down dietary protein into relatively large peptides, as well as some amino acids (AA)

- At a gastric pH of between 3.0 – 5.0, there is slow cleavage of a small terminal fragment of pepsinogen to form pepsin
- At pH < 3.0, the activation of pepsinogen to pepsin is very fast
- If the pH rises > 3.5, pepsin becomes reversibly inactivated
- Pepsin is the active proteolytic component of pepsinogen
- If the gastric pH exceeds 7.2, the pepsin enzyme activity is destroyed (irreversible inactivation)

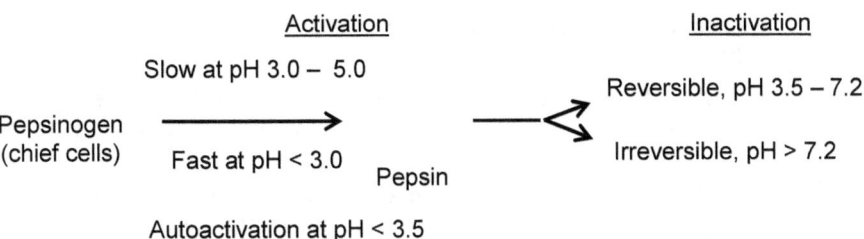

- Explain why secretion of pepsinogen is essential for the normal secretion of gastric acid, and why secretion of gastric acid is essential for the normal function of pepsinogens?
    - Pepsinogens are converted to pepsins, which is then the start of digestion of dietary proteins to amino acids (AA)
    - AA directly stimulates G–cells to ↑ gastrin, and indirectly activates Ach neurons, as well as the GRP from neurons
    - This ↑ gastrin leads to ↑ histamine released from ECL cells, which in turn stimulates the H2 receptors in the parietal cells to stimulate the secretion of H^+
    - Pepsins become inactive at pH > 4, so the low intragastric pH (↑ H^+) maintains pepsins in an active form, which then maintains the AA–stimulation of the release of gastrin from G–cells, as well as the release of Ach and GRP from neurons

CLINICAL PHYSIOLOGICAL CHALLENGE – BAO / MAO vs. pepsin output

Background: In hypergastrinemia arising from a gastrin–producing tumor, an increase in BAO is greater than the increase in MAO, such that the ratio BAO / MAO becomes > 60%.

- However, the ratio of gastric BAO / MAO (basal acid output divided by maximal acid output) is much higher than the ratio of basal to maximal pepsinogen secretion.

- Explain why does the basal and maximal outputs of pepsinogen increase with gastrinoma.
    - The Ach–responsive HCl secretion stimulates a local cholinergic reflex to release even more Ach, and thereby more pepsinogen from the chief cells.
    - When HCL empties into the duodenum, secretin is released from the duodenal S–cells, and secretin also stimulates chief cells to secrete pepsinogen.
    - In gastrinoma, there is ↑ H⁺ entering the duodenum, ↑ release of secretin from duodenal S–cells, and ↑ secretin–associated secretion of pepsinogen from the chief cells.

"All life is an experiment. The more experiments you make, the better"

Ralph Waldo Emerson

DYSPEPSIA

- Demography
  - Annual occurrence in general public is ~ 25%

- Definition
  - Dyspepsia is pain or discomfort in the upper abdomen associated with symptoms described as heartburn, indigestion, nausea, fullness, poor digestion, i.e. Rome III
  - Epigastric pain or burning ("epigastric pain syndrome")
  - Postprandial fullness ("postprandial distress syndrome")
  - Early satiation ("inability to finish a normal-sized meal or postprandial fullness)
  - Uninvestigated dysplasia
  - Blood work, ECG may be performed as needed, but dyspeptic patient has not been investigated with an esophagogastroduodenoscopy (EGD)
  - Note:
    - Positive predictive value (PPV) of alarm symptoms is low, but the negative predictive value (NPV) is 99%; so, the absence of "red flag" or "alarm" symptoms argues against the upper GI malignancy being the cause

- Types
  - Using the Rome III classification, give types of functional dyspepsia
    - Postprandial distress (PPD)
    - Epigastric pain syndrome (EPS)
    - Reflux-like
    - Ulcer-like
    - Dysmotility-like

- Clinical
  - There may also be "alarm symptoms" (suggesting possible esophageal or gastric malignancy):
    - "VBAD"
      - Vomiting
      - Bleeding – hematemesis, melena
      - Anemia
      - Dysphagia, odynophagia
    - "FWLMS"

- Family history of upper GI cancer
- Weight loss (non-intentional)
- Liver disease, jaundice, ascites
- Mass in the abdomen, or lymphadenopathy
- Previous surgery of the stomach

o Warning: exceptions
- Although the absence of VBAD and FWLML alarm symptoms is reassuring (NPV, 99%) in dyspeptic patients, the presence of upper GI tract malignancy must be excluded by EGD in several circumstances
- Age over a cut-off (guidelines vary from 45 – 55 years of age; suggestion – use age 50, or earlier if one from above is present)
- Family or personal history of cancer of the esophagus or stomach
- Personal origin from an ARGD of the world with high incidence of GCa; i.e. Japan, South America
- Personal origin from an area or group of individuals with high prevalence of *H. pylori* infection (because *H. pylori* infection may be a factor causing GCa)
- The age cut-off is determined by the point at which the incidence of ECa or GCa begins to rise; i.e. 1% at age < 50 in N. Europe, USA, Canada
- Middle-aged Caucasian male with > 10-year history of moderately severe GERD occurring ≥ 3x/week (risk of Barrett's esophagus and ECa)
- Note:
  - Odds ratio of gallstones in dyspepsia is low (~ 2.0)
  - Even if the patient is shown to have gallstones on abdominal ultrasound, that is not a sufficient proof that dyspepsia is not caused by GERD, PUD, NERD / NUD, or ECa or GCa

o There is so much overlap in symptoms that it is not possible to confidently distinguish between the usual causes of dyspepsia (i.e. poor specificity)
- Gastroesophageal reflux disease (GERD)

- Peptic ulcer disease (PUD) comprised of duodenal ulcer (DU) and gastric ulcer (GU)
  - DU
    - Classically, on an empty stomach
    - 2 – 3 hours *pc*, hen buffering acid of food has been lost, and HCl
    - Secretion is no longer high between 11 pm to 2 am
- Normal endoscopy reflux disease (NERD) and non–ulcer dyspepsia (NUD) describe the same condition of reflux–like dyspepsia and non–ulcer dyspepsia, in which the patient suffers from dyspepsia, but the EGD is normal (thus NERD and NUD are forms of "investigated dyspepsia" since an EGD has been performed)
- Overlap with IBS
  - Dyspepsia in patients with IBS, 14%
  - Reflux–like dyspepsia in IBS, 32%
  - IBS in patients with dyspepsia, 37%

- Clinical approaches
  o Age < 50 years, not in an "exception" group, no alarm symptoms → empiric anti–secretory, or
    - T & T ("test and treat" for *H. pylori*) if in a high prevalence *H. pylori* area
  o Age > 50 years, in an "exception" group, or with alarm symptom(s) → EGD
  o There are *pros* and *cons* for each approach
    - If patient is in a low *H. pylori* risk area or group, then T & T is not the preferred approach
    - For economic and availability considerations
      - "scope (EGD) and treat" approach may not be viable
      - Some evidence say that empirical anti–secretory pathway may not be the cheapest over the long run
      - Empirical approach may not give the greatest improvement in the quality of life of the patient

- Diagnosis

- What are the benefits and limitations associated with interventional or diagnostic approaches to patient with dyspepsia, who is under 50 years of age with no alarm symptoms?

Diagnostic Approach	Benefits	Limitations
o "Watchful waiting" only	– Patients with mild and transient symptoms are not prescribed with medication or investigated	▪ No clinical studies
o Empirical Anti-secretory therapy (PPI or H2RA)	– Addresses symptoms immediately – Documented effect on reflux symptoms and ulcer-related symptoms	▪ Recurrence after therapy is the rule; EGD is often only postponed, and may be false negative.
o Treat based on clinical diagnosis	– Clinically meaningful; low costs	▪ Unreliable
o Treat based on subgrouping and computer-based algorithms	– Clinically attractive; low costs	▪ Does not reliably predict EGD diagnosis or response to therapy
o H. pylori test-and-treat	– Infected patients with ulcer disease will have symptomatic benefits; reduces endoscopy rates; safe and cost-effective compared with endoscopy; possible reduced risk of later ulcer development	▪ Low benefit in those without peptic ulcer disease will not benefit. Continuing or recurrent symptoms may frustrate patients and clinician
o H. pylori test-and-scope	– Potential to reduce upper EGD rates in H. pylori–low prevalence areas	▪ Only meaningful if a decision about eradication therapy in infected patients is influenced by endoscopy result; increases endoscopy demands; not applicable in H. pylori–high prevalence areas

Diagnostic Approach	Benefits	Limitations
o Early endoscopy	– Diagnostic "gold standard"; might lead to reduced medication in patients with normal findings; increased patient satisfaction in some trials	▪ Invasive; costly; about half of EGDs will be normal; long waiting lists may lead to false negative results; not the preferred option for many patients; does not diagnose non–erosive reflux disease (NERD)

Adapted from: Bytzer, P. *Best Pract Res Clin Gastroenterol.* 2004. 18(4): page.683.

What's New: Tips

- o There is a poor correlation between dyspeptic symptoms and findings at EGD.
- o Attempts to predict the pre–EGD probability of finding a serious lesion have included the patient's age, the presence of "red flags" (alarm symptoms), a family history of esophageal/ gastric cancer, or belonging to a demographic group with such as high risk (i.e. in Canada, patients at high risk of *H. pylori* infection, "new Canadian" [immigrant] from high endemic areas), First Nations persons.
- o Barrett's patients with high pre–test probability of Barrett's epithelium include middle–aged Caucasian males, or patients with long standing history (> 5 years) of moderate to severe heartburn occurring > 3x/week. Even the presence of alarm symptoms and signs, i.e. vomiting, anemia and bleeding, dysphasia or weight loss, have a relatively low sensitivity and specificity to identify patients with high probability of having dysplasia or cancer, and therefore requires an EGD for the management of their symptoms. About two–thirds of patients with alarm symptoms and signs have normal EGD, and < 10% of dyspeptic patients with alarm symptoms will have a neoplasia (Zoggari, *et al. AJG.* 2010. 105:565-71).

> Treatment

- Empiric therapy
    - Empiric anti–secretory approach with over–the–counter (OTC) antacids, H2 receptor antagonists (H2RA), and half–dose
    - PPIs may already have been in the patient before consulting a physician
    - In guidelines, by "anti–secretory trial of therapy" is usually meant to be a standard dose of any PPI, given *po od* ½ hour before breakfast, for 4 – 8 weeks

- Test–and–treat (for *H. pylori*)
    - Prevalence of *H. pylori* in Northern Europe and Canada is about ~ 25% (~ 10% amongst locally born children)
    - Distinguish between *H. pylori* infection and *H. pylori* disease, i.e. prevalence of *H. pylori* in Canadian adults, ~ 25% prevalence of GU and DU, ~ 5% (by EGD)
    - Empiric treatment of *H. pylori* infection in investigated dyspeptics is higher, in part because DU– and GU–associated diseases are being treated, rather than just *H. pylori*–associated gastritis, the associated symptoms from which generally respond poorly to the eradication of *H. pylori*
    - *H. pylori* tests have a sensitivity of ~ 95%, so before stating that a patient has a *H. pylori*–negative duodenal ulcer, perform biopsy and non–biopsy–based tests for *H. pylori*, and for biopsy–based ulcers, ensure that at least 6 gastric biopsies were taken (antrum, 2; angularis, 2; and body 2) within more than 2 weeks of stopping acid inhibitory therapy
    - In patient with gastric ulcer, take 6 biopsies from the edge of the lesion looking for possible malignancy, as well as the 2–2–2 biopsies of the gastric antrum, angularis and body, noted above

- Test and investigate
    - Testing for *H. pylori* and reserving endoscopy for positive cases

- Investigate
    - Immediate diagnostic evaluation by endoscopy
    - Target therapy based on results

In patients with *H. pylori* infection with dyspepsia, *H. pylori* eradication decreases the mean dyspepsia score but has no effect on the patient's quality of life (Bektas, *et al.* 2009).

Please see: Thomson, A. B. R. Chapter 61. In: Therapeutic Choices. Grey, J. Ed. 6th Edition, Canadian Pharmacists Association: Ottawa, ON, 2011, Table 1: Drugs used for Dyspepsia and Peptic ulcer disease, page 821.

Please see: Thomson, A. B. R. Chapter 61. In: Therapeutic Choices. Grey, J. Ed. 6th Edition, Canadian Pharmacists Association: Ottawa, ON, 2011, Table 2: *Helicobacter pylori* Eradication Regimen, page 824-825.

Please see: Thomson, A. B. R. Chapter 62. In: Therapeutic Choices. Grey, J. Ed. 6th Edition, Canadian Pharmacists Association: Ottawa, ON, 2011, Table 1: Parenteral Drugs used in Management of Upper Gastrointestinal Bleeding, page 833.

A dyspeptic patient has **Thickened Gastric Folds**

- Explain the disease associations, histopathological features on mucosal biopsy, and medical therapy.
    - Histopathology
        - "corkscrew" foveolar hyperplasia
        - "stalactites" of mucus hanging from the folds
    - Associations
        - *Cytomegalovirus* (CMV) infection
        - *H. pylori* infection
    - Treatment
        - Cetuximab (anti–epidermal protease inhibitor)

- Longterm consequences of **acid inhibition with PPIs**
    - Peculiarities of Intragastric Acidity
        - Effects on gastric pH
        - Nocturnal acid breakthrough
        - Tachyphylaxis
        - Rebound hyperacidity upon stopping PPIs

- o Nocturnal Acid Breakthrough (pH < 4 for > 1 hour)
    - Occurs in up to 70% of GERD patients treated with PPI *bid*, especially those *H. pylori*–negative patients
- o Acid rebound
    - Occurs 7 days following cessation of 2 – 3 months high–dose PPI treatment
    - Increases BAO but more consistently MAO (but an unphysiological stimulus)
    - May last up to 11 months
    - May not be seen in *H. plyori*–positive patients
    - Mechanism uncertain – may be hypergastrinemia leading to enterochromaffin cell hyperplasia
- o Increased Risk of Enteral Infection
    - One case of bacterial diarrhea per 3,319 PPI prescriptions
    - PPI therapy may be a risk factor for *Campylobacter enteritis* (Odds ratio 11.7)
- o Bacterial Overgrowth (small intestinal)
    - Most obvious in *H. pylori*–positive patients
    - High nitrite levels
    - Low ascorbic acid levels → more *N*–nitroso compounds
- o Altered Metabolism of Alcohol
    - Bacterial overgrowth, particularly aerobes, causes acetaldehyde production from alcohol-acetaldehyde is a local carcinogen
    - Poor acetaldehyde metabolizers due to mutant ALDH2 have 2 – 3x higher *in vivo* salivary acetaldehyde levels after moderate amounts of alcohol (oriental flushers)

Dyspepsia and Pregnancy

- ➢ Demography
    - o Upper GI symptoms are common in pregnant women, and when EGD has been performed, the findings are esophagitis (34%) and gastritis (25%)
    - o Predictors of heartburn during pregnancy include young age of the mother, her parity, increasing gestational age, and the presence of heartburn before pregnancy, which occurs in 14% of mothers (Marrero, J. M., et al. Br J Obstet Gynaecol. 1992. 731-4)
- ➢ Diagnosis
    - o A symptom–based approach should be followed

- Endoscopy (EGD should be avoided unless absolutely necessary and under the advice of a high-risk obstetrician)

- What are the factors to consider when performing endoscopy in pregnant women?
    - A strong indication is always needed, particularly in high-risk pregnancies
    - Whenever possible, endoscopy should be deferred until the 2nd trimester
    - The lowest possible dose of sedative medication should be used (wherever possible FDA category A or B drugs)
    - Procedure time should be short
    - To avoid inferior vena caval or aortic compression, the patient should be positioned in the left pelvic tilt or left lateral position
    - Presence of fetal heart sounds should be confirmed before sedation and after the procedure
    - Obstetric support should be immediately available
    - No endoscopy should be performed in patients with obstetric complications (placental rupture, imminent delivery, ruptured membranes, or pre–eclampsia)

Printed with permission: Keller, J. *et al. Nat Clin Pract Gastroenterol Hepatol.* 2008. 5(8):435.

> Treatment
>   - Only calcium–containing antacids should be used for GERD symptoms, because of the following reasons:
>   - Aluminum–containing antacids cause fetal neurotoxicity
>   - Alginic acids (Gaviscon, sucralfate) cause fetal distress
>   - Magnesium–containing antacids cause renal stones, respiratory distress and cardiovascular impairment, and hypoxemia
>   - Nizatidine is not recommended for lactating mothers (FDA C, due to reports of growth retardation in rodent pups)

H. pylori INFECTION AND PEPTIC ULCER DISEASE (PUD)

> Demography

- About 50% of the world's population has *H. pylori* infection, but only about 15% develop peptic (gastric or duodenal) disease, and ~ 1% develop gastric cancer or MALT lymphoma
- So, there is a disconnection between *H. pylori* infection in the stomach, and *H. pylori*–associated diseases
- Endoscopic screening for *H. pylori*–infected subjects showed 1 – 6% PUD
- Lifetime risk of developing PUD is 20 – 40% (4 – 10x higher than *H. pylori*–negative patients)
- Modes of transmission of *H. pylori*
  - Gastro–oral vomitus–oral, fecal–oral
- *H. pylori*–positive parents
  - Spouse 68% *H. pylori*–positive
  - Children 40% *H. pylori*–positive
- *H. pylori*–negative parents
  - Spouse 9% *H. pylori*–positive
  - Children 3% *H. pylori*–positive
- Community Risk
  - Adults: ~ 25 – 30% (depending on patient's age)
  - Higher, 30% in older patients
  - > 50% First Nations Canadians, new Canadians from high *H. pylori* prevalence areas
  - New Canadians from high prevalence countries
- *H. pylori*–associated GI diseases
  - Non–investigated and investigated dyspepsia
  - Non–ulcer dyspepsia
  - Acute or chronic gastritis
  - Atrophic gastritis (AG) – acceleration with PPI of AG–IM–Dys–GCa → intestinal metaplasia (IM) → dysplasia (Dys) → GCa (non–cardia gastric cancer)

- Duodenal and gastric ulcer (DU and GU) (only ~ 20% of *H. pylori*–positive patients develop the clinical disease)
- Accentuation of effects of smoking in PUD
- Accentuation of ASA and NSAID effects on PUD
- Maltoma
- Fundic gland polyps
- Hypertrophic gastric folds
- Protective against GERD (possible)
- Halitosis
- Carcinoid tumors
- Colorectal cancer (possible association, due to hypergastrinemia)
- Pancreatic cancer (possible association)

o Possible *H. pylori*–associated non–GI diseases
  - Head — otitis media, migraines, headaches
  - CNS — Parkinsonism, CVA
  - Heart — atherosclerotic diseases
  - Lung — chronic bronchitis, COPD, SIDS
  - Blood — ITP, iron deficiency; B12 deficiency
  - Skin — idiopathic chronic urticaria, acne, rosacea
  - Growth retardation in children
  - Vomiting in pregnancy

Abbreviations: COPD, chronic obstructive pulmonary disease; CVA, cerebrovascular accident; DU, duodenal ulcer; GCa, gastric cancer; GERD, gastroesophageal reflux disease; GU, gastric ulcer; ITP, idiopathic thrombocytopenic purpura; PUD, peptic ulcer disease; SIDS, sudden infant death syndrome

Adapted from: Hunt, R. *AGA Institute Post Graduate Course*. 2006. page 333-342.; Adapted from: Graham, D. Y. and Sung, J. J. Y. *Sleisenger & Fordtran's Gastrointestinal and Liver Disease: Pathophysiology/ Diagnosis/ Management*. 2006. page 1054; and 2010, page 839.

➤ Pathophysiology

SO YOU WANT TO BE A GASTROENTEROLOGIST!

Somatostatin (SST) and gastrin are produced in the gastric antrum, and gastric acid is secreted by the parietal cells in the gastric body.

- Explain why gastric acid secretion falls with acute or chronic *H. pylori* gastritis, yet gastric acid secretion rises with antral gastritis.

  ❖ Acute or chronic *H. pylori* pangastritis
  - *H. pylori*
    - Direct
      - ↓ gene expression of parietal cell H^+ / K^+ ATPase α–subunit
      - ↓ gastrin release
      - ↓ duodenal HCO_3^-
    - Indirectly
      - Produces anti–secretory cytokines IL–1β and TNF–α
      - Activates CGRP sensory neurons → ↑ SST (somatostatin) → ↓ gastrin
      - ↓ HCl secretion for body parietal cells

  ❖ Chronic *H. pylori* antral gastritis
  - ↓ SST
    - Proinflammatory and prosecretory cytokines
    - Prosecretory H_3 agonist (N^3–methyl histamine)
  - ↑ gastrin (from ↑ SST, and from ↑ IL–8 and PAF)
  - ↑ gastrin → ↑ ECL cells in the fundus and body → ECL hyperplasia
  - ECL hyperplasia → ↑ HCL secretion from parietal cell antibodies

---

- Name the bacterial and host factors important in *H. pylori*–associated development of peptic ulcer, lymphoma and gastric cancer.
- ❖ The *H. pylori* organism
  - Adhesion and colonization
    - Genetically "distinct strains"
    - Bacterial genes encoding proteins in the motility apparatus of *H. pylori* (movement of organisms from the lumen of the stomach → the mucus layer) and genes for urease (provides for 2 pH optimum values of 3.0 and 7.2)

- Colonization occurs only in gastric epithelium or where there is gastric metaplasia
- O-glycans in the deeper portions of the glandular mucosa with colonization
- Secretory leucocyte protease inhibitor (SLPI) produced by *H. pylori* reduces colonization
- F3 ab A, a bacterial gene product, may be liquid for the host Lewis (Le) b receptor or MUC 5AC, enhances colonization
- *H. pylori* urease binds to major histocompatibility (MHC) class II molecules to ↑ apoptosis
- Trefoil protein (TFF$_1$) on gastric epithelial cells and mucus binds to *H. pylori*
- Toll-like receptors (TLRs) in pathogen-associated molecular receptors (PAMRs) family recognize *H. pylori* or their bacterial products which recognize lipopolysaccharide (LPS) or flagellin
- Cag pathogenicity island (cag PAI) is a segment of *H. pylori* DNA that provides cag E (type N secretion apparatus)
- Cag PAI
  - Allows host gastric cellular membrane translocation
  - ↑ IL-8 expression
  - SRC kinases phosphorylates tyrosine in Cag A protein
- All *H. pylori* have Vaac A gene, while half produce the protein, Vac A (vacuolating cytotoxin)
- Vac A is a ligand for the cell membrane receptor, protein-tyrosine phosphatase

❖ The host
  o Intensity of host inflammatory response
    - Outer inflammatory protein A (OipA)
    - ↑ IL-8 → ↑ neutrophil infiltration
    - Peptidoglycan act in the type IV secretion system
    - *H. pylori* neutrophil-activating protein (NAP)
      - ↑ chemotaxis of neutrophils and monocytes
      - ↑ reactive oxygen intermediates (ROIs)
    - ↑ recruitment of neutrophils and macrophages → ↑ inducible nitric oxide synthase (iNOS)
  o Host immune response
    - Polymorphism for IL-1β → ↑ IL-1 → intense mucosal inflammation (gastritis)

- IL–8, IL–10, TNF–α also ↑ gastritis
- Morphological changes in gastric epithelial cells
  - Tight junctions (TJ) complexes become broken
  - ↑ epithelial cell proliferation and apoptosis
- ↑ gene expression
- Inflammatory cytokines
  - ↑ signaling mechanism for gene expression
- ↑ mitogen–activated protein (MAP) kinases
- ↑ lost of cell redox factor–1
- ↑ activity of nuclear factor kappa B (NF–kB)
- ↑ activity of activator protein–1 (AP–1)
- ↑ oxidative stress
  - ↑ oxidation of DNA
- Nucleotide–binding oligomerization domain–1 (NOD_1) of the host
  - Sense *H. pylori*
  - ↑ NF–kB
- GI physiology
  - SST and gastrin effects on secretion of gastric HCl and duodenal HCO_3^-
  - Mucus — ↓ volume
  - ↓ mucosal hydrophobicity
- TNF–α and IFN–γ (interferon gamma)
  - ↑ effects of *H. pylori*–NRP
  - Prime neutrophils
- ↑ phagocytosis of *H. pylori*–infected gastric epithelial cells
- ↑ chemokines, i.e. ENA–78 GRO–α activates neutrophils
- ↑ cytokine induction
  - TNF–α
  - IL–6, IL–12, IL–17, IL–18
  - Heat shock protein 60 (HSP–60)
- T cell
  - ↓ IL–4 activation of STAT6 → ↑ Th1 and ↓ Th2 response
  - ↑ Th1 response
  - ↑ apoptosis
  - ↑ inflammation
  - ↑ atrophy
  - ↑ dysplasia

- ↑ IL–1β, IFN–α, TNF–α
  - ↑ Fas antigen expression → Fas–FasL (ligand) interactions → ↑ gastric epithelial cell death by apoptosis
- ↓ NFAT (↓ nuclear translocation of a transcription factor) → ↓ IL–2
- Dysregulation of Treg (regulatory T–cells)
- ↑ IgA, IgM and complements
- ↑ monoclonal antibodies to *H. pylori* cross react with gastric epithelial cells
- Innate host responses are impaired by catalases and ureases

SO YOU WANT TO BE A GASTROENTEROLOGIST!

- *H. pylori* was declared by the WHO as a carcinogen with an attributable risk for gastric cancer (GCa) of ~ 60%.
- In addition to dietary and lifestyle factors, molecular factors represent a genetic basis for non–*H. pylori* GCa
    - Cytokines (i.e. IL–1β, polymorphisms of TNF–α and IL–1)
    - Toll–like receptors (TLRs), i.e. TLR–2

- **What are the molecular factors increasing the risk of carcinogenesis from *H. pylori*?**

There are several molecular factors that increase the risk of developing GCa from an *H. pylori* infection.

- Motility
    - Proteins (Fla A, Fla B) provide spiral movement for *H. pylori*
- Buffering of gastric acid (↓ H^+ secretion)
    - Urease gene cluster (Ure A, Ure B)
- Adhesion
    - Hop protein (outer membrane proteins)
    - Adhesion
        - Bab A (encoded by gene Bab A_2)
        - Bab A binds to blood group antigen Lewis B
- Cag pathogenicity island
    - Greater (2 to 28) risk of GCa with Cag A^+ *H. pylori*
- Molecular needles
    - Type 4 secretion system (TFSS) enhances movement of Cag A^+ bacterial protein into the gastric epithelial cells
- Vacuolation
    - Vac A protein, a pore–forming vacuolating toxin, especially in the presence of Cag A^+ *H. pylori* strains, reduce the activation of T–cells, and increase the risk of GCa

➤ Causes and associations

- Causes of recurrent peptic ulcer after eradication of *H. pylori* infection:

    - *H. pylori* reappearance and almost always recrudescence but no reinfection
    - Surreptitious intake of aspirin or any NSAIDs

- Poor mucosal healing due to excessive scarring
- *H. pylori*–negative DU with abnormally high acid response
- Other conditions (i.e. gastrinoma, Crohn's disease)
- Idiopathic duodenal ulcer disease
- *H. pylori* virulence factors
    - Cag A is translocated within the epithelial cell by cag–encoded type IV secretion system (~ Tir of EPEC)
    - After injection, bacterial protein is recognized as a host–encoded protein, tyrosine–phosphorylated and activated
    - Activated Cag A triggers cortical actin reorganization by N–WASP and Arp 2/3 interactions and nuclear signals mediated by the Rho GTPases and the JNK pathway

> Laboratory

MCQ ALERT

- An MCQ scenario speaks to the need for it to be proven that a previous *H. pylori* infection has been eradicated. Given the need to be certain, the test is not falsely negative, watch out for the following:

    - UBT — falsely negative, if patient has been on PPIs, H2RA or antibiotics in a week before the test

    - Biopsy (EGD is necessary) — based techniques if the test will be falsely negative and *H. pylori* may have migrated to the gastric body; biopsy needs to be taken from the mucosa of both gastric antrum and body before you may be confident that the pathology report of "no *H. pylori* seen" signifies that the infection has truly been cured, and that the *H. pylori* are not simply hiding in the mucus adjacent to the mucosa of the gastric body

---

- If using a biopsy–based test for *H. pylori*:
  - Stop PPI for at least 1 week before having EGD biopsy
  - Take 2 EGD biopsies from the gastric antrum, 2 from the body, and 1 from the angularis
- Positive serology for *H. pylori* only indicates previous exposure; a negative serology test excludes *H. pylori*–associated disease
- Specificity is even lower with increasing age and in cirrhosis
- Determine the presence of active infection with UBT or stool antigen test

---

SO YOU WANT TO BE A GASTROENTEROLOGIST!

- Canadian guidelines recommend that a patient with dyspepsia at age 50 or over, or dyspepsia at any age with alarm symptoms (vomiting, bleeding, anemia, dysphagia, weight loss) should have an EGD to diagnose the cause of dyspepsia.
- Unfortunately, the waiting time for an EGD may be very long (~ 6 months), by that time an early gastric cancer (definition: "a cancer that does not invade beyond the submucosa regardless of lymph node involvement" [Feldman, M., et al. *Sleisenger and Fordtran's Gastrointestinal and Liver Disease*. 10th Edition. Saunders/Elsevier, Philadelphia, 2016, page 914] may possibly have advanced).

- Explain why an upper GI (UGI) barium study is not recommended for the investigation of dyspepsia, but is still understandably used in at–risk dyspeptic patients waiting for EGD.
  - It has all to do with performance characteristics: the sensitivity and specificity of an UGI to detect an advanced gastric cancer (GCa) is about 65%, and 90%, respectively. So, a negative UGI does not exclude a serious lesion, and certainly does not exclude EGCa (early gastric cancer), because the sensitivity is disappointingly low.
  - However, if the UGI shows a suspicious lesion thought to possibly be EGCa, with a specificity of ~ 90%, this information should be forwarded to the consultant and should inspire a prompt endoscopy.
  - In staging GCa, the TNM system is used.
  - Endoscopic ultrasound (EUS) is recommended to stage GCa, including early GCa because EUS has 90% accuracy to differentiate mucosal from submucosal tumor invasion (note the accuracy for restaging T and N after neoadjuvant chemotherapy is lower, ~ 50%).

> **MIND TEASER**
> - Explain why is the rate of symptom relief with *H. pylori*–triple therapy higher in functional dyspepsia with EGD, than in uninvestigated dyspepsia.
>   o EGD shows an ulcer, so pretest probably for symptom relief is higher.

- Diagnosis
    - There is a broad range of tests available to diagnose the presence of *H. pylori* infection
        - Use only upper endoscopy with biopsy for histological examination or culture to have the diagnosis of *H. pylori*
        - Associated diseases, i.e. gastritis, peptic ulcer disease intestinal metaplasia, gastric cancer or mALT lymphoma (Guarner, *et al.* 2010)
    - Culture of gastric biopsies are also used in testing for *in vitro* antibiotic sensitivity of the organism, as well as gene testing for antibiotic resistance, but the sensitivity is low
    - Rapid urease tests have better sensitivity than histology
    - Non–tissue, non–endoscopy tests include blood, breath and stool antigen testing. Urea breath test is > 75% sensitive and can be used both to diagnose an *H. pylori* infection and to confirm its eradication
    - Testing for *H. pylori* antigens in the stool is useful before and after treatment, and has > 95% sensitivity

- Diagnostic Tests for *H. pylori*
    - Invasive
        - Rapid urease test
        - Histology
        - Culture
        - PCR
    - Non–invasive
        - Antibody detection
            - Serum–ELISA (quantitative)
            - Immunoblot (qualitative)
        - 13C, 14C urea breath test (UBT)

> Performance Characteristics of **Diagnostic Tests for *H. pylori***

Tests	Sensitivity (%)	Specificity (%)
o Rapid urease test	> 90	> 90
o Histology	90 – 98	
o Culture	Varies widely	100
o Urea breath test	> 95	> 95
o Serology	90 – 100	76 – 96
o Antigen–based stool assay	94	91

Useful background: Urea Breath Test to Diagnose Active infection

- o [13C]–urea
  - Stable isotope
  - Non–radioactive
- o [14C]–urea
  - Radioactive isotope
  - Special handling and disposal

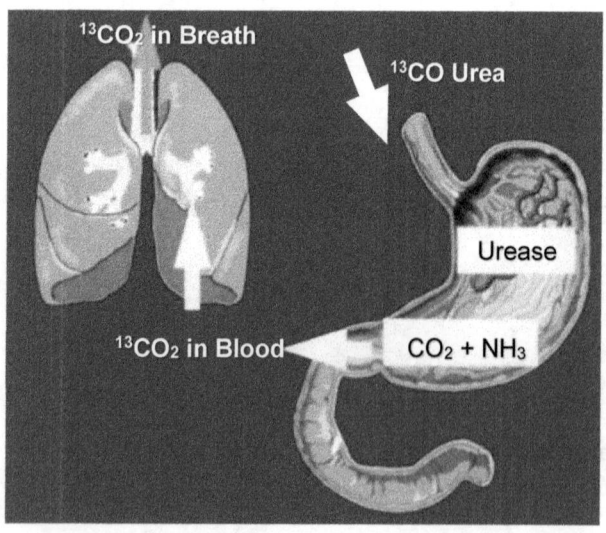

➤ Histopathology

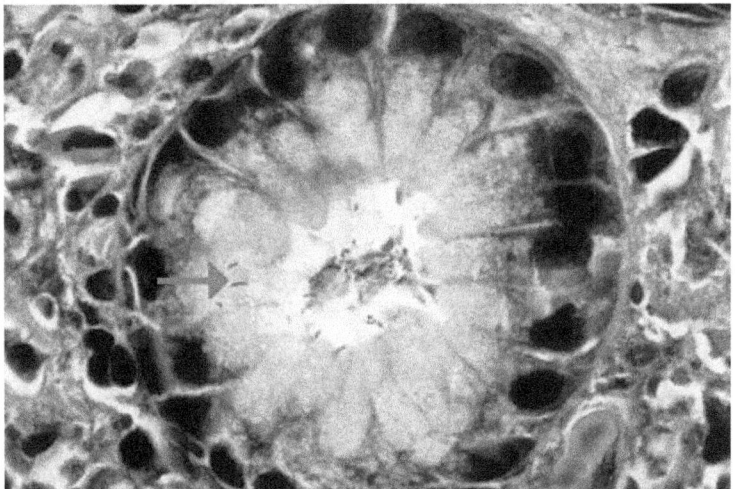

- o Gastritis is often accompanied with infection with the small curved to spiral rod–shaped *Helicobacter pylori* bacterium found in the surface epithelial mucus of most patients with active gastritis
- o Rod–shaped bacteria are seen here with methylene blue stain

➤ Treatment

- What are the recommended indications for *H. pylori* eradication therapy (ET) in patient taking NSAIDs or ASA?
    - o Reduce PUD formation
    - o Reduce recurrent PUD
    - o Reduce recurrent PUD bleeding (in ASA or NSAID high risk users; ET does not prevent further PUD bleeding in high risk ASA or NSAID users on PPI)

Abbreviation: ET, eradication therapy

Adapted from: Lai, L. H. and Sung, J. J. Y. *Best Pract Res Clin Gastroenterol.* 2007. 21(2): page 270.

- Meta-analysis
  - No statistical difference in *H. pylori* eradication rates using either triple or quadruple therapy (RR = 1.002; 95% CI 0.936 – 1.073)
  - 93% eradication rate with sequential therapy versus 74% for clarithromycin-based triple therapy, particularly in patients with clarithromycin-resistant strains of *H. pylori*
  - Superiority of a 10-day course of levofloxacin-based triple therapy vs a 7-day course of bismuth-based quadruple therapy (RR = 0.51; 95% CI: 0.34 – 0.75) for persistent *H. pylori* infection
- Rifampin has been used as an alternative to clarithromycin, with eradication rates of 38 – 91%; there may be rare but serious adverse effects (myelotoxicity and ocular toxicity)
- Furazolide used in place of clarithromycin, metronidazole or amoxicillin gives an eradication rates of 52 – 90%
- Points to consider:
  - It is useful for the physician to have an available data of the local rates of *H. pylori* resistance to clarithromycin
  - "PPI-clarithromycin-containing therapy without prior susceptibility testing should be abandoned when clarithromycin resistance rate in the region is more than 15 – 20%" (Malfertheiner, *et al. Gut.* 2012. 61: 646-664).
  - Smoking reduces *H. pylori* eradication rates by about 8%
  - Extending the duration of triple therapy with PCM or PCA from 7 to 10 – 14 days increases the *H. pylori* eradication rate by only ~ 5%
  - Bismuth-containing quadruple therapy is also an alternate first-line empirical therapy since compliance with quadruple therapy is high and particularly useful in areas of high clarithromycin resistance
- To note with *H. pylori*
  - If eEradication fails with PCM or PCA, use either the following:
    - Bismuth-containing quadruple therapy
    - Levofloxacin-containing triple therapy (PLA, PPI, levofloxacin plus amoxicillin or PCL for 10 days)
    - Sequence therapy (PA-PMC)
    - Concomitant therapy
  - *H. pylori* tests have a sensitivity of ~ 95%, so before stating that a patient has an *H. pylori*-negative duodenal ulcer, perform biopsy- and non-biopsy-based tests for *H. pylori*, and for biopsy-based ulcers, ensure that at least 6 gastric biopsies were taken (antrum, 2; angularis, 2; and body, 2) within more than 2 weeks of stopping acid inhibitory therapy and antibiotics

Please see: Thomson, A. B. R. Chapter 61. In: Therapeutic Choices. Grey, J. Ed. 6th Edition, Canadian Pharmacists Association: Ottawa, ON, 2011, Table 1: Drugs used for Dyspepsia and Peptic ulcer disease, page 821.

Please see: Thomson, A. B. R. Chapter 61. In: Therapeutic Choices. Grey, J. Ed. 6th Edition, Canadian Pharmacists Association: Ottawa, ON, 2011, Table 2: *Helicobacter pylori* Eradication Regimen, page 824-825.

Please see: Thomson, A. B. R. Chapter 62. In: Therapeutic Choices. Grey J, Ed. 6th Edition, Canadian Pharmacists Association: Ottawa, ON, 2011, Table 1: Parenteral Drugs Used in Management of Upper Gastrointestinal Bleeding, page 833.

- ❖ **Non–eradication** of *H. pylori* (failure of therapy) with standard triple or quadruple therapy
    - o Confirm perisitence of infection
    - o Confirm patient adherence to treatment recommendations
    - o If local antibiotic resistance to *H. pylori* is known, use this information to guide therapeutic decisions
    - o If initial therapy for 7 days fails, consider repeat for 14 days
    - o Consider switching PAC to PMC or PMC to PAC, use a second–round same therapy but for 14 days, or bismuth–based first line therapy, or second line therapies (with levofloxacin plus ampicillin, sequential therapy (PA–PMC), or concomitant therapy (PMCA)
    - o If eradication fails after the first and second line treatments, subsequent treatment "...should be guided by antimicrobial susceptibility testing, whenever possible"
    - o For patients who cannot take amoxicillin (penicillin allergy), use PCM or bismuth–containing quadruple therapy
    - o Concomitant therapy (CT) is comprised of PPI, clarithromycin, metronidazole, amoxicillin
        - More effective than the standard triple therapy (pooled OR is 2.86), and is less complex than ST
    - o Sequential therapy is comprised of the following:
        - PPI *bid* plus amoxicillin 1 gm *bid* for 5 days, followed by
        - PPI *bid* plus clarithromycin 500 mg *bid* plus metronidazole or tinidazole *bid* for the next 5 days
        - ST in guidelines remains to be established
- Explain why the rate of symptom relief with *H. pylori*–triple therapy lower in functional dyspepsia with EGD than in uninvestigated dyspepsia (UD)?

- In UD, there are patients who have peptic ulcer disease (GU, DU), who respond well to eradication of *H. pylori*, plus those with only *H. pylori*–associated gastritis, any symptoms of which do not respond well to *H. pylori* eradication
- In patients who had EGD and an ulcer is found, their symptom response to *H. pylori* eradication is higher than in those infected with *H. pylori* but no ulcer
- DU occurs in duodenal and antral transitional zone or in areas of gastric metaplasia
- Chronic acid peptic ulcer from the stomach contributes to focal mucosal injury and metaplasia
- Less mucosal bicarbonate secretion in vulnerable areas
- *H. pylori* infection of transitional zone or metaplastic areas lead to inflammation, epithelial destruction, coalescing erosions and ulceration (microinfarction)
- GU occurs in antral type of mucosa bordering corpus–type mucosa
- Speculations
  - Mucosal boundaries are inherently unstable
  - More acid along the lesser curvature
  - Restricted mural blood flow
  - Higher *H. pylori* density, more pronounced alteration of the mucus layer, more extensive mucosal damage
  - More mural stretching
- Who should receive the *H. pylori* eradication therapy?
  - All NSAID users
  - High risk patients
  - Patients starting NSAIDs
  - Patients stopping NSAIDs
  - Patients with GU
  - Patients with DU
  - Patients taking COX–2 inhibitors (Coxibs)
  - Patients taking aspirin (ASA)
  - Possibly patients taking antiplatelet agents
  - Possibly patients with dyspepsia while on NSAIDs, ASA or Coxibs

- Meta–analysis of *H. pylori* eradication therapy in FD
  - Anti–*H. pylori* treatment superior to placebo (p = 0.0002)

- Resolution of symptoms in 9% anti–*H. pylori* treated versus placebo treated patients (95% CI = +4 to +14%)
- No evidence of heterogeneity or of bias publication of positive results

Helicobacter pylori–negative peptic ulcer disease

➤ Demography

  o The proportion of all peptic ulcers which are *H. pylori*-negative is increasing (~ 25%)

➤ Clinical

H. pylori–negative peptic ulcers are more serious or severe than are *H. pylori*–positive peptic ulcers

- In the absence of the use of NSAIDs, what factors support this statement?

Clinical	*H. pylori*⁺	*H. pylori*⁻
o Bleeding ulcer	4%	50%
o Recurrent ulcer bleeding	11%	42%
o ASA risk ≥ grade 3	18%	~ 50%
o Mortality rate	37%	88%

Abbreviations: ASA, American Society of Anesthesiologist

- Explain the theories why *H. pylori*–negative is more serious than *H. pylori*–positive peptic ulcers (GU or DU).

  o *H. pylori* involving the gastric body may ↓ the secretion of HCl from the parietal cells

  o *H. pylori* may have an anti–secretory effect → PPI therapy more efficacious

  o The abnormalities in gastric acid secretion and in gastrin metabolism may be worse or different in *H. pylori*–negative from *H. pylori*–positive peptic ulcer disease

An understanding of gastric parietal cell secretion of HCl and G–cell secretion of stimulatory gastrin as well as D–cell secretion of inhibitory somatostatin, is important to understand the pathophysiology of dyspepsia, PUD, as well as the effects of hypergastrinemia, including Zollinger–Ellison Syndrome (ZES) of the sporadic type or MEN–1.

- Diagnosis
    - Ensure that if the diagnosis of H. pylori infection is based on UBT or gastric mucosal biopsies, anti–secretory therapy must be stopped at least 1 week before taking (mucosal gastric) biopsies and biopsies must be taken from the antrum (2), body (2), and angularis (1) areas of the stomach
    - Before deeming that the patient has H. pylori–negative peptic ulcer disease, care must be taken to exclude the following:
        - H. pylori infection using 2 different types of standard tests
        - Use of ASA, NSAIDs, coxibs, bisphosphonates (check for platelet aggregation or thromboxane B2 levels)
        - Fasting hypergastrinemia (ensure patient if not currently taking anti–secretory therapy)

Helicobactor pylori–Positive Peptic Ulcer Disease

- Pathophysiology
    - H. pylori
        - Associated with, or causative of GU and DU, as well as gastritis, gastric cancer and gastric mucosa associated lymphoid tumors (MALT lymphoma)
        - Worse chance of developing ASA or NSAID–associated GU or DU
        - Worse effects with smoking on slow healing of peptic ulcer, and with high risk of relapse of ulcer

    Note: Once associated H. Pylori infection has been cured, smoking loses these adverse effects on ulcer healing and relapse.

    - ↑ risk of ulcer relapse (80% for H. pylori⁺, 10% for H. pylori⁻)
    - Combine anti–H. pylori therapy with PPI to the following:
        - ↑ anti–H. pylori effects of antibiotics
        - Accelerate improvement of ulcer healing and symptom relief

- Optimal pH outcomes of different upper GI disorders (18 hours/day)
  - ≥ 3   GU, DU
  - 4   GERD
  - 5   *H. pylori* eradication
  - 6   Non–variceal upper GI bleeding

- Explain the postulated mechanisms of *H. pylori* causing duodenal ulcer (DU).
  - Antrum D–cells ↓ – ↓ S – ↓ inhibition of G cells – ↑ G – ↑ HCl – ↑ metaplasia — *H. pylori* infection develops in metaplasia of the duodenum
  - Urease activity of *H. pylori* enables the organism to burrow through the mucous overlying the gastric epithelium to bind to adhesions and to colonize the alkaline environment adjacent to the membrane
    - It invades the gastric mucosa, while evading the host immunity
    - Adhesions provide an interplay between bacteria and Lewis antigen (Sheu, *et al.* 2010)
    - IL–1, a TNF–α gene clusters are important in defining the extent and severity of *H. pylori*–associated gastritis
    - The common pangastritis may or may not be symptomatic, the antral predominant gastritis is associated with an increased risk of duodenal ulcer disease and gastric body associated gastritis is associated with multifocal gastric atrophy and an increased risk of gastric cancer (Shanks and El-Omar, 2009)

➢ Differentials
- What are the differential diagnoses for stomach ulcerative diseases?
  - Benign
    - Peptic ulcer disease
    - Pill–ulceration
    - Gastric erosion
  - Malignant
    - Adenocarcinoma
    - Lymphoma
    - Gastrointestinal stromal tumor (GIST)
    - Metastases

- Give the differential diagnosis for ulcerative diseases in the duodenum.

- Peptic ulcer disease
- Zollinger–Ellison Syndrome
- Crohn's disease

➢ Treatment
- Uncomplicated peptic ulcer
  - PPI of your *po bid* for 2 weeks with 2 antibiotics followed by PPI *od* for 2 weeks
  - If patient experiences frequent recurrent recurrences
    - Perform UBT to patient off PPI for 1 week
    - If UBT is positive, re–treat *H. pylori*
    - If UBT is negative, consider PPI *po od* continuously as maintenance therapy

- Complicated peptic ulcer
  - Complications, i.e. hemorrhage, obstruction, perforation
  - Treat PUD plus *H. pylori* infection as above as uncomplicated ulcer
  - Either repeat UBT off PPI therapy, and re–treat and prove the eradication of *H. pylori*, with no PPI maintenance therapy (PPI *po od*)
  - PPI maintenance therapy (PPI *od*)
    - Risk (low) of reinfection with *H. pylori*
    - Risk (low) of re–ulceration even without reinfection with *H. pylori*
    - Possibility that the original ulcer may have been caused by ASA or NSAIDs plus *H. pylori* infection

- Caution alert
  - Every patient being considered for long term use of ASA, NSAIDs or coxibs should be tested (by UBT) and treated for *H. pylori* if positive
  - Depending on patient (host) and medication considerations, some patients on long term PPI *po od*, even after eradication of any associated *H. pylori* infection

- In patients with *H. pylori*–associated non–ulcer dyspepsia, eradication of *H. pylori* results in long term symptomatic relief in about 8% of patients
- PPI – clarithromycin – metronidazole (PCM) and PPI – clarithromycin – amoxicillin (PCA) regimens are equivalent
- Only calcium–containing antacids should be used for GERD symptoms
  - Aluminum–containing antacids may cause fetal neurotoxicity
  - Alginic acid (Gaviscon, sucralfate) may cause fetal distress
  - Magnesium–containing antacids may cause renal stones, respiratory distress and cardiovascular impairment, and hypotemia

CLINICAL ALERT

- An MCQ is directed at the issue of the recommended follow–up of a dyspeptic < 55–year old whose UBT is positive and was given successful triple therapy for *H. pylori*. You are tempted to answer that the correct follow–up is to repeat UBT to determine if the infection has been eradicated.
    - Wrong! (sorry). Successful triple therapy for *H. pylori* in this setting means the patient has lost her or his dyspepsia.
- The **only circumstances are UBT that must be repeated** is
    - Persistent dyspepsia after treatment
    - Patient with complicated *H. pylori*–associated peptic ulcer (i.e. hemorrhage) must be proven by repeat testing that the anti–*H. pylori* treatment has effectively eradicated the bug (expected cure rate for triple therapy is only 80%)

ZOLLINGER – ELLISON SYNDROME (ZES)

> Clinical syndromes

- What are the characteristics and clinical syndromes of functional gut endocrine tumors?

Type of tumor	Localization	% frequency	Malignancy
o Carcinoid	– Ileum – Pancreas	90	100
o Insulinoma	– Pancreas	10	
o Gastrinoma	– Pancreas		5
o VIPoma	– Pancreas – Duodenum	60 25	50-80
o Gluucagonoma	– Pancreas	90	90
o Somatostatinoma	– Pancreas – Duodenum	56 44	90

* VIPoma – vasoactive intestinal peptide

Syndromes	Signs and Symptoms	Hormones or Peptide Markers
o Gastrinoma (Zollinger–Ellison syndrome)	- Abdominal pain - Dyspepsia, diarrhea, MEN-1	• Gastrin
o VIPoma or Verner Morrison	- Severe, watery diarrhea - Hypokalemia, dehydration	• Diarrhea • VIP
o Insulinoma	- Hypoglycemic syndrome	• Insulin
o Glucagonoma	- Rash, anemia, weight loss, diabetes - Glucose intolerance - Thromboembolic disease	• Glucagon
o Somatostatinoma	- Diabetes mellitus - Cholelithiasis - Diarrhea, steatorrhea	• Somatostatin
o GRFoma	- Acromegaly	• GRF
o Ppoma	- Weight loss, abdominal mass - Often asymptomatic	• PP
o CCKoma	- Hypersecretion of pancreatic enxymes	• CCK
o Neurotensinoma	- Flushing, diarrhea	• Neurotensin
o Ulcerogenic tumor acid syndrome with non-gastrin secretagogue	- Abdominal pain - Dyspepsia - Diarrhea	• Non-gastrin

➢ Clinical

- Give the presenting clinical features of Zollinger-Ellison Syndrome (ZES).
    - o Abdominal pain (75 – 100%)
    - o Diarrhea (35 – 73%, isolated presentation in up to 35%)
    - o Pain and diarrhea (55 – 60%)
    - o Heartburn (44 – 64%)
    - o Duodenal and prepyloric ulcers (71 – 91%)
    - o Multiple ulcers in unusual parts
    - o Stomal ulcers
    - o PUD is refractory to treatment

- Ulcer complications (bleeding, 1 – 17%; perforation, 0 – 5%, or obstruction, 0 – 5%)
- MEN–1–associated tumors (22 – 24%)

o MEN–1–associated Gastrinomas
- Parathyroid ~ 100% of the following:
  - Symptomatic hypercalcemic patients
  - Parathyroid gland removal
  - Parathyroid autograft ± cervical thymectomy
- Pancreas
  - ~ 80% of MEN–1 patients
  - 40% have asymptomatic ↑ gastrin (serum) or ZES
- Pituitary adenomas, ~ 20% (usually a lactotroph adenoma)

Adapted from: Metz, D. C. and Jensen, R. T. *Gastroenterology*. 2008. 135:1469.

Most gastrinomas occur in the "gastrin triangle".

- Name the landmarks of the gastrin triangle.

  o The triangle is made up of the following 3 junctions:

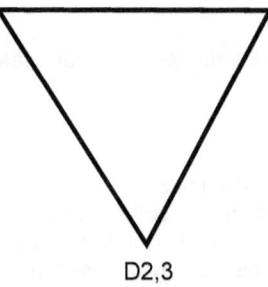

Cystic duct or CBD   Pancreatic neck or body

D2,3

Abbreviations: CBD, common bile duct; D2,3, junction of the first and second parts of the duodenum

- How to investigate patients with fasting hypergastrinemia performed after a detailed history and physical examination?

➢ Laboratory tests
  o Confirm the fasting state for gastrin measurement, and not on PPIs
  o Calcium (albumin is corrected)
  o PTH
  o TSH
  o Creatinine (excludes renal failure)
  o Chromogranin A
  o Prolactin
  o Insulin–like growth factor 1
  o Insulin
  o Proinsulin
  o Glucagon
  o Pancreatic polypeptide (PP)
  o Urinary metanephrins
  o Schilling test, serum B_{12}

➢ Provocative tests
  o Secretin infusion (increases gastrin paradoxically in ZES)
  o Ca^{+2} infusion (marked increase in serum gastrin)
  o Basal and pentagastrin–stimulated acid secretion (↑↑ BAO), BAO / MAO > 60% (ZES)
  o Food–stimulated acid secretin (G–cell hyperplasia or hyperfunction)

➢ Endoscopy
  o EGD
    - Multiple ulcers in unusual sites
    - Biopsy of the antrum for G–cell number (to distinguish between G–cell hyperplasia [↑ G–cell number] versus G–cell hyperfunction (normal G–cell number); *H. pylori* infection
    - Thick gastric folds
    - Fundic gland polyps
  o EUS for possible tumor localization (especially in the wall of the duodenum)

- ➢ Diagnostic imaging
  - o Abdominal ultrasound
  - o CT or MRI, head (pituitary fossa tumor in MEN–1)
  - o Octreotide scan
  - o MBIg scan
  - o CT scan of the abdomen
  - o MRI of the abdomen
  - o Parathyroid scan
  - o Single or multiple ulcers in usual or unusual sites
  - o Thick gastric folds
  - o Fundic gland polyps
  - o CT thick walls of the stomach and duodenum may be pancreatic mass

- ➢ **Mechanisms of Malabsorption** in Zollinger–Ellison Syndrome

  - o Acidification and dilution of small intestinal contents → disturbances in the physical – chemical events of fat digestion
    - − Irreversible inactivation of pancreatic lipase, impaired formation of micellar lipid
    - − Precipitation of bile salts (dihydroxyglycine conjugates); contributory factor by decreased formation of micellar lipid; unabsorbed bile acids may inhibit water and electrolyte transport in colon → diarrhea
    - − Acid milieu inhibits transfer of fatty acids from oil to micellar phase
    - − Excess fluid load presented to the colon → diarrhea
    - − Importance of gastric acid in items 1 – 3 underscored by the fact that diarrhea and steatorrhea are often ameliorated by measures directed at reducing acid output, i.e. gastric aspiration, vagolytic drugs, PPI and total gastrectomy
    - − Structural changes in the duodenal and jejunal mucosa
    - − Changes are highly variable with patchy lesions, including blunted mucosa with absent villi, acute inflammatory exudate in the lamina propria, edema, hemorrhage, microerosions, prominent Brunner's glands, abnormal surface epithelium

- Primary Biochemical **Screening Program for MEN-1**
  - Glucose
  - Albumin corrected total s-calcium
  - Parathyroid hormone
  - Prolactin
  - Insulin–like growth factor 1
  - Insulin
  - Proinsulin
  - Glucagon
  - Pancreatic polypeptide (PP)
  - Gastrin
  - Meal test with PP and gastrin analysis

> Pathology

Hypergastrinemia and hypersecretion of gastric acid may occur with sporatic gastrinoma, or with a gastrinoma-associated with MEN-1 (multiple endocrine neoplasia type 1).

- Give the tumors found in patients with Multiple Endocrine Neoplasia-Type I (MEN-1), and their approximate frequency % is shown.

Tumors	Approximate frequency (%)
o Parathyroid	78 – 97
o Pancreatic endocrine tumor	81 – 82
- Gastrinoma	54
- Insulinoma	21
- Glucagonoma	3
- VIPoma	1
o Pituitary tumors	21 – 65
- Prolactin–secreting	15 – 46
- Growth hormone–secreting	6 – 20
- Cushing's syndrome	16
o Adrenal cortical adenoma	27 – 36
o Thyroid adenoma	5 – 30

- What are the differences between sporadic and MEN–1–associated gastrinomas?

Clinical	Sporadic	MEN–1–associated
o Pathlogy		
– Carcinoid tumors	~ 1%	30%
– Number of tumors	Often single	Often multiple and in different sites
– Site, gastrinoma triangle	80%	Pancreas, duodenal wall
– Growth rate of metastases	Rapid	Slow
– Liver metastases at diagnosis	~ 24%	6%
o Prognosis		
– Overall survival		100% at 20 years
o Laboratory		
– Identification of source of excess gastrin	Yes	No imaged tumors may not be source of ↑ gastrin
o Clinical		
– Family history	No	Yes
o Treatment		
– Consider exploratory laparotomy with curative intent when no evidence of metastatic disease	Yes	No
– Surgical cure (duodenotomy and subtotal pancreatectomy)	50%	No definitive evidence of the benefit of surgery

> Treatment
>   - Optimal outcome is to reduce acid secretion to < 10 mEq/h measured just before the next planned dose of PPI
>   - Control the symptoms with PPI
>   - Reduce the complications of peptic ulcers
>   - Control the gastrin–producing tumor (gastrinoma)

- o In patients with metastatic gastrinoma, there are benefits of external beam radiotherapy, and some gastrinoma with somatostatin receptor–positive tumors from octreotide or lanreotide–SR for the control of symptoms
- o Therapeutic options directed at the metastatic liver disease include
  - Resection
  - Embolization of the hepatic artery ± chemotherapy
  - Radiofrequency ablation (RFA) or cryoablation ± surgical debulking
  - Systemic chemotherapy
    - Streptozocin
    - Doxorubicin
    - Temozolomide
    - Mammalian target of rapamycin (mTOR)
    - Tyrosine kinase (TK) inhibitors
    - Peptide receptor radioligand therapy
- Give the treatment of gastric hypersecretion due to ZES.

Optimal outcome is to reduce acid secretion to < 10 mEq/h, measured just before the next planned dose of PPI, so as to ↑ healing and ↓ recurrence of peptic ulcers, and their complication.

- o Tumor < 2 cm
- o Resection of tumor > 2 cm
- o Parathyroidectomy (if ↑ PTH)
  - Control of symptoms
  - Prevent complications (hemorrhage, obstruction, perforation)
  - Control gastrin–producing tumor (gastrinoma)
- o Give oral PPIs in adequatet doses
  - Achieve optimal acid control

Clinical Cautions

- o Because of prolonged hypergastrinemia in sporadic gastrinoma, there may be hypertrophy of parietal cells even when gastrin levels have returned to normal.
- o As a result, even after a curative resection for a sporadic gastrinoma, the intragastric rate of acid secretion need to be monitored and the dose of continued PIs altered to keep gastric acid secretion below 10 mEq/h as measured just before the next dose of PPI.

SO YOU WANT TO BE A GASTROENTEROLOGIST!

Normally, secretin in the blood decreases gastric antral ECL secretion of SST as well as gastrin (secretin ↓ SST or ↓ gastrin).

- Explain why the opposite effect in ZES in the secretin–stimulated gastrin test in ZES (loss of functional coupling).
    - ↑ SST reduces the release of gastrin from antral G–cells
    - The balance is such that serum gastrin falls and gastric acid secretion also falls.
    - In ZES, there is secretion of large amount of gastrin affecting the gastrin lowering effect of SST in G–cells resulting to the rise of serum gastrin level.
    - Because of the lack of effects of SST in ZES (loss of functionally coupled SST cells), there is a positive effect of exogenous secretin on serum gastrin levels.

> "The covers of the book are too far apart."
> Anonymous

ACUTE NON–VARICEAL UPPER GI BLEEDING (NVUGIB, UGIB)

- Demography
  - The overall incidence of hospitalization for UGIB was 134 per 100,000 population; incidence was higher among men than women (153 versus 117 per 100,000)
  - UGIB incidence but not mortality was associated with lower socio-economic status
  - The overall case fatality rates 30 days after hospital admission was 10.0%; fatality rates rose with age and were higher for men than women and for those with (versus without) co–morbidities.
  - Adjusted fatality rates were 13% higher for patients admitted on weekends than on weekdays, and 41% higher for patients admitted on holidays than on weekdays (the difference in mortality could be attributed to the reduced staffing and lack of availability of endoscopy on weekends and holidays in some hospitals)
  - Patients admitted on weekends or holidays suffered higher mortality than those admitted on weekdays (13% higher on weekends, and 41% higher on holidays).
  - Fatality rates decreased from 11.4% to 8.6% during the study period.
- Clinical
  - A negative NG aspirate in patient who presents with melanoma or hematochezia reduces the likelihood of an upper GI source of bleeding, but because of curling of the tube or duodenal bleeding which does not reflux into the stomach, 15 – 18% of patients with UGIB will have a non-bloody aspirate.
  - The distribution of the endoscopic type of bleeding ulcers is clear–based, 55%; flat pigmented spot, 16%; clot, 8%; visible vessel, 8%; and active bleeding, 12% (Enestvedt, B. K., et al. Gastrointest Endosc. 2008. 422-9.)
  - RCTs show that adding bolus plus infusion of PPI to endoscopic hemostatic therapy (EHT) significantly decrease bleeding (NNT, 12) surgery (NNT, 28) and death (NNT, 45) (Laine, L, et al. Clin Gastroenterol Hepatol. 2009:33-47).

- What are the clinical features of UGIB in elderly and younger patients?
  - Similarities
    - Presenting manifestations of bleeding: hematemesis (50%); melena (30%); hematemesis and melena (20%)

- Peptic ulcer disease is the most common etiology
- Safety and efficacy of endoscopic therapy
  o Differences (elderly compared to younger patients)
    - ↓ antecedent symptoms (abdominal pain, dyspepsia, heartburn)
    - ↑ prior aspirin and NSAID use
    - ↑ presence of comorbid conditions
    - ↑ hospitalization, rebleeding, death

Adapted from: Farrell, J. J. and Friedman, L. S. *Gastroenterol Clin North Am*. 2001. 30(2):377-407, viii.

➢ Causes and associations

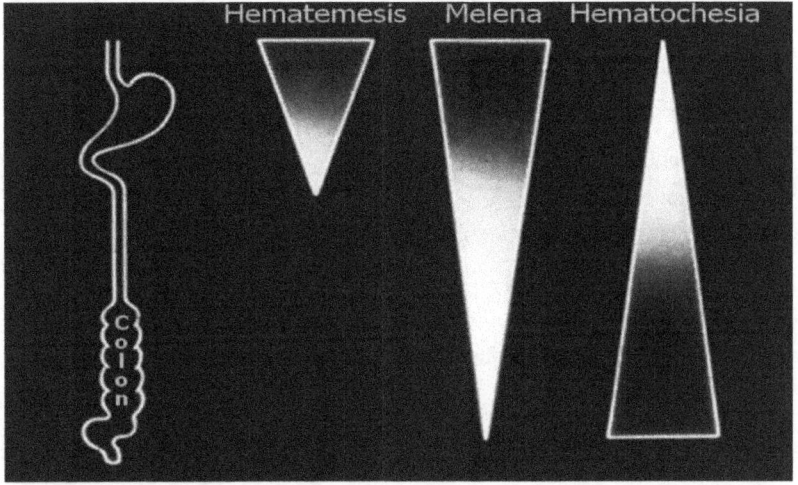

- The causes of NVUGIB (non-variceal Upper GI Bleeding)

  - Esophagus   <u>Causes of NVUGIB</u>
    - Varices   5 – 20%
    - Esophagitis   5 – 10%
    - Esophageal ulcer (Barrett's epithelium)   < 3%
    - Mallory–Weiss tear   5 – 15%
    - Neoplasm, prosthesis, vascular malformation   < 5%

  - Stomach
    - Peptic ulcer   15 – 20%
    - Erosive hemorrhagic gastritis   10 – 20%
    - Neoplasm   < 5%
    - Hiatal hernia   < 2%
    - Vascular malformation   < 2%

  - Duodenum
    - Peptic ulcer   20 – 25%
    - Stromal (anastomotic ulcer)   1 – 5%
    - Erosive duodenitis   5 – 10%

Coagulation and *in vitro* platelet function: influence of pH and peptic activity

  - At pH 6.8   –   Optimal coagulation and platelet aggregation

  - At pH 6.4   –   Doubling of coagulation time
                               –   Reduction in platelet aggregation by 50%

  - At pH 5.4   –   Coagulation is virtually abolished
                               –   Platelet aggregation virtually abolished

  - Peptic activity digests clot   –   Maximal at pH 2 – 3
                               –   Virtually abolished at pH 5

Adapted from: Patchett. *Gut.* 1989. 30:1704.; Green. *Gastroent.* 1978. 74:38.; Low. Thromb Res. 1980. 17:819.

> Diagnosis

- Name the differential diagnoses of bleeding from upper and lower GI tract in patients suffering from HIV/AIDS, excluding non–AIDS–related diagnoses.

Infections	Esophagus	Stomach	Small bowel	Colon
o Candida	+			
o Cytomegalovirus	+	+	+	+
o Herpes simplex	+			
o Idiopathic ulcer	+			+
o Cryptosporidiosis		+	+	
o Salmonella sp.			+	
o Entamoeba histolytica				+
o Campylobacter				+
o Clostridium difficile				+
o Shigella sp				+
o Kaposi sarcoma		+	+	+
o Lymphoma		+	+	+

Adapted from: Mel, Wilcox C. *Sleisenger & Fordtran's Gastrointestinal and Liver Disease: Pathophysiology/ Diagnosis/Management.* 10th Edition. Saunders/Elsevier, Philadelphia, 2016. Box 34-5, page 550.

> Risk Stratification of Initial Bleeding

- What are the patient–related adverse prognostic variables in patients with acute NVUGIB?
  o Increasing age
  o Increasing number of comorbidities (especially renal failure, liver failure, heart failure, cardiovascular disease, disseminated malignancy)
  o Shock — hypotension, tachycardia, tachypnea, oliguria on presentation
  o Melena or hematochezia
  o Increasing number of units of blood transfused
  o Onset of bleeding in the hospital
  o Need for emergency surgery
  o Anticoagulant use, glucocorticosteroids

Abbreviations: NVUGIB, non-variceal upper GI bleeding

- Give the performance characteristics of vital signs and acute blood loss.

Physical Findings	Sensitivity (%)		Specificity (%)
	Moderate Blood Loss	Large Blood Loss	
o Postural pulse increment ≥ 30/min or severe postural dizziness	7 – 57	98	99
o Postural hypotension (≥ 20 mmHg decrease in SBP)	-	-	90 – 98
o Supine tachycardia (pulse > 100/min)	1	10	99
o Supine hypotension (SBP < 95 mmHg)	13	31	98

Adapted from: McGee, S. R. 2007. Evidence–Based Physical Diagnosis. 2nd Edition. *Saunders/Elsevier,* St. Louis, Missouri. Table 15.2 page 167.

➢ **Risk factors** for ulcers and bleeding

Risk factors	
o H. pylori	– 70 – 90% in non–bleeding duodenal ulcers
	– Lower in bleeding ulcers and gastric ulcers
o NSAIDs or ASA (dose–dependent)	– Increased risk of ulcers and bleeding with doses as low as 75 mg/day of ASA
o Corticosteroid + NSAIDs	– Little increased risk when used alone
	– With NSAIDs, increased risk: • Ulcer complications is 2x • GI bleeding is 10x
o Oral anticoagulants +/- NSAIDs	– Increased risk of bleeding versus controls: • Alone is 3.3 • With NSAIDs is 12.7

- What are the clinical methods to estimate volume depletion?

Clinical	Class I	Class II	Class III	Class IV
o Blood loss (mL)	< 750	750 – 1500	1500 – 2000	> 2000
o Blood loss (% blood volume)	< 15	15 – 30	30 – 40	> 40
o Heart (beats/min)	< 100	> 100	> 120	> 140
o Blood pressure	Normal	Normal	Decreased	Decreased
o Pulse pressure	Normal or increased	Decreased	Decreased	Decreased
o Ventilatory rate (breaths/min)	14 – 20	20 – 30	30 – 40	> 35
o Urine output (mL/h)	> 30	20 – 30	5 – 15	Negligible
o Mental status	Slightly anxious	Mildly anxious	Anxious and confused	Confused and lethargic
o Fluid replacement	Crystalloid	Crystalloid	Crystalloid and blood	Crystalloid and blood

Printed with permission: Atkinson, R. J. and Hurlston, D. P. *Best Pract Res Clin Gastroenterol.* 2008. 22(2): page 234.

- Give the performance characteristics of hypotension and its prognosis.

Findings	PLR
o Systolic blood pressure < 90 mmHg	
– Predicting mortality in intensive care unit	4.0
– Predicting mortality in patients with bacteremia	4.9
– Predicting mortality in patients with pneumonia	10.0
o Systolic blood pressure ≤ 80 mmHg	
– Predicting mortality in patients with acute myocardial infarction	15.5

Source: McGee, S. R. 2007. *Evidence Based Physical Diagnosis.* 2nd Edition. Saunders/Elsevier, St. Louis, Missouri, Box 15.1 page 161.

- What are the predictive factors of poor prognosis after hemorrhage from peptic ulcer?

  ➢ Clinical
  - Age > 60 years
  - Bleeding onset in the hospital
  - Comorbid medical illnesses
  - Shock or orthostatic hypotension
  - Multiple transfusions are required

  ➢ Laboratory
  - Coagulopathy
  - Multiple transfusions are required

  ➢ Endoscopy
  - Higher lesser curve gastric ulcer (adjacent to the left gastric artery)
  - Posterior duodenal bulb ulcer (adjacent to the gastroduodenal artery)
  - Endoscopic finding of arterial bleeding or visible vessel

Printed with permission: Barkun, A., *et al*. *Ann Intern Med.* 2003. Consensus Recommendations in Managing Patients with Non–Variceal Upper Gastrointestinal Bleed. 139: 843-57, Table 19-4.

- What is the **Forrest Endoscopic Classification** of bleeding gastroduodenal ulcers?
  - 1a, spurting
  - 1b, oozing
  - IIa, no bleeding, adherent clot
  - IIb, visible vessel
  - IIc, flat pigment spot
  - III, clean ulcer–base
  - No scoring system has been validated to use to predict when rebleeding occur after endoscopic hemostatic therapy (El Munzer, *et al*. 2008). Thus, it is not recommended to routinely undertake a second–look EGD.

- Individualize such practice based on the unproven endpoints of clinically apparent recurrent bleeding, unexplained low levels of hemoglobin concentration after appropriate transfusion, hemodynamic instability, multiple patient morbidities, or a high risk bleeding lesion seen at the index of EGD.

➤ Diagnostic imaging

Gastric Ulcer: 75–year old woman with osteoarthritis presents with dyspepsia

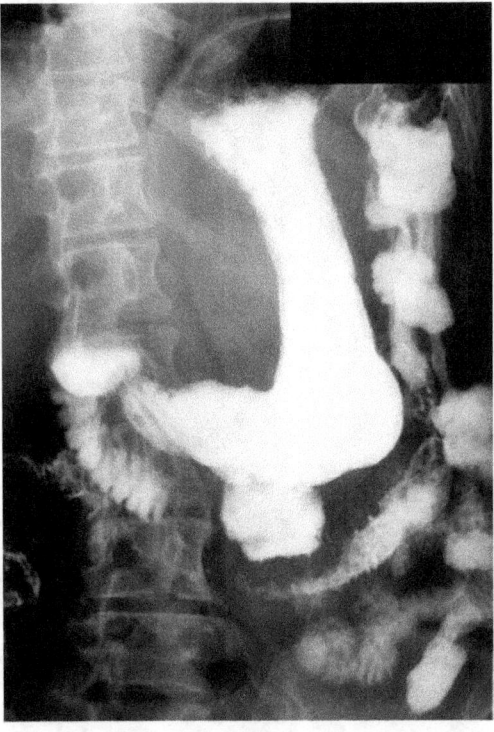

68–year old man with almost life long history of dyspepsia

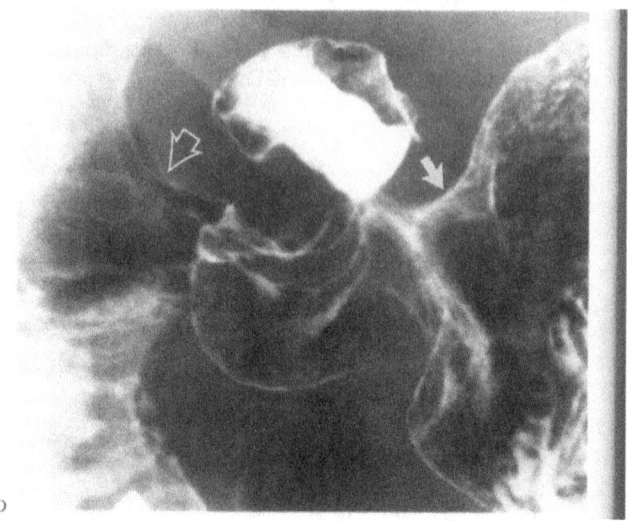

70–year old woman with 10–year history of osteoarthritis on NSAIDs for 6 months

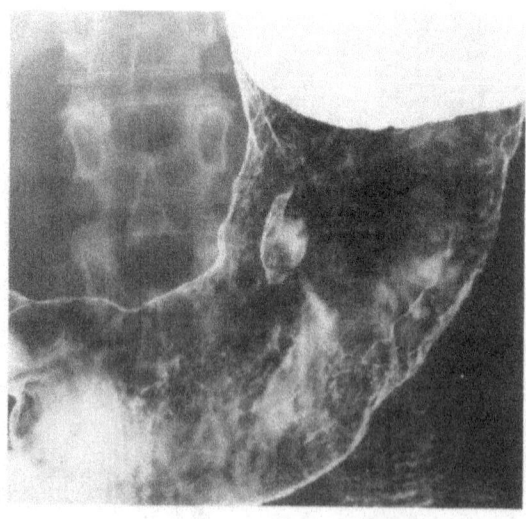

Same patient with barium study as above

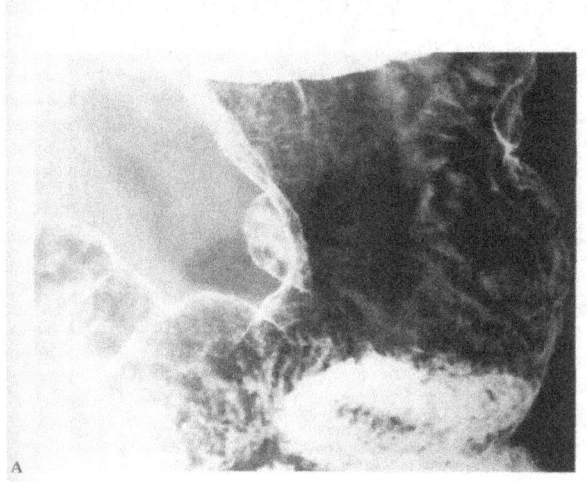

- Pathology

"Visible Vessel"

- Discrete protuberance within the ulcer crater
    - Red, blue, purple
        - High risk
    - White, black
        - Lower risk

Forrest I Non–Variceal Upper GI Bleeding

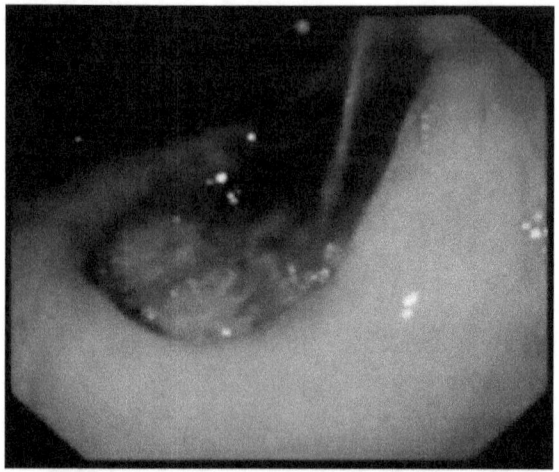

Non–Variceal Upper GI Bleeding

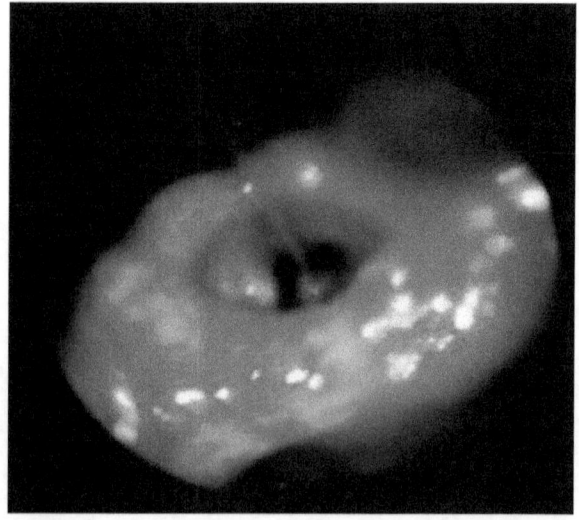

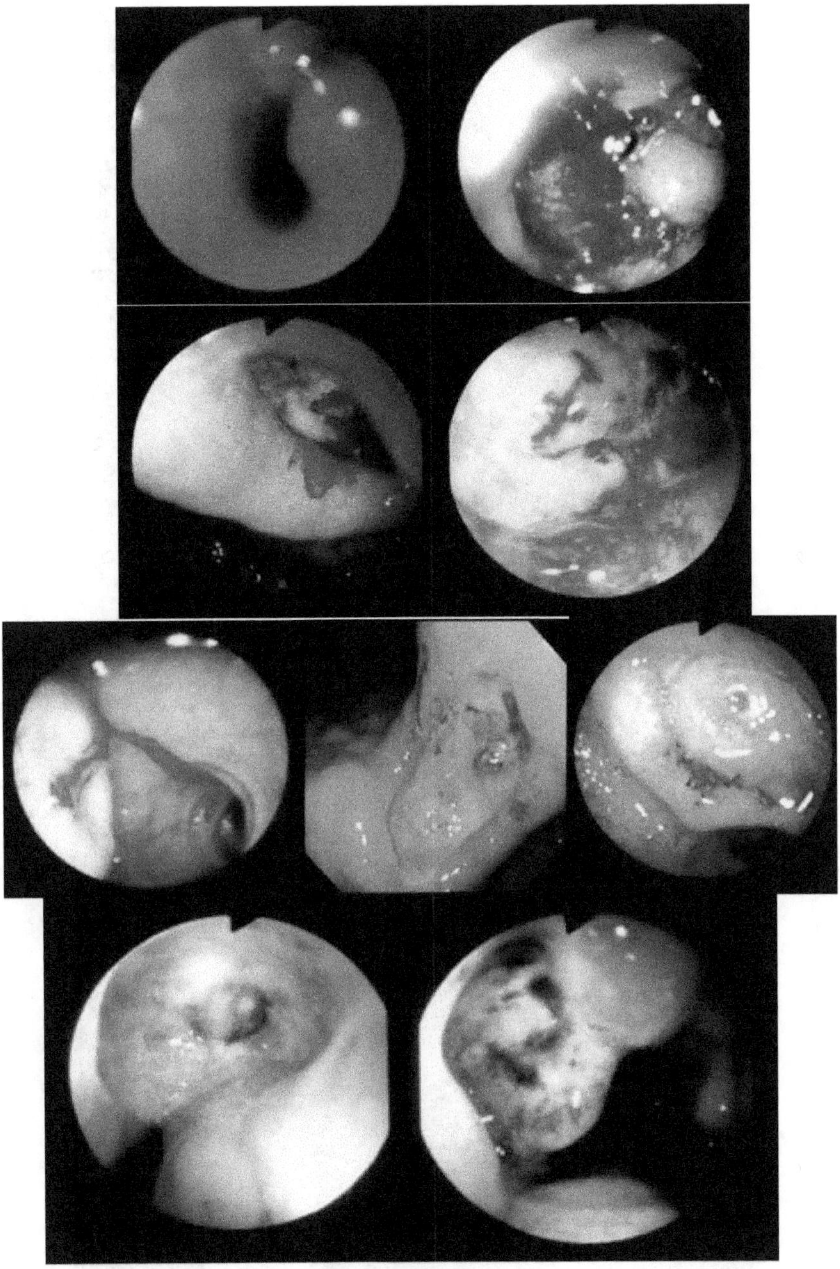

FROM COMPETENCE TO EXCELLENCE
The Stomach

© A.B.R. Thomson

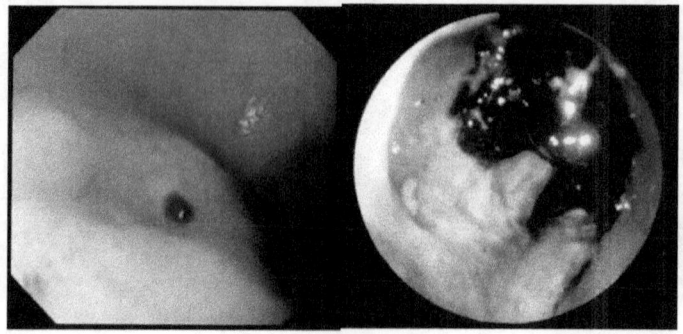

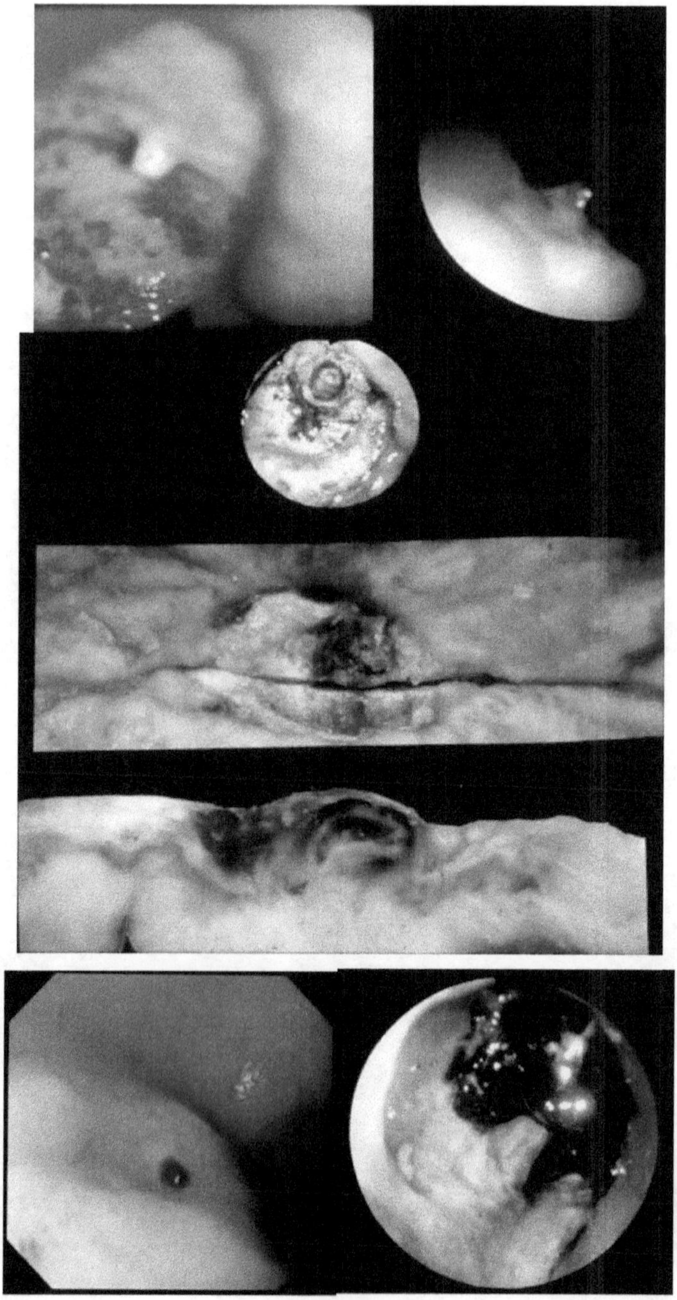

FROM COMPETENCE TO EXCELLENCE
The Stomach

© A.B.R. Thomson

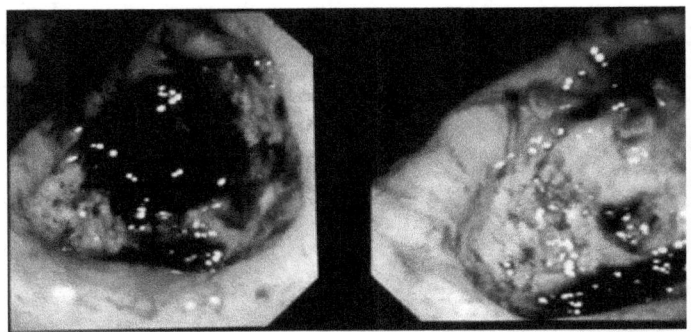

Visible Vessel Gastric Ulcer

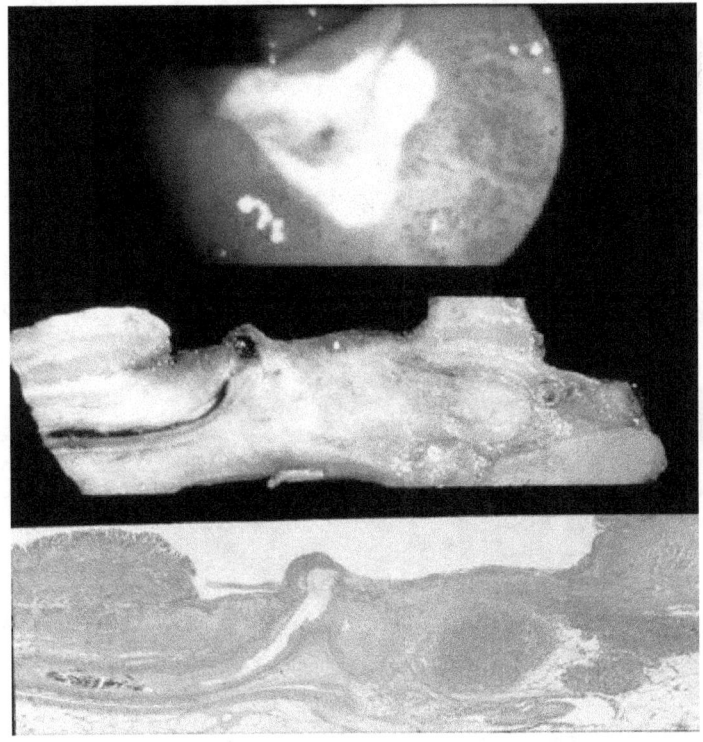

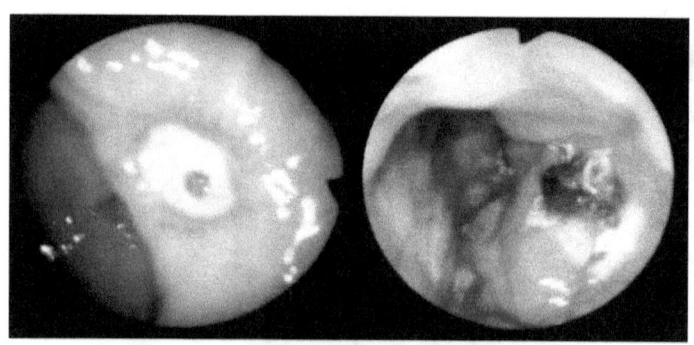
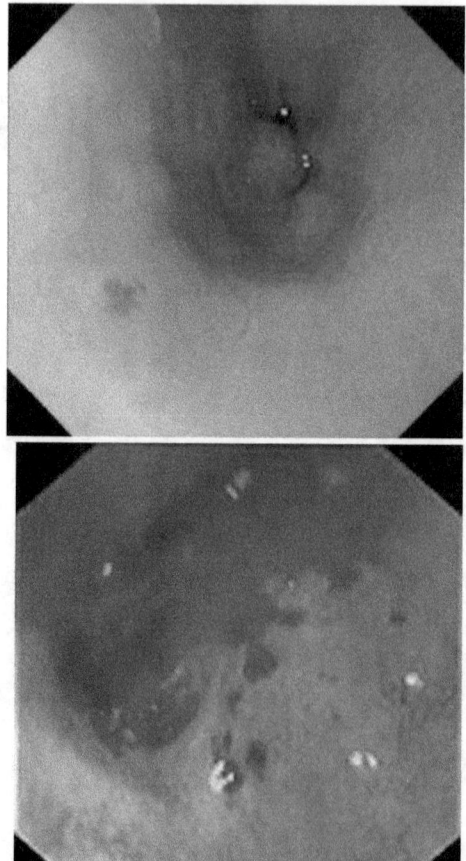

FROM COMPETENCE TO EXCELLENCE
The Stomach

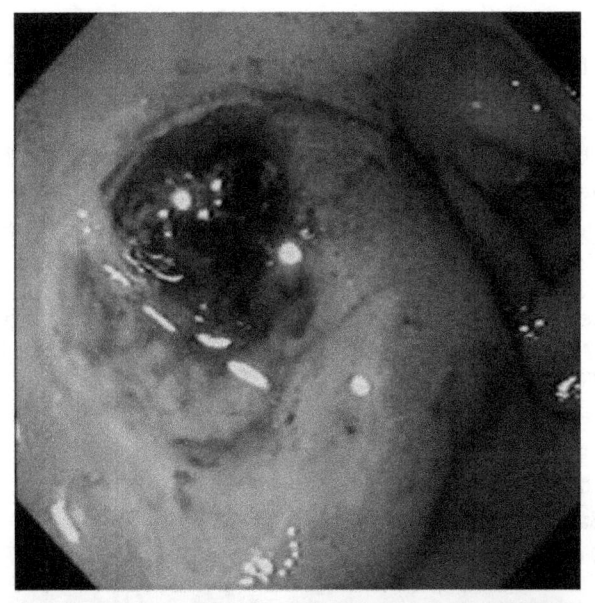
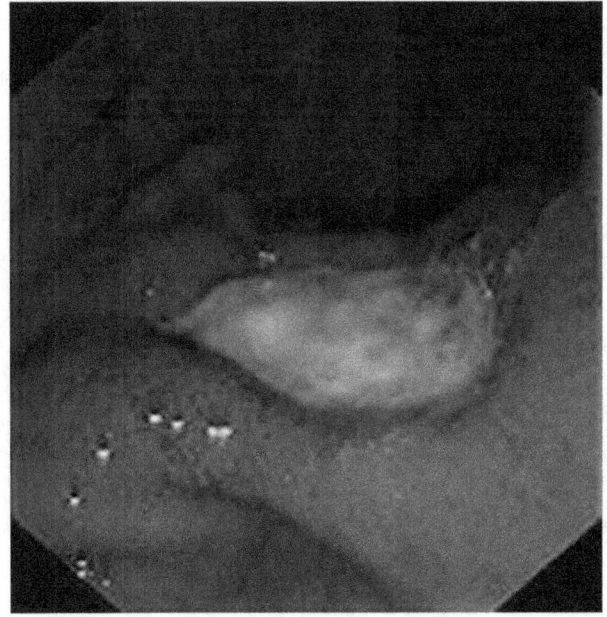

- Treatment

In patient with UGIB and signs of **chronic liver disease**, treat patient with:
  - Octreotide *sc* 50 – 100 mcg boluses, then 25 mcg/hour for up to 3 days
  - Antibiotics (fluoroquinolone) before and 7 days after UGIB, if EV is found
  - While recurrent EV bleeding is common, EGD must be performed with each presentation since just because EV are present does not mean they have bled
  - Characteristic signs of varices seen on EGD will establish whether the acute UGIB in patient with liver disease or known EV arose from the following:
    - Bleeding EV
    - Peptic ulcer disease
    - Mallory–Weiss tear
    - Portal hypertensive gastropathy
    - Gastric antral vascular ectasia (GAVE)
    - Dieulafoy lesion

- What are the rates (%) of rebleeding, surgery and mortality, without and with **endoscopic hemostatic therapy** (ET) using the Forrest classification of bleeding peptic ulcers?

EGD appearance	Prevalence	Rebleeding Rate (%) No EHT (~70% ↓)		Surgery Rate (%) No EHT (~80% ↓)		Mortality rate (%) No EHT (~50% ↓)	
		EHT°	EHT+	EHT°	EHT+	EHT°	EHT+
o Active Bleeding (Ib, oozing)*	18	55	20	35	7	11	< 5
o Visible vessel (IIa); not bleeding	17	43	15	34	6	11	< 5
o Adherent clot (IIb)	15	22	5	10	2	7	< 3
o Flat pigmented spot (IIc)	15	10	< 1	6	< 1	3	< 1
o Clean ulcer–base (III)	35	< 5	< 1	< 1	< 1	< 1	< 1

*Forrest 1a, active bleeding (spurting)
  - Overall benefit of EHT: 2/3 ↓ in risk of rebleeding, surgery, death
    - OR for the use of EHT in high risk lesions

- Recurrent bleeding, 0.46
- Need for surgery, 0.59

Abbreviation: EHT, endoscopic hemostatic therapy

Printed with permission: Atkinson, R. J. and Hurlstone, D. P. *Best Pract Res Clin Gastroenterol.* 2008. 22(2): page 235.; Enestvedt, B. K., *et al. Gastroentest Endosc.* 2008. 67:422-9.

Clinical Tips

- In the ICU patient on a mechanical ventilator, IV H2–receptor blocker or PPI through the nasogastric tube is superior to sucralfate to reduce stress bleeding (Cook, D. J., et al. *N Engl J Med.* 1998. 791-7.; Conrad, S. A., et al. *Crit Care Med.* 2005. 33:760-5.)

- Reducing the intragastric concentration of H^+ reduces the adverse effects of acid and pepsin in patients with non–variceal upper gastrointestinal bleeding (NVUGB). Depending on the risk of peptic ulcer for rebleeding endoscopic hemostatic therapy (ENT) plus an order IV PPI may be predicted (Ghassemi, *et al.* 2009)

	EHT	PPI
o Flat spot, clean ulcer base	-	po
o Adherent clots	+	IV
o Non–bleeding visible vessel	+	IV
o Arterial bleeding, venous oozing	+	IV

Abbreviation: EHT, endoscopic hemostatic therapy; NNT, number needed to treat; TIPS, transjugular intrahepatic portosystemic shunt; UGIB, upper GI bleeding

- **Endoscopic Hemostatic Treatments** (EHT) for bleeding peptic ulcer
    - Thermal Methods: contact
        - Bipolar electrocoagulation
        - Heater probe pain
        - Monopolar electrocoagulation
    - Thermal Methods: non–contact
        - Argon laser
        - Nd: YAG laser
    - Mechanical
        - Microwave
        - Hemo clips
        - Suture (sewing machine) corkscrew
        - Band ligation
    - Injection
        - Sclerosants
        - Vasoconstrictors
        - Saline

- Prognosis
    - Predictors of poor outcome
        - Age over 60 years
        - Cardiac, respiratory, hepatic or renal disease
        - Absence of recent alcohol or drug (aspirin) intake
        - Congestive heart failure
        - Ulcers (protruding vessels)
        - Hematemesis – hypotension
        - Varices
        - Transfusion > 4 units
        - Malignancy

- Patient–related adverse prognostic variables in patients with acute NVUGIB
    - Increasing age (> 60 years)
    - Increasing number of comorbid conditions (i.e. renal failure, liver failure, heart failure, cardiovascular disease, disseminated malignancy)
    - Shock — hypotension, tachycardia, tachypnea, oliguria on presentation
    - Hematochezia or melena
    - Increasing number of units of transfused blood
    - Onset of bleeding in the hospital
    - Need of emergency surgery
    - Anticoagulant use, glucocorticoids
    - Absence of recent alcohol or drug (aspirin) intake
    - Congestive heart failure
    - Protruding vessels in peptic ulcer (DU or GU)
    - Hematemesis, hypotension
    - Varices
    - Transfusion of > 4 units
    - Malignancy

- Give the **Rockall Risk Score Scheme** in assessing the prognosis of patients with NVUGIB (PUD).

Variables	0	1	2	3
Age (years)	< 60	60-79	≥ 80	≥ 80
Shock	SBP ≥ 100, PR < 100/min	SBP ≥ 100, PR ≥ 100	SBP < 100 mm, PR ≥ 100	SBP < 100, PR ≥ 100
Comorbidity	None	None	Cardiac failure, ischemic disease, any major comorbidity	Renal failure, liver failure, disseminated malignancy

Variable	0	1	2	3
o Diagnosis at time of endoscopy	Mallory–Weiss tear, or no lesion identified and no stigmata of recent hemorrhage	All diagnoses except malignancy	Malignancy of the upper GI tract	
o Stigmata of recent hemorrhage	None, or dark spot only		Blood in the upper GI tract Adherent clot Visible or spurting vessel	

Maximum score prior to endoscopic diagnosis = 7, maximum score following diagnosis = 11

Abbreviations: NVUGIB, non–variceal upper GI bleeding; PUD, peptic ulcer disease; PR, pulse rate; SHR, endoscopic stigmata of recent hemorrhage; SBP, systolic blood pressure

Adapted from: Rockall, T. A., *et al. Gut.* 1996. 38:416.; and Atkinson, R. J. and Hurlston, D. P. *Best Practice & Research Clinical Gastroenterology.* 2008. 22(2): page. 235.

Recurrent or Persistent Ulcer Bleeding

➢ Clinical

Additional factors increasing patient's risk of persistent or recurrent NVUGIB:
- o Rockwall score index EGD
- o Active bleeding (Forrest Ia, Ib)
- o DU, lesser curve of the stomach
- o Large GU and DU > 1 – 2 cm
- o CRF (end–stage renal disease) on dialysis, OR of 3

- What are the clinical endpoints suggesting recurrent NVUGIB?
  - o If you see blood in the following sites: NG tube bloody, hematemesis, melena
  - o Blood counts: ↓ hemoglobin ≥ 2 g/dL after 2 consecutive stable hemoglobin taken 3 hours apart

- Vital signs
  - 1 hour of hemodynamic stability: HR ≥ 110 bpm, SB ≤ 90 mmHg (in the absence of sepsis, cardiogenic shock) or ↑ HR / ↓ SBP within 8–hour post–index EGD despite
  - No other explanation, i.e. sepsis, cardiogenic shock
    - Continued melena, hematochezia

- What are the risk factors of persistent or recurrent gastrointestinal tract bleeding, as well as the approximate odds ratio (OR) for ↑ risk?

Risk Factors	OR
Clinical Factors	
Age ≥ 70 years	2.2
Age > 65 years	1.3
Health status (ASA class 1 vs 2 – 5)	1.9 – 7.6
Comorbid illness	1.6 – 7.6
Erratic mental status	3.2
Shock (systolic blood pressure < 100 mmHg)	1.2 – 3.7
Presentation of Bleeding	
Hematemesis	1.2 – 5.7
Red blood on rectal examination	3.8
Melena	1.6
Transfusion requirement	NA
Laboratory Factors	
Coagulopathy	2.0
Initial hemoglobin ≤ 10 g/dL	0.8 – 3.0
Endoscopic Factors	
Ulcer location is high on lesser curve	2.8
Diagnosis of gastric or duodenal ulcer	2.7
Ulcer location on superior wall of duodenum	13.9
Ulcer location on posterior wall of the duodenum	9.2
Active bleeding	2.5 – 6.5
High risk stigma	1.9 – 4.8
Clot over the ulcer	1.7 – 1.9
Ulcer size ≥ 2 cm	2.3-3.5

Printed with permission: Barkun A., Bardou M. and Marshall, J. K. 2003. *Ann Intern Med* Consensus Recommendations for Managing Patients with Non–Variceal Upper Gastrointestinal Bleed. 139: 843-57, Table 19-5.

- What are the risk factors of peptic ulcer rebleeding after successful endoscopic hemodynamic therapy?
    - Hemodynamic instability
    - Active bleeding during endoscopy (spurting more than oozing)
    - Large ulcers (either > 1 cm or > 2 cm as the threshold)
    - Posterior duodenal ulcer or high lesser curve gastric ulcer
    - Need for red blood transfusion

- Treatment
    - Stabilize ABCs
    - IV fluids
    - Transfuse PRBC to maintain hemoglobin concentration at 70 g/L (90 g/L for patient with angina or ischemic heart disease)
    - O_2 by nasal probes or mask, as indicated
    - Routine blood work, i.e. CBC, electrolytes, Cr or BUN, LEs, LFTs
    - Monitor renal function and adequacy of fluid replacement
    - Risk stratification
        - Without or before EGD   Blatchford score
        - With or after EGD   Rockall score
    - Acid inhibition
        - Continuous IV PPI — infusion may be given after EGD, to determine duration of PPI infusion
        - May be given before EGD to "down grade" Rockall risk score: 80 mg IV bolus over 30 minutes, then 8 mg/hour
            - High stigma lesion, continuous 72 hours IV infusion, followed by PPI *po*, duration depends on the lesion
            - Low risk lesion o/c IV infusion after EGD; switch to PPI *po*, for the duration depends on the diagnosis of the cause
        - Note
            - PPI infusion before EGD is recommended for patients with non-variceal UGIB

Abbreviations: EGD, esophagogastroduodenoscopy; LEs, liver enzymes; LFTs, liver function tests; PRBC, packed red blood cells

- Give the benefits of empiric therapy (pre-EGD) use of PPIs in NVUGIB.
  - Downgrade the severity of the lesion and the risk of it rebleeding or requiring surgery (i.e. changing Forrest Ib → IIa)
  - ↓ activation of platelets
  - ↓ peptic digestion of clot ↑ cost effectiveness

  - Downgrading of Rockall risk when giving IV PPIs to EGD or EHT

	IV PPI infusion	Placebo
Active bleeding on EGD	6%	15%
Need for EHT	19%	28%

  - Oral PPIs
    - Use high dose oral PPI to approximate IV PPI infusion, i.e. lansoprazole 30 mg tabs 4, then 30 mg (tabs 1) *po q* 30 minutes
  - Octreotide and somatostatin
    - Potential explanation for clinical benefits
      - ↓ splanchnic blood flow
      - ↓ gastric acid secretion
      - ↑ gastric cytoprotection
    - When to use
      - When EGD or EHT is not available, and PPI infusion or high dose *po* has not been effective

"The key to a good speech: a brilliant opening and a brilliant ending, and keep them as close together as possible"

Peter Ustinov

UPPER GI BLEEDING FROM POSSIBLE ESOPHAGEAL AND GASTRIC VARICES

In patient with UGIB and signs of chronic liver disease, give patient the following:
- Octreotide *sc*
  - For NVUGIB
    - Octreotide 50 – 100 mcg bolus, then 25 mcg/hour for up to 3 days
  - For esophageal variceal bleed (EVB)
    - 50 mcg bolus, followed by 50 mcg/hour
  - If somatostatin to be used for NVUGIB
    - 250 mcg by bolus, then 250 mcg/hour, for 3 to 7 days
- Antibiotics (fluoroquinolone) before and 7 days after UGIB if EV is found
- Endoscopy
  - Diagnosis
    - Exclude esophageal or gastric variceal blood (EVB or GVB) if with liver diseases and varices
      - Prophylactic antibiotics
      - If EVB or GVB → EBL
- Exclude risks for future rebleeding
  - ASA or NSAIDs
    - Use preventive maintenance co–therapy
  - H. pylori
    - Test and treat, then repeat UBT ± EGD biopsies when off PPI for > 7 days
  - H. pylori–negative, NSAID–negative ulcer
    - Maintenance PPI *po*, in standard dose, ½ hour before breakfast
- In fact, while recurrent EV bleeding is common, EGD must be performed with each presentation, since just because EV are present does not mean they have bled (i.e. peptic ulcers are common in patients with cirrhosis)
- Characteristic signs of varices seen on EGD establish whether the acute UGIB in patient with liver disease or known EV arose from bleeding EV, PUD, Mallory–Weiss tear of the gastroesophageal junction, portal hypertensive gastropathy, gastric antral vascular ectasia (GAVE), or a Dieulafoy vascular lesion
- Co–morbidities to be treated

- For non-variceal upper GI bleeding (NVUGIB)
  - Octreotide 50 – 100 mcg bolus, then 25 mcg/hour for up to 3 days
- For esophageal variceal bleed (EVB)
  - 50 mcg bolus, followed by 50 mcg/hour
- If somatostatin is used for NVUGIB
  - 250 mcg by bolus, then 250 mcg/hour, for 3 – 7 days

Abbreviations: ABCs, airway breathing circulation; UBT, urea breath test (for *H. pylori* infection)

- Overall benefit of PPI infusion after EHT, ~ ½ further ↓ in risk of rebleeding, surgery, death
- Timing
  - Usually within 24 hours of the index bleed
  - Earlier may be necessary in some patients
  - Best done with full GI bleeding team of experiences endoscopy nurses, staff, trainees, and available anesthesiologists and general surgeons
- Adherent clots
  - Gently wash to visualize the nature of the underlying lesion
- Use two modalities of endoscopic hemostatic treatment, i.e. injection of epinephrine plus thermal coagulation or hemostatic clips
  - Epinephrine 1:10,000 dilution, 0.5 – 2.0 mL aliquots given into 4 quadrants, within 3 mm of the bleeding site

---

Clinical Heads–Ups

Hemospray®, a nanopowder that promotes hemostasis, has been shown in preliminary studies to be 95% effective in achieving acute hemostasis in patients with oozing peptic ulcers.

- Second look on EGD
  - No scoring system has been validated to use to predict when rebleeding will occur after endoscopic hemostatic therapy (El–munzer, et al. 2008).
  - Thus, it is not recommended to routinely undertake a second look on EGD
  - Unexplained low levels of hemoglobin concentration after appropriate transfusion

- Unexplained hemodynamic instability, multiple patient morbidities
- A high risk bleeding lesion seen at the index of EGD
- A planned second look on EGD within 24 hours of the index EGD may be justified, if the following are present:
  - Poor visualization in the initial EGD
  - Possible poor EHT in the initial EGD
- An unplanned second look EGD
  - Persistent or recurrent bleeding

- Interventional Angiography: Transarterial Embolization (TAE)
  - Success of TAE for index bleed is 52 – 88%
  - Risk of rebleeding 10 – 20%
  - After EHT failure — consider TAE for high surgical risk
    - Hematobilia or bleeding into the pancreatic duct

- Surgery in NVUGIB
  - Mortality rate
    - Urgent ~ 25%
    - Elective ~ 5%
  - Recurrent (post–op) bleeding ~ 5%

CLINICAL TIP

- Explain why patient with isolated IgA deficiency should not be given blood transfusion.
  - The patient would have IgG and IgE antibodies (anti–IgA antibodies), which react against the IgA in the transfused blood, just as would happen with IV immunoglobulins.

SO YOU WANT TO BE A GASTROENTEROLOGIST!

If blood transfusion is contraindicated in patient with isolated IgA deficiency, give what is done if an urgent situation is faced and a blood transfusion is the only life saving.
  - The RBCs may be washed, removing most of the serum containing the IgA in the blood to be transfused. The washed and packed RBC may then be given safely.

OBSCURE GI BLEEDING

➢ Demography

Useful background: Obscure GI bleeding: Where in the small bowel are the lesions?

- o AVMs
  - Jejunum: 36%
  - Ileum: 34%
  - Jejunum and ileum: 30%

- o Polyps
  - Jejunum: 70% (36% proximal jejunum)
  - Ileum: 30% (16% terminal ileum)
  - Endoscopic therapy for AV malformations, angiodysplasia, angioectasia, angioma, venous ectasia (AVMs): < 10% of patients with angioectasia never bleed, and 50% will never rebleed
  - Cessation rates from AVM using push enteroscopy (PE), 57 – 85% (*AGA technical review, 2007*)
  - One year after double balloon enteroscopy for AVM, 57% required retransfusion, or are bleeding–free (Gerson, L. B. 2009. *Gastrointest Endosc Clin N Am*. Jul;19(3):481-96); other studies have shown rebleeding rates ranging from 20 – 63% (Viazis, N., *et al. Gastrointest Endosc*. 2009. 69(4):850-6.; Kafes, A. J., *et al. Gastrointest Endosc*. 2007. 66(2):304-9.; de Leusse, A., *et al. Gastroenterology*. 2007. 132(3):855-6.)

Printed with permission: Feagins, L. A. and Kane, S. V. *Am J Gastroenterol.* 2009. 104:770.

➢ Diagnostic imaging

- What diagnostic methods in determining the cause of obscure GI bleeding?

  - o Endoscopy
    - Capsule endoscopy (CE)
    - Double balloon enteroscopy (DBE)
    - Push enteroscopy (PE)
    - Intraoperative endoscopy
    - Repeat endoscopy
    - Repeat colonoscopy

- Small bowel contrast-ray
  - Small bowel single contrast
  - Small bowel double contrast (enteroclysis)
- CT or MRI
  - CT angiography (CTA)
  - CT or MRI enteroscopy (CTE or MRIE)
  - CT enteroclysis
- Angiography
  - In the presence or absence of acute bleeding
- Scintigraphy
  - Erythrocyte scintigraphy (RBC scan)
  - Meckel scintigraphy

Abbreviations: CE, capsule endoscopy; DBE, double balloon enteroscopy

Adapted from: Heil, U. and Jung, M. *Best Pract Res Clin Gastroenterol.* 2007. 21(3): page 402.

A patient has iron deficiency anemia, FOB–positive melena stools, a normal EGD with normal duodenal biopsies (excludes celiac disease), and normal colonoscopy with intubation of the terminal ileum.

- "best test" from a long list of diagnostic options for obscure GI bleeding
  - Diagnostic imaging
    - Small bowel follow through
    - Enteroclysis
    - CT or MR enteroscopy
    - RBC scan
    - Meckel scan
    - Angiopathy
  - Endoscopy
    - Capsule endoscopy
    - Push enteroscopy
    - Double balloon enteroscopy
  - And the right answer is...
    - None of the above!
    - Repeat the EGD or colonoscopy, perhaps by a more experienced operator
    - Most causes of OGIB are identified on the second EGD or colonoscopy

Pros and cons of diagnostic choices for: Obscure GI bleeding (OGIB)

- ➢ EGD or colonoscopy
  - o In patients with OGIB, 35 – 75% of the causes are revealed by second look EGD, and 6% by second look colonoscopy (Leighton, 09). Small bowel lesions account for only 5% of OGIB, and most of these (70%) are vascular lesions (Cellier, C. *Best Pract Res Clin Gastroenterol.* 2008. 329-40)

- ➢ Small bowel endoscopy
  - o Most of the lesions diagnosed by push enterostomy in patients with OGIB are within the reach of standard EGD
  - o Double balloon enteroscopy (DBE) is superior to single balloon enteroscopy (SBE). DBE can be performed in an oral or antegrade, or anal or retrograde manner.
  - o Approximate depth of endoscopic penetration of small bowel
    - Push enteroscopy   90 – 150 cm
    - Ileoscopy   50 – 80 cm
    - DBE
      - Oral   240 – 360 cm
      - Rectal   102 – 140 cm
  - o DBE has a diagnostic yield of 60 – 80% in patients with OGIB suspected to be from the small intestine, with therapeutic intervention being possible in 40 – 73%
  - o Meta–analysis has shown comparable diagnostic yield for DBE and CE (57-60%), with therapeutic potential with DBE (Pasha, S. F., *et al. Clin Gastroenterol Heptaol.* 2008. 671-6.; Chen, X., *et al. World J Gastroenterol.* 2007. 13:4372-8.)

- ➢ Capsule endoscopy
  - o Diagnostic yield of capsule endoscopy (CE) in patient with OGIB ranges from 38 – 83% (Rondonotti, E., *et al. World J Gastroenterol.* 2007. 6140-9).
  - o CE is more likely to give a positive yield when there has been more than one episode of bleeding, overt bleeding rather than occult (60% vs 46%), CE is performed within 2 weeks of the bleeding episode (91% vs 34%), bleeding occurred over more than 6 months, and bleeding has resulted to hemoglobin concentration of < 10 g/dL (Carey, E. J., *et al. Am J Gastroenterol.* 2007. 102:89-95)
  - o False negative rate for CE is 19% for tumors, and 11% overall

- CE cannot be performed in patients with stricture or obstruction, since this requires surgical removal of the capsule

➤ Meckel scan
- Meckel scan for Meckel diverticulum is performed with technetium–99m pectinate, and has a sensitivity of 64 – 100% for bleeding from ectopic gastric mucosa
- A false negative Meckel scan may be the result of a recent barium X-ray obscuring the area of uptake, too small diverticulum, too small vascular supply to the diverticulum, or too rapid bleeding from the diverticulum washing out to the technetium

➤ RBC scan
- Technetium–99m–labeled RBC scan shows slow bleeding, (0.1 – 0.4 ml/min), whereas angiography needs higher rates of bleeding (> 0.5 ml/min) to be positive
- With active bleeding, the bleeding site may be localized in 50 – 75% of patients, but the sensitivity rate falls below 50% with slower rates of bleeding

➤ Angiography
- An angiography suggests angioectasia from a vascular tuft or slow filling of a vein
- Therapeutic embolization may be performed with gelfoam or coils
- Papaverine may be infused at the time of angiography

➤ CTE
- For CT enterography (CTE), oral contrast is given and by nasojejunal tube for CT enteroclysis
- Diagnostic yield of CTE in OGIB is 45% (Huprich, J. E., et al. Radiology. 2008. 562-71.), and may be useful to distinguish fibrostenotic from inflammatory Crohn disease (Paulsen, S.R., et al. Radiol Clin North Am. 2007. 303-15.; Horsthuis, K., et al. Radiology. 2008. 64-79.).

- Compare and contrast the endoscopic findings and treatments of portal hypertensive gastropathy (PHG) and gastric antral vascular ectasia (GAVE).

Findings	PHG	GAVE
o Sites	Fundus	Antrum
o Mosaic patterns	Yes	No
o Red color signs	Yes	Yes
o Findings on gastric mucosal biopsy		
- Thrombi	No	+++
- Spindle cell proliferation	Sparse	++
- Fibrohyalinosis	No	+++
➤ Management	o ↓ portal hypertension	o Estrogens
	o β–adrenergic blockers	o Antrectomy
	o TIPS	o (TIPS doesn't help) Endoscopic laser therapy
	o Liver transplantation	o Liver transplantation

*Note: Gastric vascular ectasia (GVE) may occur anywhere in the stomach, not just in the antrum, so do not distinguish GAVE or EVE from PHG just on the site of localization

> An alcoholic is a person who drinks more than his physician! Don't believe it. TRUST, BUT VERIFY!
>
> Grandad

NON–STEROIDAL ANTI–INFLAMMATORY DRUGS (NSAIDS)

- Dyspepsia and NSAIDs
  - Risk of bleeding with NSAIDs and COXIBs is increased with the following:
    - Use of ASA and Clopidogrel
    - *H. pylori* infection
  - NSAIDs (excluding naproxen) and COXIBs increase the risk of the following:
    - Hypertension
    - Renal dysfunction
    - Fluid retention
    - Coronary artery disease events

- Pathophysiology (NSAID–induced mucosal damage)
  - Topical irritant effects on the epithelium (ion trapping; depletion of ATP via uncoupling of oxidative phosphorylation; decreased hydrophobicity of the mucus gel layer)
  - Impairment of the barrier properties — acid back diffusion
  - Suppression of prostaglandin synthesis
  - Reduction of the gastric mucosal blood flow
  - Interference with repair of superficial injury
  - Interference with hemostasis
  - Interference with growth factors

- Deleterious effects of NSAIDs

Membrane Damage	Free Phospholipids	Loss of Hydrophobicity
o Hydrolysis of phospholipids	− Lysed platelet activating factor (PAF)	• Enhanced permeability • Ulceration
o Increased lipooxygenase activity	− Free radicals − Leukotriene A4 − Peptide–leukotriene − Increased LTC4–LTD4 LTE	• Membrane damage • Increased lysosomal activity • Vasoconstriction • Ischemia • Chronic inflammation

Membrane Damage	Free Phospholipids	Loss of Hydrophobicity
o Decreased cyclooxygenase activity	– Prostaglandin deficiency	• Impaired blood flow • Impaired mucous and HCO_3^- production
o Uncoupled oxidative phosphorylation	– AMP + free radical (via xanthine oxidase)	• Membrane damage • Lysosomal activation

➤ Scoring system for drug–induced mucosal damage
  Grade 0 No visible injury
  Grade 1 < 10 (petechial) hemorrhages with no erosions
  Grade 2 10 – 25 hemorrhages with no erosions
  Grade 3 > 25 hemorrhages and/or 6 – 10 erosions
  Grade 4 > 10 erosions and/or ulcer

*Grade 0 – 2 = clinically insignificant
**Grade 2 – 4 = clinically significant

➤ Drug–associated gastritis (i.e. ASA)
 o Rapidly absorbed in the stomach when not buffered (low pKa of 3.5; at pH and 3.5, respectively, 95% and 50% is protonated and fat soluble)
 o ASA accumulates in the surface epithelial cells due to pH–partition mechanism
 o Inhibits mitochondrial oxidative phosphorylation
 o Inhibits prostaglandin formation
 o Destruction of the barrier and back–diffusion of injurious hydrogen ions (cell shedding, erosions, disruption of microvessels)
 o Tight junctions remain intact
 o Morning dose is more damaging than the evening dose, even though acidity is higher in the evening

➤ NSAID–associated GI toxicity: for individual patient
 o GI intolerance: up to 50% incidence
 o Endoscopic ulcers: 15 – 25% incidence
 o Symptomatic ulcers or ulcer complications: 2 – 4% per year
 o Ulcer complications: 1 – 2% per year

➤ Upper GI tract: Mucosal damage from NSAIDs, a spectrum of injury

- Intramucosal petechial hemorrhage
- Superficial mucosal erosions
- Chronic ulceration
  - Stomach > duodenum
- Bleeding, perforation of ulcers
  - Stomach = duodenum

CLINICAL TIPS

- Correlate gastritis on biopsy, endoscopy and its symptoms.
  - The correlation is poor between any two of these three factors.

- What findings on biopsy suggest gastritis due to NSAIDs or ASA?
  - Foveolar hyperplasia, a "corkscrew" appearance of the gastric foveolar, is suggestive of exogenous substance damage, i.e. from ASA or NSAIDs.

GAVE Stomach

- Foveolar hyperplasia, large blood vessels near the mucosal surface of the stomach – think of GAVE!
  - Fibrin thrombi
  - CD61 highlights platelets, and may help identify fibrin thrombi

---

- NSAIDs and gastroprotection
  - Concomitant PPI use reduces the risk of the development of NSAID–induced endoscopic lesions, i.e. ulcers
  - Concomitant PPI use is strongly recommended for high risk NSAID users
  - It is not known whether concomitant PPI use reduces the risk of clinically significant GI events, i.e. hemorrhage and perforation
  - PPI co–therapy in high risk NSAID users is equivalent to COX–2 therapy in preventing NSAID–induced endoscopic lesions
  - PPI use is effective as secondary prevention for ulcer complications in patients needing antithrombotic therapy with aspirin or clopidogrel
  - As alternatives to PPIs, misoprostol and H_2RAs can be used in the prevention of NSAID–related ulcers and complications, and their use is cost–effective

- PPI as co-therapy is effective in healing and prevention of recurrence of ulcers in patients maintained on long term NSAID therapy
- Dyspepsia may be associated with the use of NSAIDs, COXIBs, ASA
- Relative increased risk of ulcer and ulcer bleeding in NSAIDs > COXIBS
- Risk of bleeding with NSAIDs and COXIBs is increased with:
  - The use of the following drugs:
    - ASA
    - Clopidogrel
  - *H. pylori* infection
- NSAIDs (excluding naproxen) and COXIBs increase the risk of the following:
  - Hypertension
  - Renal dysfunction
  - Fluid retention
  - Coronary artery disease events
- Patients with cardiovascular diseases (CV) may be on aspirin (ASA) when they develop NVUGIB
- The reflex action may stop ASA to reduce the risk of recurrent ASA–associated bleeding
- This is successful from the GI perspective (recurrent bleeding is higher in patients on rather than off ASA, 10.3% vs 5.4%).
- However, this discontinuation of ASA in high CV–risk patient leads to a higher CV mortality rate (12.9% vs 1.3%) (Sung, et al. Ann. Int. Med. 2010. 152:1-9).
- Patient with both high CV– and GI–risk should be kept on ASA and gastroprotective therapy with PPI be used
- When deciding to place a patient on NSAIDs, risk stratification must consider GI and renal risks, the presence of *H. pylori*, and importantly, the cardiovascular risks (Gupta and Eisen, 2009).
- The use of NSAID plus PPI, a COX–2 inhibitor, or a COX–2 inhibitor plus PPI does not prevent damage to the small or large intestine
- The importance of cardiovascular risk of Coxibs becomes apparent with the APPROVED study. In patient with both high GI– and CV–risk, an NSAID is given with ASA and a PPI
- The vulnerable inflammatory phenotype of atherosclerosis is associated with Th1 type immune response. The traditional NSAIDs and selective COX–2 inhibitors enhance this Th1 response by reducing prostanoids and promoting pro–atherogenic cytokines and plaque instability. It is proposed

that this is the mechanism by which these classes of drugs enhance CV risk (Padol and Hunt, 2009; Rainsford, 2010)

Adapted from: Arora, et al. Clin Gastroenterol Hepatol. 2009. 7:725-735

- Risk Stratification
    - There must be risk stratification for the development of peptic ulcer bleeding because of poor association between NSAID–associated dyspepsia and peptic ulcer or peptic ulcer bleeding
    - There is numerous patient–related risk factors associated with the use of NSAIDs, COXIBs, ASA, Clopidogrel. The magnitude of the relative risks should not be compared because various studies were used, including different patient populations and risk factors
    - Treatment algorithms often refer to low, moderate or high GI risk, but actual values of the relative or absolute risks are not used to define these risk categories
    - It is reasonable to accept that low GI risk comprises a group with no risk factors other than the intake of the usual doses of the single agent (NSAID, COXIB, ASA, Clopidogrel)
    - An arbitrary definition of the risk has been provided by Lanza, et al. (Am J Gastroenterol. 2009. 104:728-738):
        - High risk
            - History of previous complicated ulcer, especially recent
            - 3 or more risk factors
        - Moderate risk
            - 1 or 2 risk factors
            - > 65 years
            - High dose of NSAID therapy
            - Previous history of uncomplicated (non–bleeding) ulcer
            - Concurrent use of any dose of the following drugs:
                - ASA
                - Steroids
                - Anticoagulant

- Who is at high risk of bleeding from NSAID–associated ulcer?

Established	Probable	Not established

- o Patient Age < 60 years   CVS disease   Sex
           Past history   Arthritis–type

- o Drug   High dose   1st 3 months of   Half life
           Toxic NSAID   treatment   Form
           Steroids   On warfarin

"The Mucosa Trial" (M = 8849)

	Misoprostol	Placebo
o Complications (*H. pylori*)	25	42
o Complication rate (%)	0.57	0.95

- o Risk of hemorrhage and perforation were reduced by approximately half using gastroprotection with misoprostol

- What is the relative risk (RR) of clinical factors associated with upper gastrointestinal clinical events (i.e. bleeding, perforation, obstruction) in the patients taking NSAIDs?

Clinical features	RR*
o Age > 60 – 75 years	2.5
o History of upper gastrointestinal symptoms	2.5
o History of peptic ulcer	2.5
o History of gastrointestinal bleeding	5
o *H. pylori*–positive	2.0
o Severe rheumatoid arthritis disability	2.5
o History of cardiovascular disease	2.5
o Medications	
– High dose of NSAIDs	7
– Multiple NSAIDs	10
– Concomitant low dose ASA	10
– Concomitant anticoagulant	10
– Concomitant corticosteroids	1.5
– Concomitant SSRIs	2.0

Abbreviations: ASA, acetylsalicylic acid; NSAID, non–steroidal anti–inflammatory drug; SSRI, selective serotonin reuptake inhibitors

*RR, relative risks associated with various risk factors; since these studies included differing patient populations and not all studies considered all risk factors, direct comparisons of the magnitudes of the risks (i.e. rows of the table) should be avoided

Adapted from: Rostom, *et al. Alim.Pharm.Therapeutics.* 2009. 29:481-496.

> "A journey of a thousand miles begins with a single step"
> Lao Tzu

- Calculate the annual risk adverse effects in a 70-year old man on a high dose of NSAIDs, who has a history of prior bleeding peptic ulcer, and is on maintenance PPI - his *H. pylori* status is unknown

The annual incidence of NSAID-induced adverse event can be estimated by multiplying the baseline absolute risk with patient-specific relative risk modifiers.

Risk Characteristics

- Baseline absolute risk for GI event (%) - 2.5 (1.5 – 4.5%)   2.5   1.5 – 4.5
- Increased in risk [B]:
  - Age > 65 years   2.5   1.5 – 5.5
  - Use of anticoagulants   2.5   2.0 – 5.0
  - Use of steroids   2.0   1.0 – 3.0
  - History of peptic ulcer disease   5.0   2.0 – 12.0
  - High dose of NSAIDS   2.0   1.5 – 3.0
  - Presence of *Helicobacter pylori*   1.5   1.0 – 3.0
- Reduction of risk [C]:
  - Therapy with PPI   0.5

> COXIBs
  - COX-2 inhibitors are "...probably as effective as a combination of non-selective NSAIDs combined with PPI in patients at risk for ulcers"
  - Considering celecoxib vs diclofenac plus PPI, "...neither treatment could eliminate the risk of recurrent bleeding in very high risk patients" (recent history of bleeding peptic ulcer, 6 months risk of ulcer 20 – 25%, risk of recurrent bleeding, 5%
  - "...COX-2 inhibitors but also non-selective NSAIDs, with the exception of full dose naproxen (1000 mg/day), have increased cardiovascular risk" (risk ratio of tomach1.42), and "...there was no significant difference in cardiovascular risk between COX-2 inhibitors and non-selective NSAIDs. Naproxen (500 mg *bid*) was the only exception (Feldman, M., et al. *Sleisenger and Fordtran's Gastrointestinal and Liver Disease*. 2010. 9th Edition. *Saunders/Elsevier*, Philadelphia. page 875).

> H. pylori
  - *H. pylori* increases the risk of ulcer bleeding 1.79 folds, NSAIDs 4.85 folds, and *H. pylori* plus NSAIDs is ~ 6 folds.
  - "Among the patients who are about to start NSAIDs therapy, eradication of *H. pylori* reduced [by about 50% but does not prevent] the subsequent risk of ulcer development"

- Thus, "...eradication of H. pylori infection alone is not sufficient for the prevention of ulcer bleeding in NSAID users with high ulcer risks"
- Although, H. pylori increases the ulcer risk in patients receiving low-dose aspirin, "co-therapy with PPI after eradication of H. pylori was still required..."

Adapted from: Feldman, M., et al. Sleisenger and Fordtran's Gastrointestinal and Liver Disease. 2016. 10th Edition. Saunders/Elsevier, Philadelphia. Table 58-2, page 893.

> Summary
  - Odds ratios (ORs) and P values for comparisons between gastroprotective strategies of patients using NSAIDs or COXIBs (COX-2 inhibitors)

  A. For all upper GI complications, refer to the following table:

	NSAID + low dose misoprostol	NSAID + PPI	NSAID + PPI + low dose misoprostol	COXIB alone	COXIB + PPI
NSAID + low dose misoprostol (0.74)					
NSAID + PPI (0.67)	0.88 (0.52 – 1.49) $P > 0.20$				
NSAID+PPI+low-dose misoprostol 0.58	0.78 (0.46 – 1.34) $P > 0.20$	0.86 (0.47 – 1.57) $P > 0.20$			
COXIBs (0.51)	0.68 (0.56 – 0.85) $P = 0.0006$[a]	0.75 (0.53 – 1.06) $P = 0.11$	0.87 (0.52 – 1.49) $P > .20$		
COXIBs + PPIs (0.36)	0.48 (0.36 – 0.65) $P < 0.0001$[a]	0.53 (0.36 – 0.79) $P = 0.0018$[a]	0.62 (0.35 – 1.09) $P = 0.093$	0.70 (0.55 – 0.91) $P = 0.0068$[a]	

NOTE: Those shown in bold are statistically significant.

B. For all upper GI complications secondary to peptic ulcer disease

NSAID + low dose misoprostol (0.61)					
NSAID + PPI (0.50)	0.81 (0.48-1.38) $P > .20$				
COXIB (0.46)	0.74 (0.55-1.00) $P = .050$	0.91 (0.55-1.50) $P > .20$			
NSAID+PPI+low-dose misoprostol (l0.29)	0.46 (0.18-1.21) $P = .117$	0.58 (0.21-1.60) $P > .20$	0.63 (0.25-1.60) $P >.20$		
COXIB + PPI (0.23)	0.37 (0.23-0.57) $P < .001^a$	0.49 (0.25-0.82) $P =.0084^a$	0.50 (0.34-0.73) $P < .001^a$	0.79 (0.29-2.09) $P > .20$	
	NSAID + low-dose misoprostol	NSAID + PPI	COXIB alone	NSAID + PPI + low-dose misoprostol	COXIB + PPI

NOTE: ORs for relative risk reduction versus nsNSAID users alone shown in parentheses.

Printed with permission: Targownik, L. E., et al. Gastroenterology. 2008. 134:937-44.

> Antiplatelet drugs
  o Low dose aspirin alone slightly decreases all the causes of mortality (RR, 0.93; 95% CI, 0.87 – 0.99) but increases the risk of major GI bleeding (odds ratio, 1.55; 95% CI, 1.27 – 1.90)
  o PPI use plus aspirin decreased the likelihood of bleeding (OR, 0.34; 95% CI, 0.21 – 0.57).
  o Low dose aspirin negates the GI mucosa–sparing effects of COX–2 inhibitor
  o Combining ASA with clopidogrel or anticoagulants, the risk for major bleeding is higher than with aspirin alone (OR, 1.86; 95% CI, 1.49 –2.31 and OR, 1.93; 95% CI, 1.42 – 2.61, respectively).
  o One of the major complications of these anti–ischemic therapies is gastrointestinal bleeding
  o Omeprazole can significantly reduce the risk of adverse upper gastrointestinal events in patients receiving clopidogrel alone
  o Patients with acute coronary syndrome, or ST elevation myocardial infarction, esomeprazole is superior to famotidine in preventing upper gastrointestinal complications related to aspirin, clopidogrel, and enoxaparin or thrombolytics

Source: Ng, F. H., et al. Am J Gastroenterol. 2012. 107:389-391.; Goldstein, J. L., et al. Aliment Phamacol Ther. 2011. 34:808.

- Prevention
  - PPIs but not H₂RAs reduce (by ~ 50%), but do not eliminate the risk of endoscopic ulcer, ulcer symptoms and recurrent ulcer bleeding
  - Eradication of an *H. pylori* infection ↓ risk of the following:
    - Endoscopic ulcer in patients starting on treatment with NSAIDs or ASA
      - Beneficial before starting NSAID therapy
      - Ulcer bleeding in patients who are already on ASA (weak data)
      - Mandatory in patients with history of peptic ulcer disease
      - In patients with NVUGIB associated with *H. pylori* infection, start the treatment as soon as oral feeding is started
  - Maintenance therapy with PPIs is "...superior to *H. pylori* eradication alone in primary or secondary prevention of endoscopic ulcers among NSAID users" (Rostom, et al. Aliment Pharmacol Ther. 2009. 29:481-96.

Adapted from *Rostom, A., et al., Aliment. Pharmacol Ther.* 2009. 29:481-496.

- What should you recommend to avoid peptic ulcers (gastric or duodenal; GU, DU) associated with the use of NSAIDs as a function of low, moderate and high gastrointestinal, as well as low and significant cardiovascular risk (CV) (i.e. required use of ASA plus NSAID)?

	Low Risk	Moderate Risk	High Risk
❖ Low CV Risk (no ASA)	o An NSAID with low ulcerogenic potential at the lowest effective dose o Consider testing or treating for *H. pylori* if starting with NSAIDs o Avoid multiple or high dose NSAIDs	- NSAID plus PPI - Misoprostol - COXIB	• COXIB plus PPI • Misoprostol
❖ Significant CV Risk (requires ASA)	o NSAID plus PPI	- NSAID plus PPI	• Avoid NSAIDs and COXIB, if at all poss (risk of myocardial infarction, stroke)

*these recommendations did not embrace the patients who require antiplatelet therapy, but the same principle is likely to apply

Printed with permission: Lanza, F. L., *et al. Am J Gastroenterol.* 2009. 104:728-38.

> **SO YOU WANT TO BE A GASTROENTEROLOGIST!**
> - In patients who require NSAIDs, it is recommended to "use the least ulcerogenic NSAIDs at the lowest effective dose"; naproxen 500 mg *bid* is effective.
> - Ibuprofen is available over–the–counter (OTC), and is often advertised as being relatively safe.
> - In patients with high GI risk plus high cardiovascular risk, ibuprofen is not recommended, even if PPI co–therapy is used.
>
> - In this clinical scenario, why ibuprofen is <u>not recommended</u>?
>   - Aspirin reduces cardiovascular (CV) risk
>   - In high risk CV patients, ASA must be taken
>   - Ibuprofen reduces the serum concentration of ASA
>   - The lower serum concentration of ASA reduces the CV protection
>   - So, **do not** combine ibuprofen with ASA in high CV risk patient

> Endoscopy

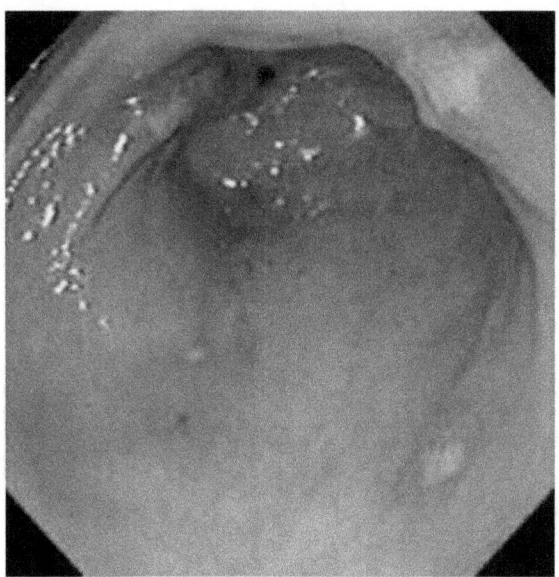

NSAID–induced ulceration

BARIATRIC SURGERY

➤ Indications

- What are the indications for bariatric surgery?
    o BMI > 40 kg/m^2
    o BMI > 35 kg/m^2 plus comorbid complications

➤ Benefits

- Name the benefits of bariatric surgery.
    o ↓ all–cause mortality rate (CV, CRC), as well as other obesity–related cancers
    o ↓ diabetes
    o ↓ NAFLD histology score in > 80% (↓ fibrosis in 60%)
    o ↑ quality of life for patient

➤ Types

- What are the major types of bariatric surgery?
    o Restriction procedures
        - Vertical banded gastroplasty (VBG)
        - Laparoscopic adjustable gastric banding (LAGB)
        - Sleeve gastrectomy (SE)
    o Malabsorption–producing procedures
        - Biliopancreatic diversion (BPD)
        - BPD plus duodenal switch (BPD–DS)
    o Mixed procedures
        - Roux–en–Y Gastric Bypass (RYGB)
        - Expected weight loss
            ▪ RYGB
                - First 6 months: 10 – 15 lbs per month

- 2 years
  - 65% of excess body weight
  - 35% of initial body weight
- LAGB
  - 2 years
    - 45% of excess body weight
    - 25% of initial body weight

- Draw the main types of bariatric surgery used for weight loss.

Roux-en Y Gastric Bypass (RNYGB)

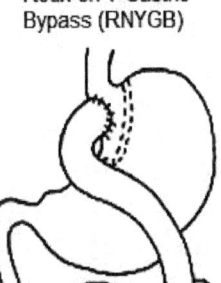

Vertical banded gastroplasty (VBG)

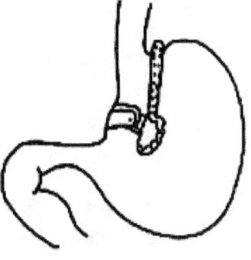

Laparoscopic adjustable gastric band (LAGB)

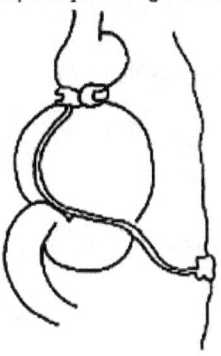

Biliopancreatic diversion (BPD) with duodenal switch

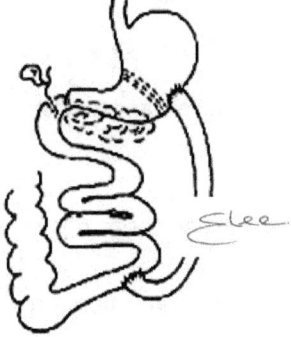

Adapted from: *Sleisenger and Fordtran's Gastrointestinal and Liver Disease.* 2010. 9th Edition. Figure 7-1, Page 116.

- Complications
    - Post-operative complications of bariatric surgery are often subdivided into 3 phases:
        1. 1 – 6 weeks
        2. 7 – 12 weeks
        3. 13 – 52 weeks

SO YOU WANT TO BE A GASTROENTEROLOGIST!

Patients with partial gastrectomy and Roux–en–Y anastomosis may develop nausea, vomiting, bloating and early satiety. These symptoms are due to the stasis of food in the gastric remnant as well as the distal Roux jejunal efferent limb, especially, if the Roux limb is > 45 cm. This is called the "Roux–en–Y stasis syndrome".

- Explain the pathophysiology of **Roux-en-Y stasis syndrome**.
    - The transection of the jejunum prevents the pacemaker wave generated in the duodenum from passing distal to the level of the transection
    - Ectopic pacemakers in the Roux limb cause retrograde contractions

---

Gems and Pearls

- URSO ↓ risk of gallstones by 40% after R–en–Y gastric bypass
- Vertical banded gastroscopy (VBG) → pseudoachalasia

- Name the complications common to all bariatric surgical procedure.
    - CNS
        - Psychiatric disturbance
    - Lung
        - Atelectasis and pneumonia
        - Deep vein thrombosis
        - Pulmonary embolism

- GI
  - Anemia
  - Diarrhea
  - Ulceration
  - GI bleeding
  - Stenosis
  - Gallstones
- Metabolic
  - Bone disease
  - Too rapid weight loss
- Surgical
  - Wound infection
  - Failure to lose weight
  - Mortality (0.5 – 1%)
  - Post–operative stomach

Adapted from: Klein, S. 2006. *AGA Institute Post Graduate Course*. page 175.

- Name the bariatric procedures and its complications, and give complications common to all bariatric surgical procedures.

> Specific procedures
  - Gastric bypass (Roux–en–Y)
    - Anastomotic leak with peritonitis
    - Stomal stenosis
    - Marginal ulcers (ischemia)
    - Staple line disruption
    - Internal and incisional hernias
    - Nutrient deficiencies (usually iron, calcium, folic acid, vitamin B12)
    - Dumping syndrome
  - Gastroplasty
    - GERD
    - Stomal stenosis
    - Staple line disruption
    - Band erosion

- Gastric banding
  - Band slippage
  - Erosion
  - Esophageal dilation
  - Band infections
- Biliopancreatic diversion
  - Anastomotic leak with peritonitis
  - Protein–energy malnutrition
  - Vitamin and mineral deficiencies
  - Dehydration

Post–Operative Stomach

➢ Pathophysiology

- What are the late non–nutritional complications of gastric surgery?
  - Stomach
    - Marginal ulcer
    - Post–gastrectomy carcinoma
    - Bezoar
    - Bile reflux gastritis
  - Duodenum
    - Afferent loop syndrome
    - Blown duodenual stump
  - Jejunum
    - Jejunogastric intussusception

- Explain the mechanisms or causes of iron and B12 deficiency–associated anemia, diarrhea, metabolic bone disease, and recurrent gastric ulceration in patient having had Billroth II partial gastrectomy for peptic ulcer disease (PUD), gastric cancer (GCa) or morbid obesity (bariatric surgery) and Roux–en–Y.

- Iron
  - Pre–surgery iron deficiency
  - Decreased intake from post–op symptoms (anorexia, early satiety)

- Decreased acid leads to decreased pepsin and decreased meat (iron) digestion
- Decreased acid inhibits acid-mediated solubilizing and reducing of inorganic dietary iron (Fe^{3+} [ferric], Fe^{2+} [ferrous])
- Decreased absorption of Fe^{2+}, Ca^{2+}, BII, bypassing site of maximal absorption (duodenum)
- Can be slow bleeding at surgical site
- Bile gastritis

- Gastric stump cancer: Vitamin B12 (cobalamine)
  - Pre-surgery deficiency
  - Decreased intake
  - Loss of stimulated and coordinated release of "R" factor
  - Decreased intrinsic factor
  - Loss of HCl or pepsinogen to liberate Vitamin B12 from the food
  - Bacterial overgrowth syndrome

- Metabolic bone disease
  - Pre-existing osteoporosis ↓ Ca^{2+} solubilization
  - ↓ vitamin D or Ca^{2+} intake
  - ↓ absorption due to ↓ solubility of Ca^{2+}
  - Bypass of the site of maximal absorption of Ca^{2+} (duodenum)
  - Binding Ca^{+2} (unabsorbed fatty acids)

- Diarrhea
  - Medications
    - Magnesium-containing antacids, PPIs
  - Stomach
    - Early dumping syndrome
    - Retained antrum (↑ gastrin)
    - Hypergastrinemia → HCL hypersecretion (↑ volume, mucosal damage); loss of PPY from the ileum, loss of inhibition of gastrin → ↑ gastrin

- Small bowel
  - Bypasses the duodenum
  - Bacterial overgrowth syndrome (BOS, small intestinal bacterial overgrowth [SIBO])
- Colon
  - PPI–associated collagenous colitis
- Unmasked conditions
  - Unmasked celiac disease
  - Unmasked lactose intolerance
  - Unmasked bile acid wastage
  - Unmasked monosaccharide transporter defect
  - Primary or secondary (unmasked) pancreatic insufficiency

- Peptic ulceration (stomal or marginal ulcer, previous PUD)
  - ↑ gastrin — ZES, incomplete vagotomy, gastric retention, afferent loop syndrome
  - *H. pylori* infection
  - NSAIDs, ASA use
  - "Stump" cancer
  - Ischemia at the site of anastomosis
  - Bile gastritis

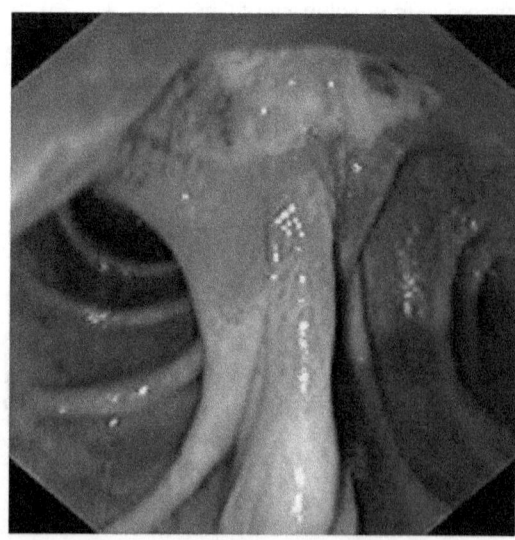

- ➢ Diagnostic Imaging
  - o Post–gastric surgery
    - Fundoplication
    - Billroth I or II
    - Roux–en–Y
    - Stomal ulcer or cancer
    - Blown duodenal stump
    - Bile (reflux) gastritis
    - Jejunogastric intussusceptions
    - Gastric remnant bezoar
  - o Stomal (marginal) ulcer
    - Usually within 2 cm of the stoma, the efferent limb of the jejunum after gastroenterostomy
    - Findings include:
      - Ulcer crater
      - Giant ulcer
      - Thick jejunal folds
      - Rigid efferent limbs
    - May develop jejunocolic fistula
  - o Afferent loop syndrome
    - Dilation of the afferent limbs may have non–filling of the limbs
    - Destruction of the afferent limb after Billroth II anastomosis
    - Obstruction due to the following:
      - Recurrent ulcer or tumor
      - Adhesions
      - Intend herniation
  - o Jejunogastric intussusceptions
    - Tubular filling defect in the gastric remnant after gastroenterostomy
    - Valvulae conniventes in tubular structure, representing efferent of afferent loop
  - o Stomal cancer (stump carcinoma, post–gastrectomy carcinoma)
    - Lobulated mass in gastric remnant (filling defect)
    - Effects of mass:
      - Obstructs outlet of stomach
      - Produces mass effect on transverse colon
  - o Bile reflux gastritis
    - Filling defect in gastric remnant
    - Thick (edematous) gastric folds
    - Narrowing or deformity of the gastric remnant and perianastomotic jejunum

- o Thickened Folds
  - Zollinger–Ellison syndrome
    - Single or multiple ulcers in the usual or unusual sites
    - Thick gastric folds
    - Fundic gland polyps
    - Thick walls of the stomach or duodenum may be pancreatic mass
  - Differentials
    - Lymphoma
    - Nodular, irregular, thick folds with variable size
    - Adenocarcinoma mass
    - Ménétrier's disease
      - Proximal stomach
      - Thick gastric folds
      - Usually proximal half of stomach
      - Specifically, the greater curve
      - Pliable (stomach canal is distended)

➢ Treatment

The gastroenterologist is often involved in Phase 2 and 3 medical problems.

- Name the Phase 2 and 3 post–operative (7 – 52 weeks) medical care of patient with bariatric surgery.
  - o Nutrition
    - Eat slowly (< 1 oz per 10 minutes)
    - Eat solids, wait for 30 minutes, then take beverage
    - Beware of possible new food intolerance, i.e. red meat
    - Avoid snacks and high calorie fluid drinks, i.e. coal "pop"
    - Identify and correct any vitamin D deficiency
    - Beware of alcohol use disorder (10% in second post–op year)
    - Anticipate the possible deficiencies of the following:
      - Thiamine
      - Copper 2 mg/day
      - Zinc 8 mg/day
      - Calcium (use calcium citrate *po*, which does not need gastric acidity for dissolution)

- Medications
  - Medications need to be crushable, or in liquid form
  - If anti-diabetic therapy, use metformin *po* (only small changes in the blood sugar)
  - Reassess the need of treatment for GERD (GERD symptoms may improve with weight loss)
  - Reassess the need for contraception
    - ↑ fertility in weight loss
    - Menses may return
    - Consider the use of non-oral hormonal regime
  - Reassess the need of drugs for obesity-associated arthralgias
    - ↓ need or NSAIDs is possible
    - Use acetaminophen if arthralgias persist
    - Return of post-psychiatric issues

- Be on lookout for the following disorders:
  - Psychiatric disorders
    - Emotional liability
    - Self-destructive behavior
    - Bulimia
    - Somatization (nausea, vomiting)
  - GI disorders
    - Dyspepsia due to the development of stoma
    - Nausea and vomiting
  - Cholelithiasis
    - 22% in 6 months post-op
    - Consider ursodeoxycholic acid (UDSA) or ursodiol (USAN) 300 mg *bid* for 6 months
  - Dumping syndrome
    - Avoid food causing the symptoms (i.e. sugar, pop)
    - Eat slowly, "by the clock"
    - Take liquids at end of rather than during a meal
  - Prolonged vomiting
    - Only slowly advance intake to solid foods
    - Stomal strictures
    - Marginal ulcers
    - Small bowel obstruction, i.e. from internal hernia
    - Food intolerances
    - Somatization
    - Overrating

- New onset of heartburn, regurgitation, dysphagia
    - Gastric outlet obstruction from slippage of band, i.e. may occur if the patient has had previously
    - An unrecognized or unrepaired hiatus hernia
- Hematemesis
    - Marginal ulcer
    - Mallory–Weiss tear from vomiting
    - Severe esophagitis from partial gastric outlet obstruction
    - Band erosion through the wall of the stomach
- Slowing of initially satisfactory weight loss
    - Recidivism
    - Development of new and poor eating habits
    - Development of gastrogastric fistula
- Expected weight loss
    - RYGB
        - First 6 months 10 – 15 lbs per month
        - 2 years
            - 65% of excess body weight
            - 35% of initial body weight
    - LAGB
        - 2 years
            - 45% of excess body weight
            - 25% of initial body weight

- Endoscopic treatment
    - Be smart! Review the operative notes and any relevant post–operative imaging studies to be aware of the "lay of the land".
    - Visualization may require the use of a narrower pediatric gastroscopy or colonoscopy.
    - ERCP of the biliopancreatic limb and retrograde evaluation of the by–passed stomach is especially difficult after RYGB (Roux–en–Y gastric bypass).
    - This difficulty is increasing with the more use of "distal bypass", with anastomosis of the biliopancreatic limb only 150 cm proximal to the ileocecal value.
    - Retrograde evaluation may be made easier with use of the following:
        - Shapelock™ enteroscopy guide
        - Deep small bowel enteroscope
            - Double balloon
            - Spiral enteroscopy

- o RYGB
  - "gastritis" is common, but clinical significance is unclear
  - ~ 1/3 of symptomatic RYGB have a normal EGD
  - ~ 1/4 will have stenosis of stoma, usually 1 month after surgery
- Give the endoscopic treatment of complications after bariatric surgery.
- ❖ Stoma
  - o Narrowing (symptomatic stomal stenosis)
    - Bougie dilators or balloons, using guide wire through–the–scope placement (TTS)
    - Optimal aperture diameter is 10 – 15 mm
    - If multiple dilators are needed, dilate slowly (up to 3 mm [3 French sizes] at each session, every 1 – 2 weeks until symptoms resolve
  - o Reduction in size of enlarged stomas and pouches
    - Aim for stomal diameter of ~ 12 mm
    - Objective is to reduce or eliminate symptoms, i.e. slowing of the expected weight loss from surgery; during syndrome)
    - Use sclerosants, suturing devices, clips
- ❖ Marginal ulcer (MU) bleeding
  - o Usually on jejunal side of gastrojejunal anastomosis
  - o Early MU in 10%, late in 1%
  - o Risk of MU associated with smoking, *H. pylori* infection, NSAIDs use
  - o If bleeding occurs early after surgery, perform EGD in the OR
- ❖ Leaks
  - o Fistulae, dehiscence of staple line, gastric leaks
    - Tissue apposition
      - Fibrin glue
      - Biomaterial (from pig intestine)
      - Clipping
    - Stents
      - Self–expanding plastic stents (SEPS)
      - Self–expanding esophageal metal stents (SEMS)

- ❖ Band erosion
  - o Nd:YAG laser
  - o Scissors
  - o Cutters (endoscopic)

> **SO YOU WANT TO BE A GASTROENTEROLOGIST!**
>
> Weight loss after RYGB may be partial due to the restriction of food intake, and partially from the associated malabsorption.
>
> - Give the changes in GI peptides occurring after RYGB, contributing to the improved insulin secretion, glucose tolerance, and weight loss.
>   - o Malabsorption in the jejunum leads to ↑ delivery of nutrients to the ileum
>   - o ↑ nutrients in the ileum lead to the following:
>   - ↑ Peptide YY (PYY)
>   - ↑ Glucagon–like peptide–1 (GLP–1)
>   - ↑ Glucose–dependent insulinotropic polypeptide (GIP)
>
> With rapid weight loss after bariatric surgery, a woman's menses may stop. In any situation when menses stop, you would suspect pregnancy and arrange pregnancy testing.
>
> - Explain why this index of suspicion should be high in post–bariatric surgery female patient.
>   - o Fertility improves in post–surgical weight loss

Obesity
- o Many different approaches are used to lose weight, which vary widely in their success in helping patient to achieve their ideal body weight
- o Basal energy expenditure is approximately 0.8 kcal/min, or 1150 kcal/day
- o Recommended daily energy intake, ~ 22 – 25 kcal/kg
- o Maintaining achieved purposeful weight loss is usually difficult
- o Optimal waist circumference
  - – Women   < 35 inches/88 cm
  - – Men   < 40 inches/102 cm
- o BMI (weight [kg]/height [m^2])

Definition	BMI, kg/m²
Normal	< 25
Overweight	25 – 29.9
Obese	≥ 30
Severe obesity	≥ 40 (or > 35 plus comorbidities)

- Give two processes rendering maintenance of weight loss so challenging.
    - Recidivism in proper calorie and food group intake
    - Reduction in the basal energy expenditure because of weight loss, requiring an even further reduction in energy intake even though the ideal body weight has been achieved with the initial short term dieting

- Give evidence–based classes of pharmaceuticals used to treat increased BMI.

    - Centrally acting
        - Anti–depressants
        - Anti–epileptics
        - Serotonin 2 receptor agonist
        - Non–adrenergic sympathomimetics
        - Cannabinoid receptor antagonists
    - ↓ food intake
    - ↓ pancreatic lipase
    - Control of hyperglycemia
    - Dietary supplements

- **Orlistat®**
    - Inhibits activity of pancreatic lipase
    - 120 mg *po bid*, continued loss of weight at 1 year, as % of initial body weight
        - "placebo" (lifestyle changes)   5.5 – 6.6
        - Orlistat plus lifestyle changes   8.5 – 10.2
        - Therapeutic gain   1.9 – 4.7

- What are the adverse effects of Orlistat®?
    - Nuisance
        - Cramps
        - Borborygmi
        - Flatus
        - Oil spotting on underclothes
        - Fecal incontinence
    - Nutrition
        - ↓ absorption of fat soluble vitamins A, D, E
    - Liver
        - Development of liver injury
        - $3/10^5$ orlistat users
    - Kidney
        - Oxalate–induced acute renal injury

- Explain the mechanisms of the development of acute **oxalate–induced renal injury** in patients taking Orlistat®.
    - Orlistat → ↓ digestion of triglyceride (TG) → ↑ TG in stool → ↑ binding of Ca^{2+} → less Ca^{2+}–oxalate and ↑ luminal oxalate → ↑ absorption of oxalate → ↑ oxalate excretion by the kidney with ↑ deposition of oxalate in the renal parenchyma
    - Note: Ca^{2+}–oxalate in the lumen of the intestine requires fatty acids removed from dietary TG for the Ca^{2+} to become bounded (Ca^{2+}–FA), the oxalate to be absorbed by the intestine, and excreted into the urine
    - The above pathophysiology of oxalate damage to the kidney is due to the problem that orlistat blocks pancreatic lipase, so fewer rather than more FAs are present in the intestinal lumen to bind to Ca^{2+} in Ca^{2+}–oxalate

- **Serotonin agonist** (lorcaserin)
    - Selective agonist of serotonin 2C receptor → ↓ food intake
    - 10 mg po bid
        - % of patients losing ≥ 5% of baseline weight in 1 year:
            - Lorcaserin (Lor)   48%
            - Placebo (PL)   20.3%
            - Therapeutic gain (TG)   ~ 18%
        - % of patients maintaining weight loss in second year:
            - Lor   68%
            - PL   50%
            - TG   ~ 18%
    - Target weight loss is ~ 3 kg – 4 kg/year

- ↓ SBP/DBP, HR, total or LDL cholesterol, CRP, fibrinogen, fasting glucose and insulin concentrations in blood
  - No lorcaserin-associated cardiac valvular disease (i.e. seen with fenfluramine), because lorcaserin is a selective agonist of the serotonin 2C receptor, rather than the 2B serotonin receptor

Abbreviations: CRP, C-reactive protein; DBP, diastolic blood pressure; SBP, systolic blood pressure

- Noradrenergic sympathomimetic drugs, phentermine and diethylpropion
  - Only for short term use (no more than 3 months)
  - ↑ satiety
    - ↓ food intake by acting on nerve terminals
    - ↑ release of norepinephrine
    - ↓ uptake of norepinephrine

- Anti-depressants
  - Bupropion
    - SR 300 – 400 mg/day
    - Especially useful for the prevention of weight gain when smokers stop smoking
    - Alters the metabolism of norepinephrine
  - Fluoxetine
    - 60 mg *po* per day
    - Selective serotonin reuptake inhibitor (SSRI)

- Antiepileptics
  - Insufficient evidence to recommend use at this time for weight loss

- Cannabinoid-1 receptor antagonist
  - Clinically meaningful weight loss is off-set by psychiatric AEs
  - Not approved for use

- Diabetes-treating drugs
  - Metformin — very modest weight loss when used or for the prevention of diabetes (~ 2.5% of the initial body weight)
  - Other oral diabetic drugs result only the minimum weight loss

- Dietary supplements
  - Non-evidence-based use

GASTRIC EMPTYING AND GASTROPARESIS

- ➤ Definition
    - o "gastroparesis" is used interchangeably with delayed gastric emptying
    - o Usual causes related to impaired motility (gastroparesis) and mechanical obstruction

Useful background

- o Vomiting center is on the blood side of the blood brain barrier
- o Some patients with severe, intractable gastroparesis, i.e. occur with severe type I diabetes, may improve with near–total gastrectomy and Roux–en–Y anastomosis
- o Slowed gastric emptying and delayed small intestinal transit occur in patients with cirrhosis
    - The assessment of gastric emptying includes the measurement of emptying, accommodation and contractility (Smout and Mundt, 2009, Szarka and Camilleri, 2009).
    - Accommodation of the proximal stomach is activated by the vagally mediated relation
    - There is no cephalic phase, but the accommodation reflex is imitated in the cricopharynx, stomach and duodenum (Vanden Berghe, et al. 2009).
    - If the pylorus is obstructed and food does not enter the duodenum, the amplitude of the accommodation reflex will be less and the patient will feel full
    - Symptoms of gastroparesis may be troublesome, but curiously there is no good association between measures of gastric emptying and severity of symptoms
    - The physical subscore of the Short–Form I2 as a measure of quality of life, and the Hospital Anxiety and Depression Scale correlated with gastroparesis severity as measured by the Gastroparesis Cardinal Symptom Index, and did not correlate with gastric emptying delay or symptom duration (Bielefieldt, et al. 2009).
- o Usual causes related to impaired motility (gastroparesis) and mechanical obstruction
- o Diabetes is one of the most common etiologies of gastroparesis
- o In order to appreciate the rational approach to the investigation and management of disorders of gastric emptying, it is first necessary to understand the complex, integrated process of gastric filling, accommodation, grinding or mixing and emptying

- Explain the process of gastric emptying.
  - The time for gastric emptying or the half life (t ½) for emptying, depends on the number of factors, including amount and composition of the ingested food
  - Usual causes related to impaired motility (gastroparesis) and mechanical obstruction
  - "gastroparesis" will be used interchangeably with delayed gastric emptying, and implies a process rather than a mechanism
- ❖ Intake of food begins the following processes:
  - Release of peptides acting on the following sites:
    - ENS
    - Vagal function
      - Afferent
      - Efferent
    - ICCs
    - Smooth muscles
  - Fundic receptive relaxation
  - Body grinding and mixing ("trituration")
  - Antral peristalsis
  - Antropyloric duodenal coordination
  - Emptying of 2 – 4 ml of chime, containing particles < 4 mm, by the varying resistance of pylorus and antrum

- ❖ Neural component

Important components for gastric motor functions:
  - Autonomic nervous system (ANS)
  - Enteric nervous system (ENS)
  - Interstitial cells of Cajal (ICCs)
  - Smooth muscle cells
  - Peristaltic reflex
  - Involvement of afferent vagal neurons and vagovagal reflexes
    - Nucleus of tractus solitarius
    - Vagal dorsal motor nucleus
    - Vagal efferents

Afferent and efferent neural connections between the stomach and central nervous system (CNS)

- 1) Low threshold mechano– and chemoreceptors stimulate visceral sensations, i.e. stomach emptiness or fullness, and symptoms, i.e. nausea and discomfort
- 2) Vagus nerve contains afferent nerves with A–delta and C–pain fibers with cell bodies in the nodose ganglia with connections to the nucleus tractus solitarius (not shown)
- Changes in the gastric electrical rhythm, excess amplitude contractions, or stretch on the gastric wall are peripheral mechanisms that elicit changes in the afferent neural activity (via vagal and/or splanchnic nerves) that may reach consciousness to be perceived as visceral perceptions (symptoms) emanating from the stomach
- 3) These stimuli are mediated through vagal pathways and become conscious perceptions of the visceral sensations, if sensory inputs reach the cortex
- 4) The splanchnic nerves also contain afferent nerves with A–delta and C fibers that synapse in the celiac ganglia with some cell bodies in the vertebral ganglia (T5 – T9)
- 5) Interneurons in the white rami in the dorsal horn of the spinal cord cross to the dorsal columns and spinothalamic tracts and ascend to the sensory areas of the medulla oblongata
- These splanchnic afferent fibers are thought to mediate high threshold stimuli for visceral pain
- 6) In contrast to visceral sensations, somatic nerves, i.e. from the skin, carry sensory information via A–delta and C fibers through the dorsal root ganglia and into the dorsal horn and then through the dorsal columns and spinothalamic tracts to the cortical areas of the somatic representation for somatic pain

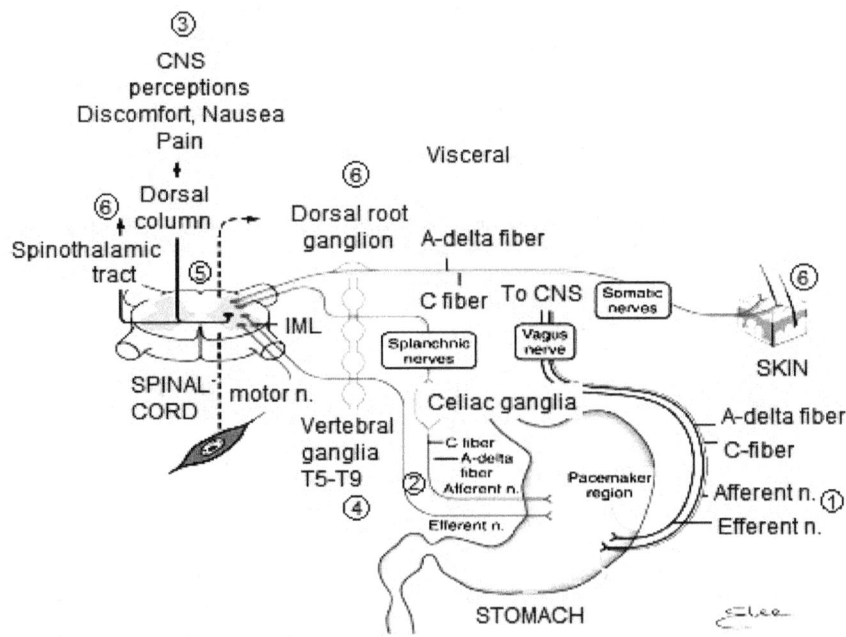

Abbreviations: IML, intermediolateral nucleus; n, nerve

Adapted from: Feldman M., et al. Sleisenger and Fordtran's Gastrointestinal and Liver Disease. 2016. 10th Edition. Saunders/Elsevier, Philadephia. Figure 49-17, page 824.

➢ Pathophysiology

- What are the neuromuscular functions of the stomach or accommodation, grinding and mixing as well as emptying?

- Smooth muscle cells
    o Receptors in the excitable membrane of the smooth muscle cells
        - Muscarinic
        - Central and peripheral dopamine (D2)
        - 5–HT3 / 5–HT4
        - Motillin
        - α–adrenergic
        - Somatostatin
        - Phosphodiesterase

- These receptors bind to amines and peptides reaching the smooth muscle cells from neurocrine, paracrine and endocrine pathways
- The excitable membrane of the smooth muscle cells fires spontaneously, causing action potentials that cause the muscle cell to contract
- The muscle cells are joined as a syncytium providing electrical coupling of the neighboring muscle cells
- The contraction due to the spontaneous depolarization, action potential and syncytial coupling causes contraction in the circumferential and longitudinal axes

- Electrophysiology of the smooth muscle

Sites	RMP, mV	PP/SP
o Fundus	- 50	-
- Effect of inhibitory vagal input	Receptive relaxation (↓ fundic tone)	
o Corpus or antrum - Effect of Ach or stretch	- 60 / - 70	↑ amplitude and duration of PP, occurrence of PP, occurrence of AP → low or high amplitude contractions

- o Pylorus
    - Electrical barrier between slow wave of the distal antrum (3 cpm) and duodenum (12 cpm), i.e. the duodenal slow wave is 12 cpm

Abbreviations: AP, action potential; PP, plateau potential; RMP, Resting membrane potential; CPM, contractions per minute

- Peristaltic reflex
  - Responsible for the "law of the intestine"
  - Ascending contraction: stimulus in the lumen, usually due to the distention by the presence of food
    - Transmitters of excitation of the smooth muscles
      - Acetylcholine
      - Serotonin acting on 5–HT4 receptors on cholinergic interneurons
      - Tachykinins
        - Substance P (SP)
        - Substance K (SK)

- o Descending contraction: inhibition of the smooth muscles below the area of stimulation causes descending inhibition
  - Resistance to the movements of food bolus pulsed distally into the relaxed area by the ascending contraction and the proximal smooth muscle excitation
  - Transmitters of inhibition of the smooth muscles
    - Nitric oxide (NO)
    - Vasoactive intestinal peptide (VIP)
    - Somatostatin
    - Gamma–aminobutyric acid (GABA)
    - Endogenous opiates
  - Pylorus (antroduodenal junction)
    - 0.6 – 1.6 cm long, maintains an area of high resting pressure
    - 3x per minute phasic contractions sweep across the antroduodenal junction, emptying 1 – 2 mm particles
    - Phasic pyloric contractions are mediated by NO, Ach and opiates
- o Muscle activity: circular, oblique and longitudinal muscle layers of the stomach leading to the following:
  - Relaxation of fundus (accommodation)
  - Contraction of antrum (chemical digestion, shearing and pulverization, propulsion, rates pulsion, sieving, emptying of 1 – 2 mm particles)

- Parasympathetic nervous system (PNS) and sympathetic nervous system (SNS)
  - o PNS
    - Stimulatory vagal nerves
    - ↑ gastric contraction
    - ↑ gastric secretion
  - o SNS
    - Inhibitory

- Enteric nervous system (ENS)
  - o "Stimulation of excitatory enteric neurons leads to the depolarization of IM–ICCs"
  - o "The depolarization (of IM–ICCs) causes positive chronotropic effects on the frequency of gastric slow waves", and also increases the contractile response of smooth muscles to slow wave depolarizations" (Feldman M., et al. Sleisenger and Fordtran's Gastrointestinal and Liver Disease. 2010. 9th Edition. Saunders/Elsevier, Philadelphia. page 793)

- Thus, the ICC networks provide the control of frequency and propagation velocity for the circular muscle contractions that comprise gastric peristalsis waves" (Feldman, M., *et al. Sleisenger and Fordtran's Gastrointestinal and Liver Disease.* 2010. 9th Edition. Saunders/Elsevier, Philadelphia. page 792).

- Autonomic nervous system (ANS)
    o Parasympathetic pathways
        - Dorsal motor nucleus (DMN)
        - Nucleus ambiguous (NA)
        - Tractus solitarius (TS)
    o Vagus efferents pass to myenteric plexus (MP) in the wall of stomach
    o Sympathetic pathways
        - From intermediolateral columns in T5 – T10 levels of spinal cord from
            - Celiac ganglia to splanchnic efferents
                - Myenteric ganglia   norepinephrine
            - Splanchnic efferents to the following sites:
                - Submucous ganglia ⎱ norepinephrine and somatostatin
                - Circular muscles ⎰
                - Blood vessels   norepinephrine and NPY
                - Pyloric sphincter
                - Non–sphincteric muscle

- Enteric nervous system (ENS)
    o Main networks
        - Submucosal (SM)
        - Myenteric
        - Deep muscular
            - Interstitial cells of Cajal (ICC)
            - Plexi involved in pacemaking
            - Muscle propulsion (MMC)
                - Sensation
                - Secretion

Abbreviations: MMC (IMMC), interdigestive migrating motor complex

- ICC (pacemaker cells), slow waves, plateau or action potentials

- ICCs in the deep muscular plexus junction in conjugation with the ENS
- ICCs in myenteric plexus do not depend on the ENS
- ICCs in pylorus are associated with inhibitory neural activity in this region, and thereby, are important in the context of rate of gastric emptying
- ICCs arise from c–kit–positive mesenchymal cell precursors
- This increased activity of the plateau or action potentials causes gastric peristaltic contractions
- The fundus does not have MY–ICCs or a slow wave, so the fundus does not participate in the linking of slow wave to the plateau or action potentials, and therefore has no role in producing peristaltic contractions
- IM–ICCs in the fundus
    - Sensory cells for mechanoreception
    - Innervated by inhibitory vagal neurons which regulate tone and receptive relaxation in the fundus
- Electrode placed on the anterior wall may be used to detect the myoelectrical activity of the slow waves arising from the pacemaker region
- This recording of the gastric myoelectrical activity is employed clinically as the electrogastrogram (EGG)

- Migrating myoelectrical [motor] complex (MMC)
    - ICCs at the junction of the gastric fundus and body at the proximal part of the greater curve of the stomach have innate activity and spontaneously produce a slow wave (pacesetter potential, gastric myoelectrical activity)
    - ICCs present in multiple layers of the stomach wall
        - Myenteric (MY–ICCs)
        - Intramuscular (IM–ICCs)
        - Submuscular
        - Subserosal
    - Slow waves occurring at 3 cpm move circumferentially and distally at 14 mm/second towards the antrum
    - MY–ICCs (ICCs in the myenteric plexus between the circular and longitudinal muscle layers) generate the slow waving
    - The slow wave of the gastric myoelectrical activity has an uptake
    - When this uptake of the slow wave depolarizes, there is a reduction in the threshold for the circular smooth muscles to contract

- When the membrane potential reaches the threshold potential, the force of contraction quickly increases (steep slope of the voltage–contraction curve)
- The slow wave becomes linked with the plateau or action potentials
- "Action potential are superimposed on the plateau potentials in the terminal antrum and pylorus (Feldman M., *et al. Sleisenger and Fordtran's Gastrointestinal and Liver Disease*. 2010. 9th Edition. Saunders/Elsevier, Philadelphia. page 792)
- Action potentials are associated with increased amplitude of the contraction of the smooth muscle
- Cyclical contractile activity
- Phase 1
  - Quite, little contractile activity
- Phase 2
  - Random, irregular contractions
  - Peristaltic reflex
- Phase 3
  - Bursts of "regular, high amplitude phasic contractions ("activity front") that last from 5 – 10 minutes and migrate from the antrum to the ileum (Feldman M., *et al. Sleisenger and Fordtran's Gastrointestinal and Liver Disease*. 9th Edition. Saunders/Elsevier, Philadelphia, 2010, page 794) in 90 – 120 minutes
  - Motilin is of importance to Phase 3 contractions
  - Cyclical contractile activity beginning phase 3 of MMC seen in stomach and small bowel, as well as in the following areas:
    - Lower esophageal sphincter (LES)
    - Sphincter of Oddi (SOD)
    - Gallbladder

- GI peptides
  - Released by food (see fasting and fed neuromuscular activity)
  - Act on the following sites:
    - ICCs
    - Smooth muscle
    - ENS
    - Vagal function
      - Afferent
      - Efferent

- Name the GI peptides involved in gastric emptying.
  - CCK
    - Released from enteroendocrine cells in the duodenal mucosa in response to fatty acids (from digested triglycerides) in the duodenum
    - Activation of CCK receptors → sensation of fullness → ↓ food intake
  - Polypeptide–YY (PYY)
    - Released from the enteroendocrine cells in the ileocolonic mucosa
    - ↓ gastric emptying and small bowel rate of transit ("ileal brake")
    - ↓ histamine–sensitive component of gastrin release
    - ↓ appetite, ↓ food intake
  - Corticotropin–releasing factor (CRF)
    - Acts through the central pathways in periventricular nucleus
      - Central dopamine 1 and 2
      - Vasopressin (AVP) pathways
    - Responds to emotional stress
  - Stem cell factor (SCF)
    - ↓ SCF with ↑ BS (increased blood sugar), i.e. hyperglycemia
    - ↓ SCF → ↓ ICCs and ↓ contraction of the smooth muscles

- Explain the process and **mechanisms of gastric emptying** of food and fluids.
    - Intake of food
        - Begins the processes of fundic receptive relaxation
        - Body grinding and mixing ("trituration")
        - Antral peristalsis
        - Antropyloruduodenal coordination
        - Emptying of 2 – 4 ml of chimes containing particles < 4 mm by varying resistance of pylorus and antrum
    - Receptive relaxation
        - Vagus and NO
            - Ingested food and fluid stretches the fundus and stimulate mechanoreceptors and chemoreceptors
            - Secretin is released from enterochromaffin cells
            - Intrinsic primary afferent neurons (IPANs) in the submucosa or myenteric plexus of the stomach
            - Activated mechano– / chemoreceptors stimulate IM–ICCs
            - IM–ICCs activate vagal efferent and vagovagal reflexes
            - Nucleus of the tractus solitarius, periventricular nucleus and dorsal motor nucleus of the vagus are stimulated
            - Inhibition of the vagal excitatory neurons
            - NO and vasoactive intestinal peptide (VIP) are released and are inhibitory to the normal tone of the smooth muscle of the fundus
            - End result is for filling of the fundus to result in receptive relaxation, which begins before mixing and grinding in the gastric body
    - Other factors
        - Distension of the antrum
        - Capsaicin–sensitive afferent vagal nerves mediated by the following:
            - 5–hydroxytryptamine (5–HT_3)
            - Gastrin–releasing peptide (GRP)
        - Duodenal CCK_A receptors
        - Duodenum
        - Colon
        - Perfusion of the duodenum
            - Acid
            - Lipid
            - Protein

150

- o Body contractions
  - Relaxation of the fundus and proximal portion of the gastric body is replaced by contractions of the fundus and proximal corpus
  - This pushes food into the rest of the body and antrum, where mixing and grinding occur
  - This initial postprandial interval of receptive relaxation, mixing and grinding is called the "lag phase"
  - Lag phase duration depends on the composition of the meal (usually about 45 – 60 minutes)

- o Emptying
  - Trituration of solid food into particles, 1 – 2 mm, begins the linear phase of gastric emptying
  - Gastric peristaltic waves arise from the electrical activity of ICC, plateau and action potentials
  - These peristaltic waves sweep waves through the body of the stomach at 3 cpm
  - Clearance of pyloric sphincter and contraction of the duodenum during the emptying of particles > 2 mm
  - Antral contraction waves pump, pulsatile "squirts" of food and fluid into duodenum
  - Depending on the strength of contraction (10 – 40 mmHg) and duration of antral peristaltic wave, and the resistance provided by pyloric sphincter and duodenal contraction, usually 3 – 4 kcal/min is emptied into the duodenum
  - About 50% of a meal will be emptied in 90 min ($T_{1/2}$ of gastric emptying), and 95% emptied in 4 hours
  - Non–caloric and caloric liquids are emptied first without lag phase and in a "mono–exponential emptying" pattern, then digestible material during the linear phase due to lower amplitude pressure waves
  - The rate of gastric emptying may be modified by the amount and composition of ingested food and fluids
    - Volume
    - Viscosity
    - Osmolarity
    - Nutrient density
    - Fats

For further details, please refer to: Feldman M., *et al. Sleisenger and Fordtran's Gastrointestinal and Liver Disease*. 2010. 9th Edition. Saunders/Elsevier, Philadephia. Table 48.1, page 800.

- Name the key factors involved in **modulation of rate** of gastric emptying.
    - Vagus contains afferent nerves with A–delta and C pain fibers with cell bodies in the nodose ganglia with connections to the nucleus tractus solitarius (not shown)
    - Low threshold mechano– and chemoreceptors stimulate visceral sensations, i.e. stomach emptiness or fullness and symptoms, i.e. nausea and discomfort
    - These stimuli are mediated through vagal pathways and become conscious perceptions of visceral sensations, if sensory inputs reach the cortex
    - Splanchnic nerves also contain afferent nerves with A–delta and C fibers that synapse in the celiac ganglia with cells bodies in the vertebral ganglia (T5 – T9)
    - Interneurons in the white rami in the dorsal horn of the spinal cord cross to the dorsal columns and spinothalamic tracts, and ascend to the sensory areas of the medulla oblongata
    - Splanchnic afferent fibers are thought to mediate high threshold stimuli for visceral pain
    - In contrast to visceral sensations, somatic nerves, i.e. from the skin, carry sensory information via A–delta and C fibers through the dorsal root ganglia and into the dorsal horn, and then through the dorsal columns and spinothalamic tracts to the cortical areas of somatic representation
    - Changes in the gastric electrical rhythm, excess amplitude contractions, or stretch on the gastric wall are peripheral mechanisms that elicit changes in the afferent neural activity (via vagal and/or splanchnic nerves) that may reach consciousness to be perceived as visceral perceptions (symptoms) emanating from the stomach
    - Vagal and splanchnic nerve activity modulate the neuromuscular activities of the stomach
    - The balance between excitatory and inhibitory nerves to the stomach leads to a slower or faster gastric emptying
    - There is slow wave gastric myoelectrical activity during fasting
    - In the postprandial period, there is summation of the slow wave activity linked to plateau and action potential activity
    - Only a large meal, hypoglycemia and reduced fundic accommodation (relaxation) speeds up emptying to the stomach (reduced $T_{1/2}$ of emptying)
    - All other gastroduodenal, ileal and colonic neuromuscular factors, as well as meal–related factors delay gastric emptying (longer $T_{1/2}$)

- Gastric emptying may be slowed by either bradygastria (1 cpm) of low or high amplitude, or by tachygastria (6 cpm), where the gastric dysrhythmia is not coordinated with opening of the pylorus
- Receptive relaxation for liquids is in the fundus, same with solids, as well as in the gastric body and antrum
- With the intake of food and fluid, the stomach initially stretches, without any increase in its basal intraluminal pressure of about 10 cm H_2O
- "accomodation" of intragastric volume is mediated by the afferent and efferent pathways of the vagus nerve
- Relaxation is effected through stimulation of an inhibitory, nitrergic neuron
- Inhibitory motor neuron may also be stimulated by Ach and serotonin

Abbreviations: IML, intermediolateral nucleus; n, nerve

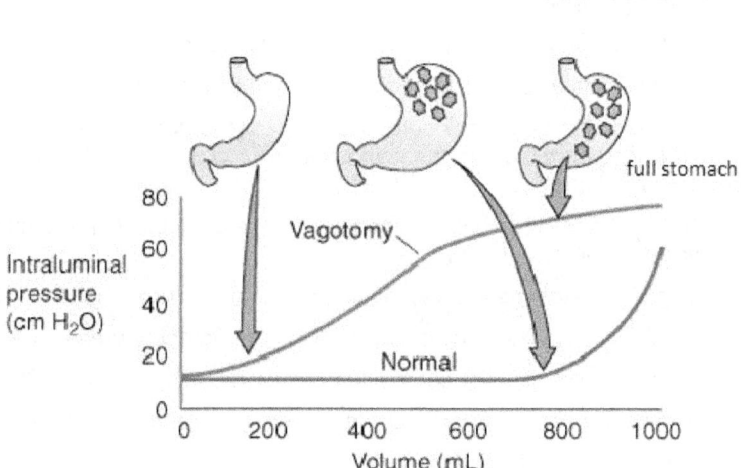

- Mechanoreceptors are also stimulated by the following:
  - IM–ICCs in the walls of the fundus
  - Vagovagal reflexes
  - Activated vagal afferent neurons
  - Distention of the antrum, duodenum, colon
  - Chemicals in the lumen: lipid, protein or H^+ in the duodenum
- Gastric enterochromaffin cells release serotonin (5–HT)
- 5–hydroxytryptamine–3 (5–HT3), gastrin–releasing peptide (GRP), and CCK_A receptors act on the capsaicin–sensitive gastric afferent vagal nerves
- 5–HT activates gastric intrinsic primary afferent neurons (IPANs) in the gastric submucosal and myenteric plexus
- IPANs signal afferent vagal neurons (vasovagal reflex) and also signal reflexes and sympathetic nervous system (SNS)
- Afferent vagal neurons connect to the nodose ganglia (cell bodies) and nucleus tractus solitarius (NTC), as well as to ICCs connecting to the circular muscles
- NTC connects to the hypothalamus and the cortex
- Pain stimulates splanchnic and spinal primary afferent neurons
- These primary afferent neurons connect to the dorsal horn of the spinal cord, and from there to the spinothalamic and spinoreticular tracts in the dorsal column
- NO and vasoactive intestinal peptide (VIP) are released and stimulate the vagal inhibitory neurons
- Vagal excitatory neurons are inhibited
- CCK activates CCK_A receptors in the vagal afferent neurons
- Vagal afferent neurons ascend to the nucleus tractus solitarius (NTS)
- Nerves from the NTS ascend to the periventricular nucleus (PN)
- PN participation leads to satiety
- Vagal dorsal motor nucleus (DMN–V) connect to the descending vagal efferent neurons
- Descending vagal efferent neurons reduce gastric emptying
- The net effect of CCK is to inhibit gastric emptying
- This represents the duodenal "brake"

- Explain the pathophysiological processes involved in the gastroparesis associated with type I diabetes.

❖ Abnormal function of the fundus
  o In response to the distention of fundus phasic contraction, ↓ accommodation due to failure of recovery of ↓ tone of the fundus during fasting (postprandial) period
  o Possible defect in the NO pathway, ↓ (50%) of IMMC during fasting associated with antral contraction and the clearance of undigested solids > 1 – 2 mm

❖ Abnormal function of the antrum
  o ↑ lag time for emptying of the stomach
  o ↓ frequency of the distal antral contractions (< 1/minute) causing hypomotility
  o ↑ isolated pyloric pressure waves (IPPN) or "pylorospasm"
  o ↓ proximal gastric contraction with failure of food in stomach to be redistributed; entering again the antrum for trituration and emptying
  o Abnormal electrical slow wave rhythms possibly due to ↑ prostaglandins
    - Brachygastria
    - Tachygastria
    - Mixture of brachygastria and tachygastria
  o Vagal dysfunction, i.e. autonomic neuropathy, hyperglycemia in type 1 diabetes
  o ↓ ICC in deep muscle plexus, i.e. in diabetes, possibly due to ↓ insulin and IGF–1 → smooth muscle cell produces ↓ stem cell factor
  o ↑ oxidative stress (i.e. in diabetes)
  o ↓ inhibitory NO–containing neurosis
  o ↑ phosphodiesterase–5 activity
  o Associated neuropathic or myopathic abnormalities of the small bowel motility

- Explain the pathophysiological defects and pharmaceutical approach in diabetic gastroparesis.

Symptoms	Pathophysiology	Pharmaceutical Approach
o Early satiety and postprandial fullness	– Defective accommodation from ↓ in NOS neurons	• NO donors
o Nausea and vomiting	– Gastroparesis secondary to enteric nervous system neuropathy – Abnormal pacemaker activity	• Prokinetic agents • Gastric • ↓ pacing
o Epigastric pain	– Sensory neuropathy in the gastric wall	• Tricyclic antidepressants • Neurostimulation
o Persistent nausea	– Tachygastria or bradygastria from the abnormal pacemaker activity	• Control of blood glucose • Domperidone

Adapted from: Owyang, C. *Gastroenterology*. 2011. 141:136.

- ➤ Causes and Associations
  - o Idiopathic (36%)
  - o Metabolic
    - – Diabetes (29%)
    - – Thyroid disease
  - o GI disorders
    - – Previous gastric surgery (13%)
    - – Gastric outlet obstruction (mechanical causes)
    - – GERD
  - o Autoimmune disease
  - o Neurological disease
  - o Post–viral gastroparesis (may improve spontaneously)

- Drugs
  - Narcotics
  - Anticholinergics
  - Diabetic–treating drugs
  - GLP–1
  - Amylin analogs (pramlintide)
  - Cannabinoids
- Eating disorders
  - Rumination syndrome
  - Effortless repetitive regurgitation of recently ingested food into the mouth within 15 min of starting a meal, followed by rechewing and reswallowing of the food, or spitting out of the ruminated food
  - Anorexia nervosa
  - Bulimia
- Cyclic vomiting syndrome
  - Abdominal pain and nausea, sudden onset of vomiting lasting for several hours over 3 – 5 days, then followed by vomiting for 3 – 4 months

➤ Clinical
  - Usual causes related to impaired motility (gastroparesis) and mechanical obstruction
  - Sometimes, the term "gastroparesis" will be used interchangeably with delayed gastric emptying

• What are the clinical tests for the components of gastric emptying?
  - Emptying
    - Scintigraphy
    - Capsule technology
    - Breath tests
    - Volume recovery tests
    - Ultrasonography
    - CT or MRI technology

- o Antral contractions
  - Antroduodenal manometry
  - Capsule technology
- o Myoelectrical activity
  - Electrogastrography (EGG)
    - Tachygastrias (> 3.7 cpm)
    - Bradygastrias (< 2.5 cpm)
- o Gastric relaxation
  - Barostat
    - Measurement of the intragastric tone and volume (not pressure)
  - Single photon emission CT (SPECT)
    - Scintigraphy, ultrasonography, MRI

SO YOU WANT TO BE A GASTROENTEROLOGIST!

Assessment of gastric neuromuscular function is divided into tests:

- o Gastric emptying rates (scintigraphy, breath tests, ultrasound, CT/MRI imaging and capsule technology)
- o Gastric contractions (antroduodenal manometry or capsule technology) and gastric myoelectrical activity

Electrogastrography (EGG) shows the amplitude and frequency of the gastric electrical rhythm (bradygastria or tachygastria, or a mix dysrhythmia).

- Gastric neuromuscular disorders based on gastric emptying test (GET) and EGG.

Conceptual framework of the categories of gastric neuromuscular disorders (useful for research purposes).

Tests	1	2	3	4
- GET	Ab–N	N	N	Ab–N
- EGG	Ab–N	Ab–N	N	N

Abbreviations: Ab–N, abnormal; EGG, electrogastrography

Adapted from: Feldman, M., et al. Sleisenger and Fordtran's Gastrointestinal and Liver Disease. 2016. 10th Edition. Saunders/Elsevier. Table 49-2, page 829.

- Diagnosis
  - A gastric emptying study performed with solid and liquid test meal will correctly establish whether the gastric emptying was slow at the time of testing
  - However, there is usually a poor correlation between the patient's symptoms, the T1/2 of emptying provided by the emptying study, or their response to prokinetic medications
- Treatment

- Wat are the **treatment** for delayed gastric emptying?
  - Meal Factors
    - Small, frequent, fluid, neutral pH and temperature, isotonic, low energy density
    - Low fat meals
    - Low non–digestible fiber
    - Frequent, small meals
    - Liquid meals (including enteral nutrition) *po*, or percutaneous endoscopically placed jejunostomy tube (PEJ)
    - Certain amino acids (i.e. L–tryptophan–[cheese])
    - Avoid offending foods and beverages
    - Vitamin B_6 (thiamine) (FDA A)
    - Ginger
    - Soda crackers (unproven benefit)
  - "prokinetics"
    - Metoclopramide
      - 1% risk of tardive dyskinesia
    - Domperidone
      - Domperidone (withhold treatment if the baseline ECG shows corrected OT > 450 ms (F) to 470 ms (M)
    - Cisapride
      - Metabolized by CYP450 3A4:AEs
      - Antibiotics
        - Macrolide
        - Antifungals
        - Phenothiazine

- Caution
    - Long QT (QTc > 0.45 sec) syndrome → SCD (sudden cardiac death)
- Erythromycin: 250 mg *po tid*, as needed, or maintenance
    - Induces high amplitude gastric propulsive contractions
    - Use is limited by tachyphylaxis
- Azithromycin
    - AEs: ototoxicity
    - Long QT syndrome → SCD
- Anti–emetics
    - Phenothiazines (do not give with cisapride → ↑ risk of QTc > 0.45 sec → SCD)
    - Antihistamines
    - 5–HT3 antagonists, i.e. ondansetron
    - Trial of tricyclic antidepressants (TCAs)
- Botulinum toxin injection into the pylorus
    - Unproven value

- Complications to be corrected
    - Dehydration
    - Hypokalemia
    - Metabolic alkalosis
    - Hyperglycemia (in diabetic)

- Treat other factors
    - Underlying diseases or condition causing or aggravating gastroparesis
    - Rectal or colonic distention
    - Pregnancy
    - Ascites
    - Hyperglycemia
    - Avoid circular oral motion
    - Avoid medications, which may relax the smooth muscles and thereby aggravate gastroparesis

- Surgery
  - Decompression
    - Venting gastrostomy
    - Jejunostomy
  - Conversion
    - Previous partial gastrectomy → subtotal gastrectomy or near–total gastrectomy and Roux–en–Y gastrojejunostomy

- Endoscopic therapy
  - Decompression with enterostomy tube
  - Percutaneous endoscopic gastrostomy (PEG) and PEG with jejunal extension tube (PEG–J), jejunostomy (surgical, endoscopic, radiographic)

- Gastric electrical stimulation ("humanitarian use device")
  - For diabetic gastroparesis, but not for idiopathic or post–surgical)

- Miscellaneous
  - Acupuncture – "P6" acupuncture point
  - Gastric electrical stimulation

Adapted from: Quigley, E. M. M. *Sleisenger & Fordtran's Gastrointestinal and Liver Disease: Pathophysiology/Diagnosis/Management.* 2006. page 1007.

- Hormonal therapy use is controversial in patients with bleeding from angiodysplasia, but may be of use in patients with angiodysplastic bleeding and hereditary hemorrhagic telegangiectasia (HHT), van Willebrand disease, or renal failure

- Explain the mechanism(s) of prokinetic drugs used for the treatment of symptoms of gastroparesis.

  - Metoclopramide
    - Central or peripheral dopamine receptor antagonist (D_2)
    - 5–HT3 receptor antagonist
    - 5–HT4 receptor agonist

  - Domperidone
    - peripheral D_2 antagonist

- o Cisapride - muscarinic (acetylcholine) receptor agonist
  - 5–HT3 receptor antagonist
  - 5–HT4 receptor agonist

- o Ondansetron - 5–HT3 receptor antagonist

- o Erythromycin - motilin receptor agonist

- o Tegaserod - cholinergic 5–HT4 partial agonist

- o Bethanechol - muscarinic receptor agonist

- o Anticholinergic (buscopan for tachygastria)

- o α–adrenergic antagonists - α–adrenergic antagonist

- o Botulism toxin injections - phosphodiesterase inhibitors (Viagra)

- o Octreotide injections - somatostatin receptor antagonist

*The FDA category for use in pregnancy is noted in brackets

CLINICAL PHYSIOLOGICAL CHALLENGE – Gastroparesis

Case: A 29–year old diabetic lady develops bloating and fullness after meal. She is diagnosed with possible gastroparesis, and is referred to you for management. You recommend alterations in her diet. Explain the choices of prokinetic drugs.

Questions:

- Explain the pathophysiology of gastroparesis (not just in this patient).
- What tests for gastric function is used in this patient to document the suspected presence of gastroparesis.
- Explain the basis for the dietary recommendations of gastroparesis.
- What are the receptors on gastric smooth muscles targeted for her pharmaceutical treatment?

Clinical Gems:
- o Acupuncture may be of benefit for relief of nausea and vomiting (Ezzo, J. M., *et al. Cochrane Database Syst Rev.* 2006. 2: CD002285.
- o Ginger (> 1 g/day) and thiamine (especially for nausea in pregnancy, pyridoxine [Diclectin] 10 mg *po bid* plus tabs II *q hs*), are alternatives for the treatment for nausea, which have proven benefit.

- o Treat the complications
    - GERD, esophagitis
    - Dehydration, electrolyte disturbances
    - Malnutrition
- o Miscellaneous
    - Acupuncture – "P6" acupuncture point
    - Gastric electrical stimulation

Adapted from: Koch, K. L. *Sleisenger & Fordtran's Gastrointestinal and Liver Disease: Pathophysiology/ Diagnosis/Management.* 2016. 10th Edition. Saunders/Elsevier, Philadelphia. Table 49-6, page 837.

SO YOU WANT TO BE A GASTROENTEROLOGIST!

Acupuncture with electrical stimulation (acustimulation) represents one of the alternate forms of electrical therapy for gastroparesis.

- What are the other forms of gastric electrical therapy?

    - o Gastric electrical stimulation (GES)
        - High frequency (12 cpm)
        - Short duration (300 <u>micro</u>seconds)
    - o Gastric pacing (to "entrain" the normal gastric slow wave rhythm)
        - Low frequency (3 cpm)
        - Long duration (300 <u>milli</u>seconds)
    - o Sequential
        - Sequential pacing using a microprocessor
        - Activation of electrodes in a series around the distal 2/3 of the stomach

Antral Filling and Pyloric Pump

- Explain the physiological function of the antrum and pylorus.
    - Food contents of the fundus are mixed with saliva, gastric acid and pepsin
    - Body and antral peristaltic waves grind the food into 1 – 2 mm solid particles (titurition)
    - Period of grinding of solid food into small particles before emptying begins the lag period
    - Antral peristalsis occurs at the rate of 3/minute
    - With coordinated relaxation of pyrolus, 2 – 4 ml of chymes containing the 1 – 2 mm solid particles are emptied through the pylorus, usually in little pulsatile "squirts"
    - Amount of material emptied across the pyrolus ("stroke volume") is set not by volume but by calories
    - Rate of caloric emptying is 3 – 4 kcal/min
    - This caloric emptying rate, and the rate of emptying of the volume which contains the calories is determined by the amplitude (normally 10 – 40 mmHg) and length of the peristaltic contraction
        - Intragastric pressure
        - Pressure gradient across the pyloric sphincter
    - Some gastric peristaltic contractions may push chymes into the antrum, and then stop
    - Other peristaltic contractions continue to the pyrolus
    - If the pylorus is closed, the chyme pushed as far as the pyrolus will return to the gastric body for more grinding (mixing, titurition)

- Food–related factors
    - Response to ingestion of liquids
        - Receptive relaxation for liquids is in the fundus, as occurs with solids, as well as in the gastric body and antrum
        - Liquids are emptied faster than solids
            - Liquids do not require grinding before passing through the pylorus
        - Water empties faster than calorie–dense liquids

- Response to ingestion of solid food
  - With intake of food and fluid, the stomach initially stretches, without any increase in its basal intraluminal pressure of about 10 cm H_2O
  - This "accomodation" of intragastric volume is mediated by the afferent and efferent pathways of the vagus nerve
  - Relaxation is effected through stimulation of an inhibitory, nitrergic neuron
  - Inhibitory motor neuron may be stimulated by Ach and serotonin
  - When the volume of the stomach distends beyond the ability of the stomach to accommodate (usually about 800 ml), the intragastric pressure rises, and the patient begins to feel "full"

➤ Body contractions

- Name the key physiological factors involved in gastric motor activity.
  - Neurons of the ENS are close to MY–ICCs and IM–ICCs
  - Excitatory neurotransmitters include Ach and substance P
  - Inhibitory neurotransmitters, including NO and VIP
  - Spread of the slow wave and smooth muscle contraction is integrated by IM–ICCs
  - IM–ICCs are electrically coupled by gap junctions to the smooth muscle cells
  - MY–ICCs produce slow electrical waves depolarizing the smooth muscle membrane depolarization
  - IM–ICCs slow wave activates the voltage–dependent L–type calcium channels in the smooth muscle cell membrane
  - Depolarization during the upstroke of the slow wave redepolarizes to the value of the RMP, and the contraction ends
  - MY–ICCs initiate, while IM–ICCs mediate neurotransmission by:
    - Integrate slow wave and smooth muscle activities
    - Coordinate the spread of slow waves
  - Relaxation of the fundus and proximal portion of the gastric body is replaced by contractions of the fundus and proximal corpus
  - This pushes food into the rest of the body and antrum, where mixing and grinding occur
  - This initial postprandial interval of receptive relaxation, mixing and grinding, is called the "lag phase"
  - Lag phase duration depends on the composition of the meal (usually about 45 – 60 minutes).

- Emptying
    - Trituration of solid food into particles 1 – 2 mm in size begins the linear phase of gastric emptying
    - Gastric peristaltic waves arise from the electrical activity of ICC, plateau and action potentials, which sweep through the body of the stomach at 3 cpm
    - Clearance of pyloric sphincter and contraction of the duodenum present in the emptying of the particles > 2 mm
    - Antral contraction waves pump pulsatile "squirts" of food and fluid into the duodenum
    - Depending on the strength of contraction (10 – 40 mmHg) and duration of antral peristaltic wave, the resistance provided by pyloric sphincter and duodenal contraction usually 3 – 4 kcal/min is emptied into the duodenum
    - About 50% of a meal will be emptied in 90 min ($T_{1/2}$ of gastric emptying), and 95% has been emptied by 4 hours
    - Non–caloric and then caloric liquids are emptied first without lag phase and in a "mono–exponential emptying" pattern, then digestible material during the linear phase as a result of lower amplitude pressure waves
    - The rate of gastric emptying may be modified by the amount and composition of the ingested food and fluids
        - Volume
        - Viscosity
        - Osmolarity
        - Nutrient density

For further details, please refer to: Feldman M., *et al. Sleisenger and Fordtran's Gastrointestinal and Liver Disease*. 2010. 9th Edition. Saunders/Elsevier, Philadelphia. Table 48.1, page 800.

- TICCs in the deep muscular plexus junction in conjugation with the ENS
- ICCs in the myenteric plexus do not depend on ENS
- ICCs in the pylorus are associated with inhibitory neural activity in this region, and thereby are important in the context of the rate of gastric emptying

- Explain the key physiological factors involved in the modulation of the rate of gastric emptying.
    - Vagal and splanchnic nerve activities modulate the neuromuscular activities of the stomach

- Vagal stimulates while splanchnic inhibits
- The balance between excitatory and inhibitory nerves to the stomach leads to slower or faster gastric emptying
- There is slow wave gastric myoelectrical activity during fasting
- GI peptides are involved in gastric emptying
- In the postprandial period, there is summation of the slow wave activity linked to plateau and action potential activity
- Only a large meal, hypoglycemia and reduced fundic accommodation (relaxation) speeds the emptying of the stomach (reduced $T_{1/2}$ of emptying)
- All other gastroduodenal, ileal and colonic neuromuscular factors, as well as meal–related factors, delay gastric emptying (longer $T_{1/2}$)
- Gastric emptying may be slowed by either bradygastria (1 cpm) of low or high amplitude or by tachygastria (6 cpm), where gastric dysrhythmia is not coordinated with opening of the pylorus

- What are the factors alternating the rate of gastric emptying?
❖ Gastric emptying is influenced by the following:
  - Food
    - Caloric density
    - Viscosity
    - Acidity
    - Contents of fat > protein > carbohydrate
    - Fatty acids in the duodenum or ileum
    - Osmolality
    - Fiber
    - Tryptophan
    - Volume
  - Motility–related factors
  - Hormones

- ❖ Motility–related Factors
    - o Fundic accomodation
    - o Antral peristaltic contraction
    - o Pressure gradient between stomach and duodenum
    - o Degree of anthropyloruduodenal coordination
    - o Pylorospasm
    - o Presence of dysmotility (i.e. tachygastria)
    - o Amount of duodenogastric reflex

- • What are the hormone–related factors modifying gastric emptying?
    - o Peptides CCK, CCK_A receptors, GLP–1, PYY, CRF, SCF, dopamine, and GLP–1

- ❖ Glucagon–like polypeptide–1 (GLP–1)
    - o GLP–1 is released in proportional response to hyperglycemia
    - o Hyperglycemia releases insulin (incretin effects of GLP–1) effects:
        - – ↓ antral contractions
        - – ↑ gastric dysrhythmias
        - – ↓ sensation of fullness from fundic distention
        - – ↓ gastric emptying
    - o Hypoglycemia and GLP–1 or hyperglycemia (> 220 mg/dL)
        - – ↑ dysrhythmias
        - – ↑ contractility
        - – ↑ emptying
        - – ↑ dysrhythmias

- ❖ CCK and the "Ileal Break"

    Fatty acids in the ileum stimulate an enterogastric reflex (the "ileal break") to slow gastric emptying
    - o Ileal break involves PYY, CCK and GLP–1
    - o Duodenal mucosal receptors for FA, AA and carbohydrates limit the rate of gastric emptying to ~ 150 kcal/hour
    - o Fat in the ileum slows small bowel emptying through the release of GLP–1 and –2, as well as PYY

- ❖ Body mass index (BMI)
    - o As BMI increases, gastric emptying becomes faster
    - o Medium and long chain fatty acids (FA) release CCK
    - o CCK slows gastric emptying
        - – ↓ fundic tone
        - – ↓ antral contraction
        - – ↑ pyloric tone

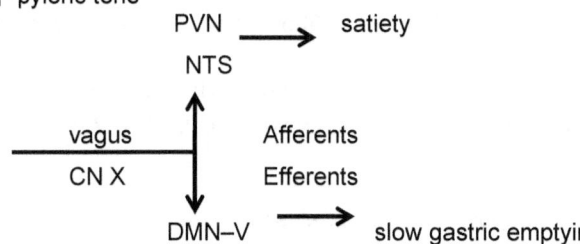

Abbreviations: DMN–V, dorsal motor nucleus of the vagus; NTS, nucleus tractus solitarius; PVN, paraventricular nucleus

- o Usual causes related to impaired motility and mechanical obstruction
- o The term "gastroparesis" is used interchangeably with delayed gastric emptying implying a process rather than mechanism

Causes of Gastric Scarring and Slowed Gastric Emptying

Gastric emptying is slowed by mechanical structural gastric narrowing

- Name the causes of gastric narrowing seen on diagnostic or endoscopic examination of the stomach.
    - o Benign
        - – Peptic ulcer disease and scarring
        - – Ingestion of lye (corrosive agents)
        - – Granulomatous
            - – Infection: Tuberculosis
            - – Syphilis
    - o Inflammation
        - – Crohn disease
        - – Sarcoidosis
        - – Eosinophilic gastroenteritis
    - o Malignant
        - – Carcinoma
        - – Lymphoma
        - – Metastases

Diabetes and Gastroparesis
- Demography
  - 30 – 50% of outpatients with long standing type 1 or type 2 diabetes mellitus have slow gastric emptying
  - The risk of developing gastroparesis among subjects with T1DM was elevated over 30–fold, whereas the risk in subjects with T2DM was increased almost 8–f fold, relative to age– and sex–matched controls
  - Subjects with T1DM were 4x more likely to develop gastroparesis than those with T2DM
  - Incidence of gastroparesis among those with diabetes is still rare

Source: Chong, R. S., et al. Am J Gastroenterol. 2012. 107:82-88.

- Pathophysiology
- Explain the pathophysiological processes in gastroparesis in the diabetes.
  - Abnormal function of the fundus
    - In response to the distention of fundic phasic contraction, ↓ accommodation due to failure of recovery of ↓ tone of fundus during the fasting (postprandial) period, possibly due to a defect in the NO pathway, ↓ (50%) of IMMC during fasting associated with antral contraction and clearance of undigested solids, > 1 – 2 mm
  - Abnormal function of the antrum
    - ↑ lag time of emptying the stomach
    - ↓ frequency of the distal antral contractions (< 1/minute) causing hypomotility
    - ↑ isolated pyloric pressure waves (IPPN), "pylorospasms"
    - ↓ proximal gastric contraction, with failure of food still in stomach to be redistributed, again entering the antrum for trituration and emptying.
    - Abnormal electrical slow wave rhythms, possible from ↑ prostaglandins
      - Brachygastria
      - Tachygastria
      - Mixture of brachygastria and tachygastria
    - Vagal dysfunction, i.e. autonomic neuropathy, hyperglycemia in type 1 diabetes
    - ↓ ICC in deep muscle plexus, i.e. in DM, possibly due to ↓ insulin and IGF–1 → smooth muscle cell produces ↓ stem cell factor
    - ↑ oxidative stress (in DM); ↓ inhibitory NO–containing neurosis
    - ↑ phosphodiesterase–5 activity
    - Associated neuropathic or myopathic abnormalities of small bowel motility

SO YOU WANT TO BE A GASTROENTEROLOGIST!

Patients with partial gastrectomy and Roux–en–Y anastomosis develop nausea, vomiting, bloating and early satiety due to the stasis of the food in the gastric remnant as well as in the distal Roux jejunal limb, especially, if the Roux limb is > 45 cm. This is called the "**Roux–en–Y stasis syndrome**".

- Explain the pathophysiology and non–surgical treatment of Roux–en–Y stasis syndrome.
    - The transection of the jejunum prevents the pacemaker wave generated in the duodenum from passing the distal to the level of the transection
    - Ectopic pacemakers in the Roux limb cause retrograde contractions leading to ↑ filling of gastric remnant and Roux limb

SO YOU WANT TO BE A GASTROENTEROLOGIST!

Gastroparesis is usually postsurgical, idiopathic ischemic, or associated with diabetes.
- Name the abnormalities seen in T1 **diabetics** contributing to gastroparesis.
    - ➢ Episodes of hyperglycemia (from poor control of blood sugars)
        - ↓ stem cell factor (SCF) → ↓ interstitial cell of Cajal (ICCs)
        - Body
            - ↑ dysrhythmias
        - Antrum
            - ↓ motility (contractions)
        - Pylorus
            - ↑ motility (pylorospasm, leading to non–coordinated antral contraction and pyloric sphincter relaxation)
        - Metabolic end–products
            - ↑ glycosylation end products
            - ↓ neural function
            - ↓ smooth muscle function
        - Fundus
            - ↓ relaxation (possible neuropathy of vagus nerve)
        - Antrum
            - ↓ MMC
            - ↓ postprandial motility
            - ↑ dysrhythmias
            - ↓ phase 3 contractions → ↓ emptying of non–digestible food (i.e. fibers)
    - Abnormal distribution of food in the fundus

NAUSEA AND VOMITING

- Definition
  - Symptom of unpleasant sensation experienced prior to vomiting
- Pathophysiology
  - Initial event leading to vomiting is the loss of intestinal slow wave activity
  - Loss of slow wave activity is linked to propulsive peristaltic contractions
  - Normal peristaltic contractions of the stomach and small intestine decline, and are replaced by retrograde contractions, beginning in the ileum and progressing upwards towards the stomach
  - These retrograde contractions are accompanied by contraction of the external intercostal muscles and diaphragm against a closed glottis
  - Valsalva–like action increases intra–abdominal pressure
  - Diaphragmatic crural muscle and lower esophageal sphincter relax
  - The increase in intra–abdominal pressure forces gastric contents up into the esophagus
  - Larynx moves upward and forward, while the UES relaxes
  - Gastric contents are vomited
  - The closed glottis protects the airway and prevents aspiration
- Causes

Causes of nausea: "N-A-U-S-E-A" (A simple aide de memoire)

N	Neurologic CNS, vestibular
A	Alcohol and drugs
U	Usually accompanies systemic illness
S	Stress and psychiatric conditions
E	Enteral conditions
	Endocrine conditions
A	"anticipating" causes

Adapted from: Maclean, C. Chapter 55. In: Therapeutic Choices. Grey, J. Ed. 6th Edition, Canadian Pharmacists Association: Ottawa, ON. 2011. page 724-734.

- Classify the causes of nausea and vomiting, and give examples.

Please see: Malagelada, J. R. and Malagelada, C. Nausea and Vomiting. *Sleisenger & Fordtran's Gastrointestinal and Liver Disease: Pathophysiology/ Diagnosis/ Management.* 2006. page 145.

Post–Operative Nausea and Vomiting

➢ Mechanisms

- Explain the mechanisms for the development of **post–operative** nausea and vomiting (PONV).
    - Release of serotonin from bowel handling stimulates $5HT_3$ receptors on afferent serotonergic pathways that stimulate the brainstem
    - Reduced blood flow to brainstem during surgery
    - Activated cerebral cortical pathways

➢ Risk factors

- What are the risk factors for PONV?
    - Patient
        - Post–puberty females
        - Non–smokers
        - Previous PONV
    - Drug
        - Use of volatile anesthetics
        - Intra–operative use of opiates
        - High dosage of neostigmine
    - Surgery
        - Prolonged surgery
        - Intra–abdominal surgery
        - Major gynecological surgery

- Give the methods to reduce the risk of PONV.
  - Avoid opioids
  - Avoid nitrous oxide
  - Avoid high dose of reversal agent
  - Adequate hydration
  - High oxygen concentration
  - Propofol anesthetic

Printed with permission: Gan, T. J., *et al. Anesth Analg.* 2003. 97(1):62-71.; and Williams, K. S. *Surg Clin North Am.* 2005. 85(6):1229-41.; and adapted from: Kovac, A. L. *J Clin Anesth.* 2006. Jun: 18(4):304-18.

➤ Differential diagnosis of vomiting in newborn.
  - Inherited
    - Congenital duodenal atresia
    - Pyloric stenosis
    - Meconium ileus
    - Hirschsprung disease
  - Intake
    - Food allergy
    - Milk protein intolerance
  - Infection
    - Gastroenteritis
  - Mechanical
    - Volvulus
  - Idiopathic
    - Gastroesophageal reflux
    - Overfeeding

> Treatment

- Give the causes and classes of medication used to treat **vomiting**.

Classes of Causes	Common Disorders	Class of Medication

❖ Middle ear	o Motion sickness
	o Meniere's disease
		Antihistamines (dimenhydrinate, short acting)
		- Gravol 50 – 100 mg *po, pr, IM, IV* every 4 – 6 hours *prn* (max 400 mg/day)
		- Benadryl
		  - 25 – 50 mg *tid qid prn po*
		  - 10 – 50 mg *tid – qid prn po IM* or *IV*
		- Hydroxyzine
		  - Atarax 25 – 100 mg *tid – qid prn po* or *IM*
		
		Anticholinergics
		Scopolamine patches (transderm V) 1.5 mg (1 patch) every 72 hours *prn*

❖ Gastrointestinal causes	o Gastroparesis o Dyspepsia	Prokinetics (benzamides, dopamine antagonists) - Domperidone 10 mg *qid po* ½ hour *AC* and *HS* - Metoclopramide 10 – 20 mg *tid – qid prn po* or *SC* or *IV*

❖ Stimulation of CTZ	o CNS conditions
	o Drugs
	o Uremia
		Dopamine antagonist
		Please see above
		Serotonin antagonists
		- Ondansetron (Zofran ®)
		  - 4 – 8 mg *od – tid po* or *IV*
		- Granisetron (Kytril ®, Apo–Granisetron)
		  - 1 – 2 mg *od – bid po*
		  - 10 mcg/kg *IV* over 5 minutes

Classes of Causes	Common Disorders	Class of Medication

	o PONV, DIN, CINV, migraine, vertigo	Phenothiazines
		- Chlorpromazine
		   ▪ 10 – 25 mg every 4 – 6 hours *prn po*
		   ▪ 25 – 50 mg every 3 – 4 hours *prn IM, IV*
		- Perphenazine
		   ▪ 2 – 4 mg every 8 hours *prn po* or IM or IV
		- Prochlorperazine
		   ▪ 5 – 10 mg *tid – qid prn po* or *pr*
		   ▪ 5 – 10 mg *bid – tid prn IM* or *IV*
		- Promethazine
		   ▪ 12.5 – 25 mg every 4 – 6 hours *prn po, IM,*

Abbreviations: CINV, chemotherapy–induced nausea and vomiting; CTZ, chemoreceptor trigger zone; PONV, post–op nausea and vomiting; DIN, drug–induced nausea

Clinical Pearl: If non–pharmacological approaches fail, and the above approach is not also effective, then combine two or more anti–emetics from different pharmacological classes

- Name the smooth muscle and the corresponding CNS receptors responsible for the mechanism(s) of action of the 12 drugs used in the treatment of refractory nausea and vomiting.

    o GI receptors
       - See previous answer on mechanism of action of prokinetic drugs
    o Central
       - H–1 receptor antagonists (inner ear) – diphenhydramine, promethazine
       - Cannabinoids – dronabinol, nabilone
       - Neurokinin (NK) –1–antagonist – aprepitant, talnetant, osanetant
       - Neuroleptic – chlorpromazine, haloperidol
       - Benzodiazepines
       - 5–HT3 antagonist – ondansetron
       - Metoclopramide
           ▪ D2 antagonist
           ▪ 5–HT3 or 5–HT4
       - Tricyclic antidepressants
       - Steroids (i.e. dexamethasone and Mannitol; nausea and vomiting due to increased intracranial pressure)

- Gastroparesis
  - Vomiting center is on the blood side of the blood brain barrier
  - Some patients with severe, intractable gastroparesis, i.e. may occur with severe T1DM, may improve with near-total gastrectomy and Roux-en-Y anastomosis
  - Slowed gastric emptying and delayed small intestinal transit occur in patients with cirrhosis

- Name the non-prescription drugs, dietary and lifestyle modifications, therapeutic options for the treatment of nausea and vomiting during **pregnancy**.
  - Avoidance of precipitating factors
    - Meal factors
      - Small, frequent, fluid, neutral pH and temperature, isotonic, low energy density, low fat meals
      - Certain amino acids (i.e. L-tryptophan – [cheese])
      - Avoid offending foods and beverages
      - Vitamin B6 (thiamine) (FDA A)
      - Ginger
      - Soda crackers (unproven benefit)
      - Avoid offending foods and beverages
      - Frequent, small meals, low in fat
    - Stimulation of P6 acupuncture point

  - Treat other factors
    - Underlying disease and condition causing or aggravating gastroparesis
    - Rectal or colonic distention
    - Pregnancy
    - Ascites
    - Hyperglycemia
    - Avoid circular vectoral motion
    - Avoid medications which may relax the smooth muscles and thereby aggravate gastroparesis

  - Gastric electrical stimulation
  - Treat complications

- GERD, esophagitis
- Dehydration, electrolyte disturbances
- Malnutrition
  o Miscellaneous
    - Acupuncture – "P6" acupuncture point
    - Gastric electrical stimulation

Adapted from: Quigley, E. M. M. *Sleisenger & Fordtran's Gastrointestinal and Liver Disease: Pathophysiology/Diagnosis/Management.* 2006. page 1007.; Keller, J. *et al. Nat Clin Pract Gastroenterol Hepatol.* 2008. 5(8): 433.

- What are the drugs used for nausea and vomiting in pregnancy and the corresponding FDA pregnancy use category?

Drugs	FDA category	Usual dosage
o Vitamin B_6 (thiamine)	A	10 – 25 mg 3x daily
o Doxylamine	B	12.5 mg 2x daily
o Prochlorperazine	C	5 – 10 mg *tid*
o Metoclopramide	B	10 – 20 mg 4x daily (*qid*)
o Domperidone, cisapride	C	1 – 20 mg *tid* or *qid*
o Ondansetron	B	4 – 8 mg *tid*
o Promethazine	C	12.5 – 25.0 mg *qid*

Adapted from: Thukral, C. and Wolf, J. L. *Nat Clin Pract Gastroenterol Hepatol.* 2006. 3(5): page 258.; and Printed with permission: Keller, J., *et al. Nat Clin Pract Gastroenterol Hepatol.* 2008. 5(8): page 433.

SO YOU WANT TO BE A CLINICAL PHARMACOLOGIST!

- Name the antiemetics reported to **prolong QTc** and/or PR interval.
    - Butyrophenone
        - Droperidol
    - Serotonin antagonist
        - Dolasetron (Anzemet®)
        - Granisetron (Kytril®, Apo–granisetron®)
        - Ondansetron (Zofran®)
    - Cisapride

- Name of antiemetics for which the dose must be adjusted for.
    - Age
        - Droperidol
    - Kidney malfunction
        - Metochlopramide
        - Dolasetron

Adapted from: Maclean, C. Chapter 55. In: Therapeutic Choices. Grey, J. Ed. 6th Edition, Canadian Pharmacists Association: Ottawa, ON. 2011. page 724–734.

- Explain the **drug interactions of antiemetics**.

Antiemetic	Other Drug Interaction	Mechanism
❖ ↑ effect of other drugs		
o Antihistamines	- Digoxin	▪ ↑ absorption
o Serotonin antagonists (Dolasetron)	- Anti–depressant	▪ ↓ CYP 2D6
❖ ↓ effects of other drugs		
o Serotonin antagonists (Dolasetron)	- Tramadol	

❖ Action of other drugs on effect of antiemetics

Other drugs	Antiemetic	Mechanisms
o Cimetidine	- Serotonin antagonist Dolasetron	- ↑ blood level of active metabolite
o Rifampin, phenytoin, carbamazepine	- Ondansetron	- ↓ blood level of active metabolite
o Rifampin	- Dolasetron	- ↓ blood level of active metabolite

➢ **Pregnancy and lactation**

- What are the treatment for nausea and vomiting during pregnancy and breastfeeding?

    o Diet and lifestyle modifications
      - Avoidance of precipitating factors
      - Frequent, small meals high in carbohydrate and low in fat
      - Stimulation of P6 acupuncture point
      - Ginger
      - Vitamin B6

    o If non–pharmacological measures fail

    ↓

    - Doxylamine 10 mg plus pyridoxine (vitamin B6) (Diclectin DR®) tab 1 *bid po* plus tabs II *qhs*

    ↓

    - Dimenhydrinate
      - With no diclectin, 50 – 100 mg every 4 – 6 hours *po* (Gravol®)
      - With 4 diclectin/day, then dimenhydrinate max 20 mg/day
      - Promethazine 12.5 – 25 mg every 4 – 6 hours *po* or *pr*

    ↓

    - Benzamide (metoclopramide)
    - Phenothiazine
    - Ondansetron (Zofran®)

*Note: If one treatment fails, move to next step; continue to reassess patient for possible dehydration and need for *IV* saline and systemic (*SC, IM, IV*) pharmacological therapy.

Caution: Ensure patient is not pregnant, and in this situation, do not use corticosteroids as an antiemetic during the first trimester (concern about risk of oral cleft abnormalities).

- Give 4 drugs that may be used for nausea and vomiting in pregnancy and the corresponding FDA pregnancy use category.

Drugs	FDA category	Usual dosage
o Domperidone, cisapride	C	1 – 20 mg *tid* or *qid*
o Doxylamine	B	12.5 mg 2x daily
o Metoclopramide	B	10 – 20 mg 4x daily (qid)
o Ondansetron	B	4 – 8 mg *tid*
o Prochlorperazine	C	5 – 10 mg *tid*
o Promethazine	C	12.5 – 25.0 mg *qid*
o Vitamin B$_6$ (thiamine)	A	10 – 25 mg 3x daily

Adapted from: Thukral, C., and Wolf, J. L. *Nat Clin Pract Gastroenterol Hepatol.* 2006. 3(5): page 258.; and Printed with permission: Keller, J., *et al. Nat Clin Pract Gastroenterol Hepatol.* 2008. 5(8): page 433.

"Your present circumstances don't determine where you can go; they merely determine where you start."

Nido Qubein

VASCULAR LESIONS

Gastric Varices (GV)

- What is the **SARIN** classification of gastroesophageal varices (GEV) or isolated gastric varices (IGV)?

    - GEV1
        - GV in continuity with EV
        - Extend 2 – 5 cm below the GE junction
        - Easiest to obliterate with cyanoacrylate

    - GEV2
        - GV in continuity with EV
        - GV extends to the cardia and fundus

    - IGV1
        - No EV
        - GV in fundus
        - Most difficult to obliterate with cyanoacrylate

    - IGV2
        - No EV
        - GV in gastric body, antrum, and pylorus

    - Bleeding risk
        - GEV2 or IGV1 > GEV1, IGV2 (unless the patient is matched for CTP score, in which case, the risk of bleeding is similar in each type of varix)

Clinical Tips: To glue or to band gastric varices (GV)

- Cyanoacrylate injection of GV is superior to EVL or sclerotherapy
- "Band Ligation of EV greater than 10 mm in diameter usually is unsafe" (Feldman, M., *et al. Sleisenger and Fordtran's Gastrointestinal and Liver Disease*. 2010. 9th Edition. Saunders/Elsevier, Philadelphia. page 1512).
- EVL of GV in the cardia of stomach is safest
- If bleeding occurs from IGV1 after TIPS, consider transhepatic embolization of fundal GV

> **SO YOU WANT TO BE A HEPATOLOGIST!**
> - Gastric vascular ectasia (GVE), including those that occur in the antrum (GAVE), are associated with thrombi in the vessels, fibrohyalinosis, and proliferation of spindle cells
> - When patients with GVE bleeding are supplemented with iron, but become transfusion dependent, thermoablative therapy may be given (i.e. argon plasma coagulation or cryotherapy), or oral estrogen–progesterone combination therapy may be given
> - If this fails and bleeding continues, surgical approaches may need to be considered, such as antrectomy or liver transplantation
> - Note
>   - TIPS, or any other maneuver to reduce portal pressure is not a successful therapy in GVE or GAVE
>
> - Explain why liver transplantation (LT) is an effective therapy for both PHG and GHE or GAVE.
>   - Pathogenesis of PHG is portal hypertension corrected by LT
>   - Pathogenesis of GVE or GAVE is unknown, but is presumably related to the process causing thrombi in the microvasculature of the stomach
>   - It is speculated that GVE or GAVE is caused by some products produced in the failing liver, and which is not appropriately cleared in the presence of liver failure
>   - LT corrects liver failure, and improves EVE or GAVE

- Primary prophylaxis
  - EGD surveillance for 1 – 2 years
  - Non–selective beta blocker (NSBB)
    - Start when:
      - ↑ EV size
      - Development of red wales
  - Possibly (one study) cyanoacrylate ("glue") injection for large GV

Outcomes	"Glue"	NSBB or placebo
– Probability of first bleed from GV	28%	45%
– Actuarial probability of survival	90%	72%

  - Do not use sclerotherapy, or TIPS, shunt for primary prophylaxis of GV
  - EV + GV, treat as EV; isolated GV, glue or TIPS

- For acute bleeding GV, or for secondary prophylaxis, "glue" GV with n-butyl–2–cyanoacrylate, or 2–octyl cyanoacrylate
- TIPS may also be effective for the following:
  - Bleeding GV
  - Secondary prophylaxis
- Liver transplantation may be considered in selected patients

Abbreviation: TIPS, transjugular intrahepatic portosystemic shunt

> Endoscopy

A 29–year old man presents with an upper GI bleed, jaundice, and sudden onset of severe epigastric pain radiating to the back. There are no extrahepatic signs of chronic liver disease. Describe the endoscopic findings, give differential diagnosis of the causes, and your management.

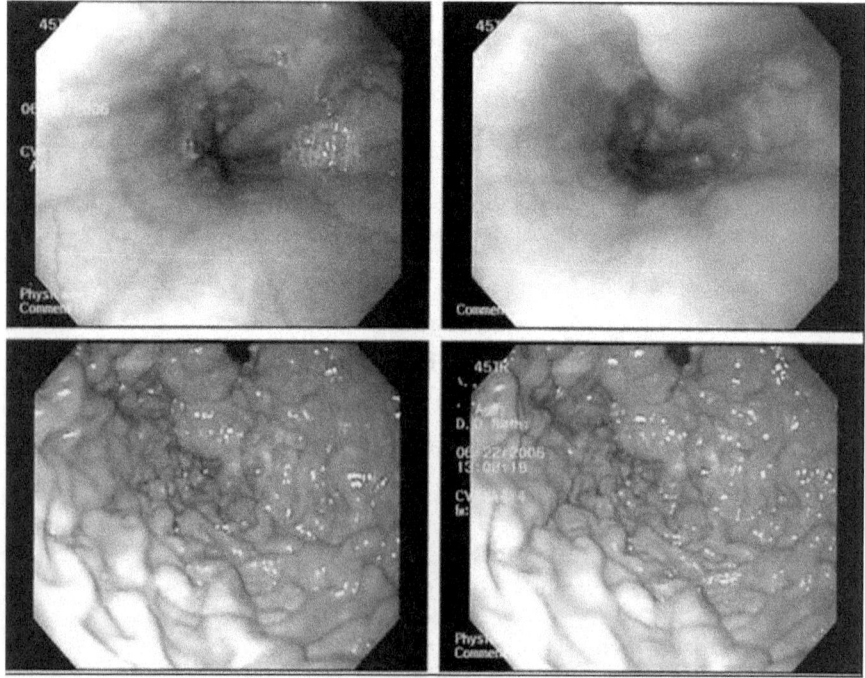

A 48-year old man with a B cell lymphoma involving the tail of the pancreas presents with an upper GI bleed. Describe the endoscopic findings, give the differential diagnosis, speculate on the mechanism and outline the management.

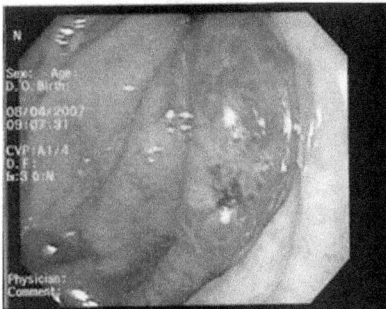 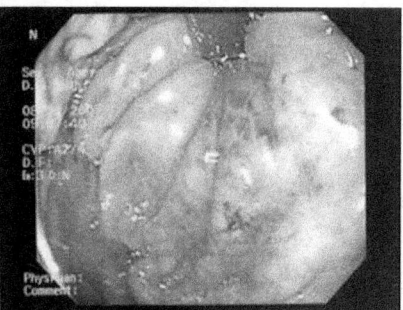

Portal Hypertension Gastropathy (PHG)

➢ Definition
- o Endoscopic findings of mosaic–like appearance (snake skin) of gastric body or fundus, with or without red spots, in patient with portal hypertension with or without cirrhosis

➢ Pathogenesis
- o Portal hypertension with or without cirrhosis
- o ↑ risk after endoscopic homostatic therapy (EHT) for EV

➢ Endoscopy
- o Mosiac or snake skin–like appearance of gastric body or fundus
- o May show spectrum of red spots
  - Small, faint red
  - Large, bright red
  - Hemorrhagic gastritis, diffuse

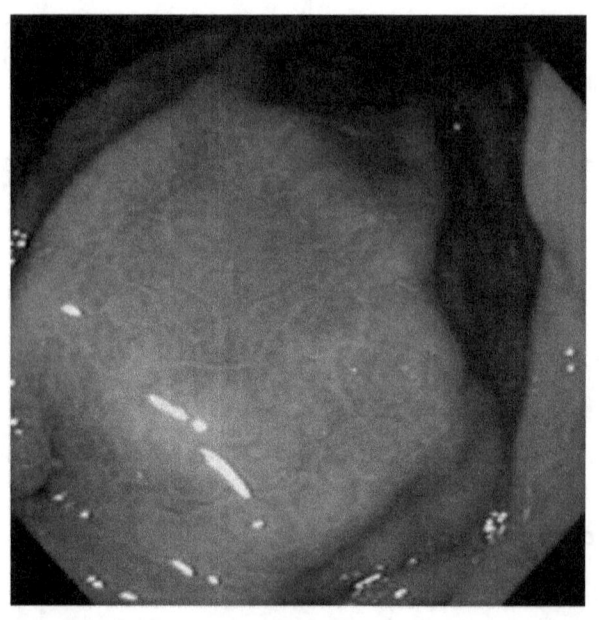

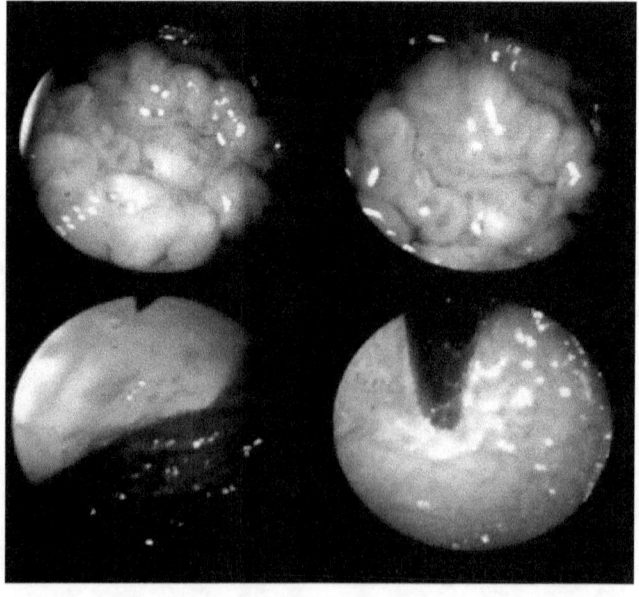

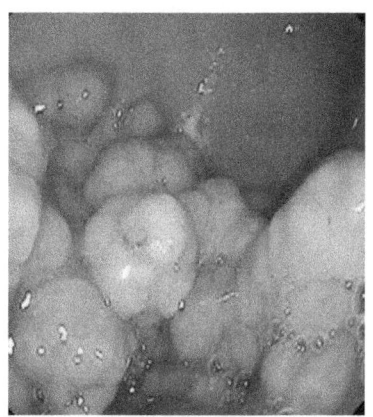

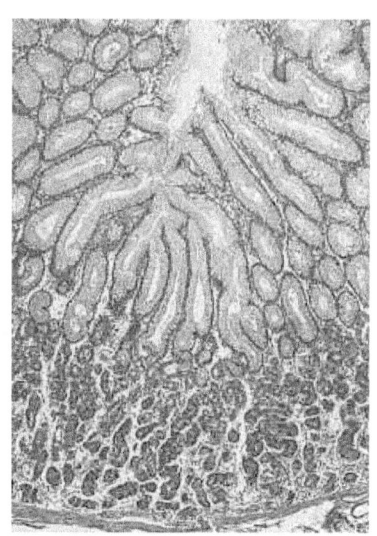

Portal Hypertensive Gastropathy

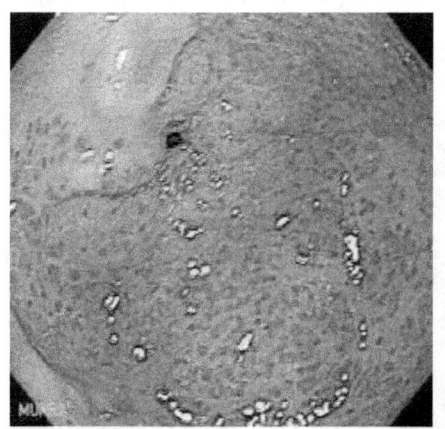

Corkscrew appearance of foveolae

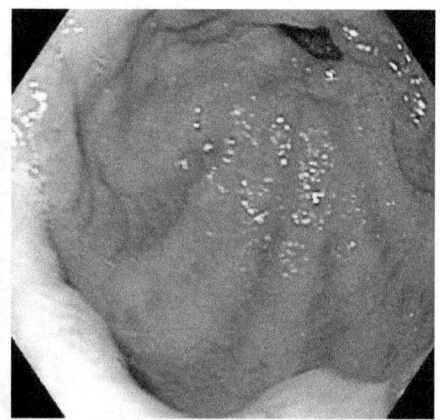

Reactive changes in foveolar epithelial cells; loss of mucus, enlarged nuclei

- Histopathology
  - Submucosal capillaries and venules
    - Dilated
    - No fibrin thrombi
    - Tortous
    - Intima
    - Thickened
    - Perivascular stromal fibrosis
  - Dilated mucosal capillaries and venules
  - Dilated submucosal veins
    - Tortuous
    - Initimal thickening
    - Congestion
  - Perivascular stromal fibrosis
  - No fibrin thrombi, and minimal inflammation
  - Note:
    - Endoscopic biopsies must be deep (biopsy–within biopsy) to detect submucosal changes

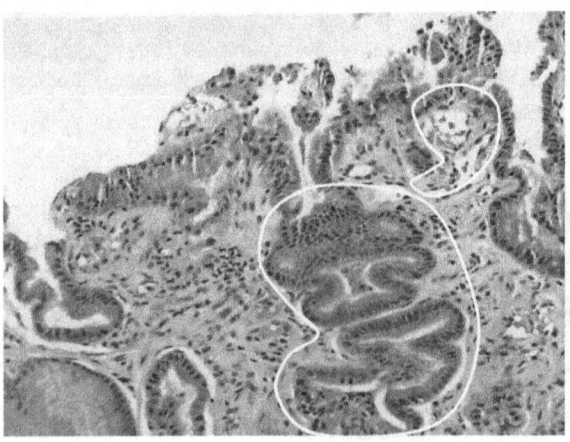
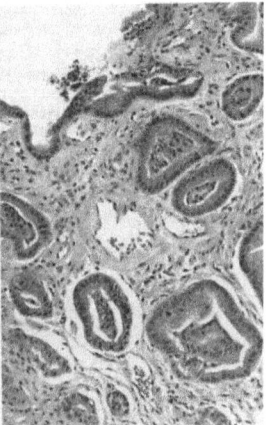

- Sclerotic, ecstatic capillaries in the lamina propria
- Mosaic pattern in gastric body from mucosal vascular ectasia
- Punctate redness in the fundus
- Nodular antrum, erosions, folds radiating to the pylorus
- Vascular ectasia of capillaries in the lamina propria, with sclerosis
- Foveolar hyperplasia

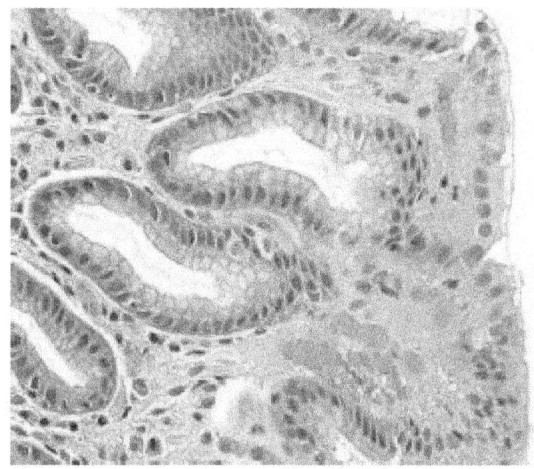

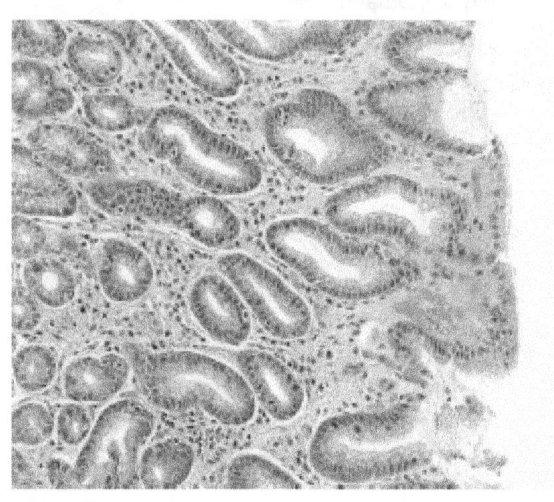

Provided kindly by Dr. Aducio Thiesen, University of Alberta

- Treatment
    - Reduction in portal pressure
        - β–blockers
        - TIPS
        - Shunt surgery

Gastric Dieulafoy Lesion

- Definition
    - Endoscopic finding of a mucosal defect, 2 – 5 mm in length, within 6 cm of the gastroesophageal junction and along the lesser gastric curvature, with a protruding muscular large caliber artery of persistent caliber (i.e. not dilated)

- Demography
    - ~ 5% of all upper GI bleeds
    - M > F = 2:1
    - Median age of 54

- Endoscopy
    - Mucosal tear 2 – 5 mm in length
    - Within 6 cm of gastroesophageal junction
    - Along lesser curve of stomach
    - Protruding large muscular artery of persistent caliber
    - Overlying mucosa may show the following:
        - Erosion
        - Bleeding
        - Clot
    - May also occur in other parts of the GI tract

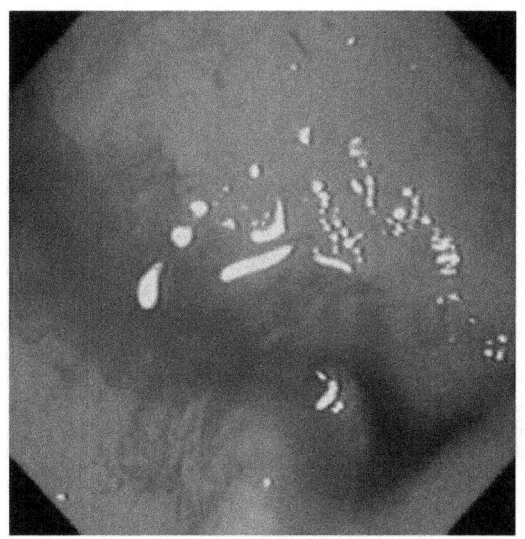

- Treatment
  - Endoscopic hemostatic therapy

Gastric Antral Vascular Ectasia *(GAVE, Watermelon Stomach)*

- Definition
  - Parallel red stripes on the crest of mucosal folds in gastric antrum, radiating towards pyloris, and comprised of fibrin thrombi in dilated mucosal capillaries and submucosal blood vessels

- Demography
  - F > M = 3:1
  - Mean age is 69

- ➢ Differential

- • Differentiate GAVE from PHG).

Features	GAVE	PHG
o Location	Predominantly antrum	Predominantly body
o Endoscopic appearance	Linear red stripes resembling watermelon	Diffuse mosaic vascular pattern, cherry red spots, scarlatina rash
o Endoscopic ultrasound	Thin atrophic gastric wall with thickening limited to antral region	Diffusely thickened gastric wall with dilated veins
o Characteristic histology	Dilated mucosal capillaries with thrombi Spindle cell proliferation Fibrohyalinosis	Vascular ectasia, perivascular stromal thickening
o Associated conditions	Autoimmune and connective tissue diseases, also cirrhosis	Cirrhosis with portal hypertension
o Management	Endoscopic laser therapy, antrectomy	Portal decompression, shunting, transplantation

*Note: Gastric vascular ectasia (GVE) may occur anywhere in the stomach, not just in the antrum, so do not distinguish GAVE or GVE from PHG just on the site of localization

- ➢ Clinical
  - o GI bleeding
  - o Associated conditions
    - Heart
      - Cardiovascular disease
    - Liver
      - Cirrhosis
      - Primary biliary disease
      - Autoimmune hepatitis (AIH)
    - Stomach
      - Atrophic gastritis
      - Intestinal metaplasia
    - MSK
      - Scleroderma
      - Raynaud phenomenon
    - Renal
      - Chronic renal disease
    - Blood
      - Bone marrow transplantation

- Endoscopy
  - Parallel line as red stripes on top of the central mucosal folds radiating towards the pylorus
  - Note
    - Vascular ectasia may occur in parts of the stomach other than the antrum called gastric vascular ectasia (GVE)

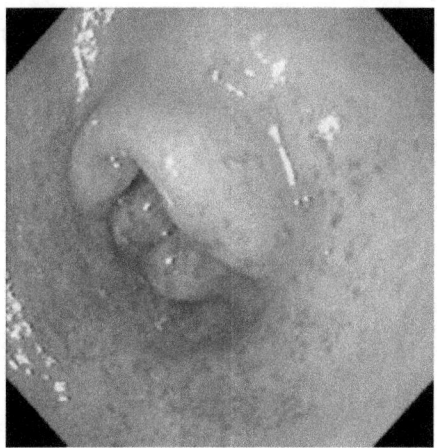

- Histopathology
  - Mucoal capillaries
    - Fibrin thrombi
    - Dilated capillaries
  - Submucosa
    - Dilated, tortous vessels
  - Lamina propria
    - Fibromuscular hyperplasia
  - Minimal inflammation
  - Fibrin thrombin in the following areas:
    - Dilated mucosal capillaries
    - Submucosal blood vessels
  - May be associated with the following conditions:
    - Atrophic gastritis
    - Intestinal metaplasia
  - Gastric wall thick in antrum, but thin (atrophy) in body

- Large blood vessels near the mucosal surface of stomach
  - Fibrin thrombi
  - CD61+ highlights platelets, and may help identify fibrin thrombi
- Thick–walled, ecstatic vessels in the foveolar compartment
- An organizing fibrin microthrombus
- Foveolar hyperplasia
- Chronically inflamed body–type mucosa replaced by intestinal (goblet cell) epithelium

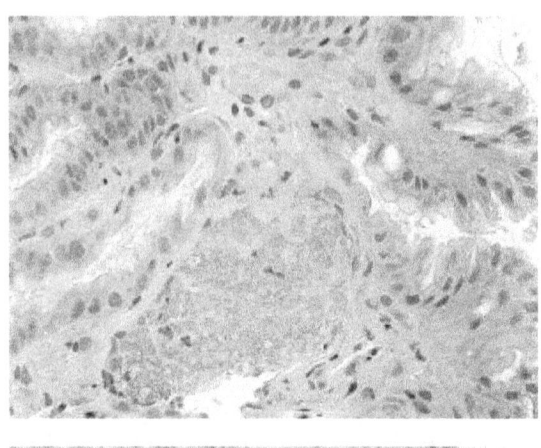

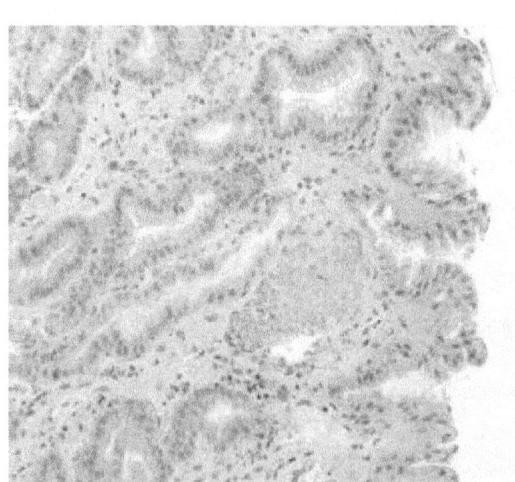

Provided kindly by Dr. Aducio Thiesen, University of Alberta

ACUTE GASTRITIS AND GASTROPATHIES

- ➢ Terminology
  - o Autoimmune metaplastic atrophic gastritis (AMAG)
  - o Carditis, inflammation of gastric cardia
  - o Diffuse corporal atrophic gastritis (DCAG), autoimmune metaplastic atrophic gastritis (AMAG, or type A gastritis), environmental multifocal atrophic gastritis (EMAG)
  - o Gastritis cystica profundal (CGP)
  - o Multifocal atrophic gastritis (MAG, or metaplastic atrophic gastritis)
    - Patchy
    - Gastric body and antral mucosa
    - Often associated with the following conditions:
      - *H. pylori* infection
      - Hyperplastic, hypersecretory gastropathy (HHG, or Ménétrier's disease)
  - o APG, *H. pylori* gastritis
  - o Phlegmonous gastritis (PG)

- ➢ Types

- Name the types of gastritis.

Types of Gastritis	Etiologic Factors	Gastritis Symptoms
o Non–atrophic	– *Helicobacter pylori*	<ul><li>Superficial</li><li>Diffuse antral gastritis (DAG)</li><li>Chronic antral gastritis (CAG)</li><li>Interstitial – follicular</li><li>Hypersecretory</li><li>Type B</li></ul>
o Atrophic Autoimmune	– Autoimmunity	<ul><li>Type A</li><li>Diffuse corporal</li><li>Pernicious anemia–associated</li></ul>
o Multifocal Atrophic	– *Helicobacter pylori* – Dietary – Environmental factors	<ul><li>Type B</li><li>Environmental</li><li>Metaplastic</li></ul>

- Special Forms
  - Chemicals
    - Chemical irritation (reactive)
    - Bile (reflux)
    - NSAIDs
    - Other agents (type C)
  - Radiation
    - Radiation injury
  - Lymphocytic (endoscopic)
    - Idiopathic (varioliform)
    - Immune mechanisms
    - Gluten (Celiac disease–associated)
    - Drugs (ticlopidine)
    - *H. pylori*
  - Non–infectious
    - Crohn's disease
    - Sarcoidosis
    - Wegener granulomatosis and other vasculitides
    - Foreign substances
    - Idiopathic (isolated granulomatous)
  - Eosinophilic
    - Food sensitivity (allergic)
  - Other infectious
    - Bacteria (no *H. pylori*)
    - Phlegmonous
  - Gastritis
    - Viruses
    - Fungi
    - Parasites

- ➢ Causes

- What are the causes of histologically diagnosed gastritis?
- Drugs, chemicals, radiation
  - Medications
    - Aspirin, NSAIDs, COXIBs
    - Bisphosphonates, K⁺ tablets
  - Drugs, chemicals

- – Alcohol, bile, cocaine, chemotherapy, radiotherapy, red peppers, pickles
- Infection
    - Bacterial — *H. pylori*, *Mycobacteria*
    - Viral — CMV, HSV
    - Fungal
    - Parasitic
- Graft–versus–host disease (GVHD)
- Autoimmune gastritis (pernicious anemia)
- Ischemia
    - Atherosclerosis
    - Sepsis
    - Burns
    - Shock
    - Mechanical ventilation
- Associated with liver disease – GAVE, PHG
- Trauma or foreign body
    - Nasogastric or gastrostomy tubes
    - Bezoar
    - Prolapse or sliding hiatal hernia or paraesophageal hernia
    - Cameron ulcer (ulcer in hiatal hernia)
- Infiltration and tumor
    - Lymphocytic or collagenous
    - Granulomatous
    - Eosinophilic
    - Tumor
- Miscellaneous
    - Gastritis cystica profunda
    - Ménétrier's disease (hyperplastic, hypersecretory gastropathy, HHG)

Adapted from: Lee, E. L. and Feldman, M. *Sleisenger & Fordtran's Gastrointestinal and Liver Disease: Pathophysiology/Diagnosis/ Management.* 2006. page 1068.; and Printed with permission: Francis, D. L. 2008. *Mayo Clinic Gastroenterology and Hepatology Board Review*: 67.

➢ Pathological types

- Give the characteristics of **distinctive gastritides**.

- ***H. pylori* gastritis** (HPG)
    o Active gastritis (acute gastritis)
        - Neutrophils, lymphocytes, plasma cells in the mucosa and submucosa
    o Epithelial damage
        - ↓ surface mucin
        - Nuclear changes
        - Lymphoid follicles
    o May be associated with the following conditions:
        - Environment multifocal atrophic gastritis (EMAG)
        - Lymphocytic gastritis (> 5 lymphocytes per 100 cells)

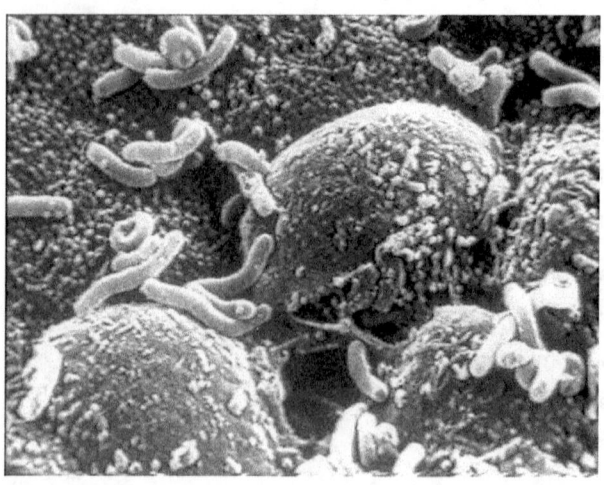

- Give the patterns of gastritis or gastropathy.

Pathologic Diagnosis	Pathologic Findings	Etiology	Possible Endoscopic Findings	Probable Clinical Associations
o Acute gastritis	– Neutrophilic inflammation	H. pylori	Normal; large folds, erosions	Acute gastroenteritis
		Streptococcal species, other bacteria	Erythema, distended stomach, exudate	Perforation, gangrene
o Chronic and active chronic gastritis, common pattern	– Mixed inflammation +/- foveolar hyperplasia – Erosion or ulcer – Intestinal metaplasia, atrophy	H. pylori H. heilmannii, autoimmune	Normal erythema, nodularity, and friability; thin body folds with prominent vessels; prominent mosaic mucosal surface pattern	None, dyspepsia, duodenal or gastric ulcer, adenocarcinoma, MALT lymphoma, pernicious anemia
o Lympho-cytic gastritis	– Common pattern and increased intraepithelial lymphocytes	Hypersen-sitivity to gliadin, other proteins; autoimmune	Chronic erosive gastritis (nodules with central ulceration), giant body folds	Celiac sprue, Ménétrier's disease, autoimmunity, H. pylori
o Granulo-matous gastritis	– Multifocal active chronic inflammation – Ulcers or fissures – Granulomas	Crohn, sarcoid, idiopathic, fungi, Mycobacterium, spirochetes, parasites, drugs, vasculitis; foreign body	Variable; thickened folds, ulceration	Depends on underlying disease
o Eosino-philic gastritis	– Sheets of eosinophils	Idiopathic, food and drug allergy, parasites	Prominent antral folds, hyperemia, nodularity, ulcer; normal	Pain, nausea, vomiting, early satiety, weight loss, anemia
o Hyper-trophic lympho-cytic gastritis	– Lymphocytic gastritis with extreme foveolar hyperplasia	Ménétrier's disease	Giant body folds	Pain, weight loss, vomiting, +/- protein loss

Pathologic Diagnosis	Pathologic Findings	Etiology	Possible Endoscopic Findings	Probable Cli Associatio
o Acute erosive gastropathy	- Microvascular ischemia (erosions) - Minimal focal inflammation	Alcohol, NSAIDs, other drugs, hypovolemia, stress, uremia	Erosions, subepithelial hemorrhages	Bleeding
o Reactive gastropathy, common pattern	- Foveolar hyperplasia, +/- - Erosion or ulcer - No inflammation except near ulcer	NSAIDs, bile reflux, uremia	Same as acute erosive gastropathy	
o Reactive gastropathy with features suggestive of bile reflux	Common pattern with subnuclear vacuoles	Bile reflux	Erythema, friability, bleeding	Vomiting bile pain, usually post–Billroth II
o Reactive gastropathy with features suggestive of radiation or chemo-therapy	Common pattern with cellular and nuclear enlargement Vacuolization, macronucleoli	Radiation, chemotherapy	Ulcers, predominantly antral	Perforation,
o Congestive gastropathy	Common pattern with superficial vascular ectasia +/- microthrombi	Portal hypertension	Antral erythema, red spots, mosaic pattern	Cirrhosis, bleeding, sp vein thrombo
		Watermelon stomach	Linear erythema on folds radiating from pylorus	Proximal ga: atrophy, ane
		Scleroderma		Sclerodacty CREST syndrome
o Hypertrophic-gastropathy	Massive foveolar hyperplasia with little or no inflammation	Ménétrier's disease	Giant body folds	Pain, weight loss, vomitin +/- protein lo

Adapted from: Carpenter, H. A. *et al. Gastroenterology*. 1995. 108:917-924.

- Diagnostic imaging
    - Thickened folds: smooth and nodular
    - Body and antrum

SO, YOU WANT TO BE A GASTROENTEROLOGIST!

A patient with dyspepsia has an upper GI barium study.

- Mention the gastric radiological features seen in dyspepsia with an infectious etiology.
    - *H. pylori* infection — Gastric folds
        - Thick
        - Polypoid
        - Areae gastricae
            - Enlarged
    - Non–*H. pylori* causes — Antral erosions

- Pathology

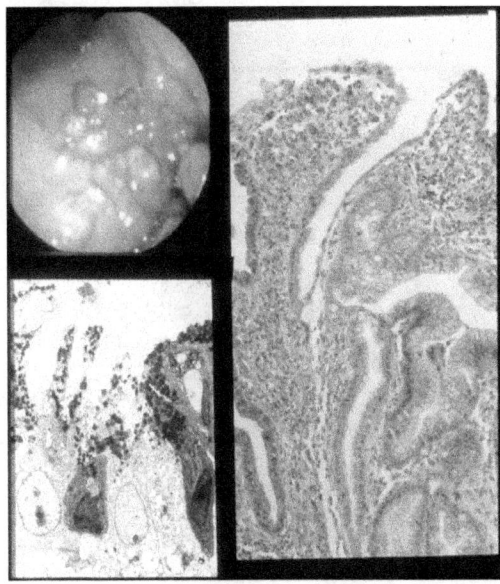

A 70–year old woman is treated for 12 weeks with PPI for a benign pre–pyloric ulcer. She is now asymptomatic. Endoscopy is repeated. Describe the endoscopic findings, and provide your management.

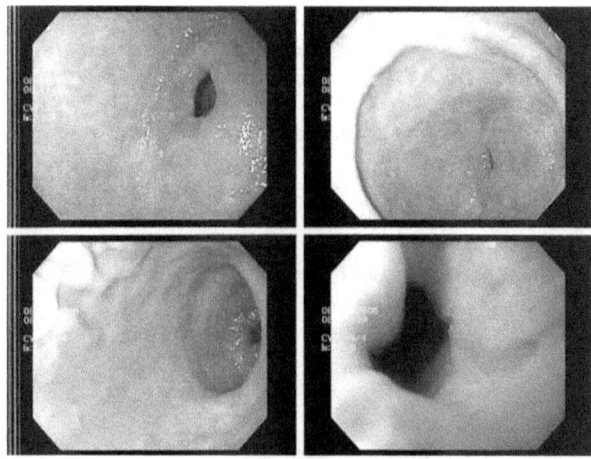

Erosive gastritis

A 63–year old woman with a previously drained choledochal cyst with hepatojejunostomy. A Billroth I procedure was performed 20 years ago for resistant PUD. She now presents with dyspepsia. Give the endoscopic findings and differential diagnosis.

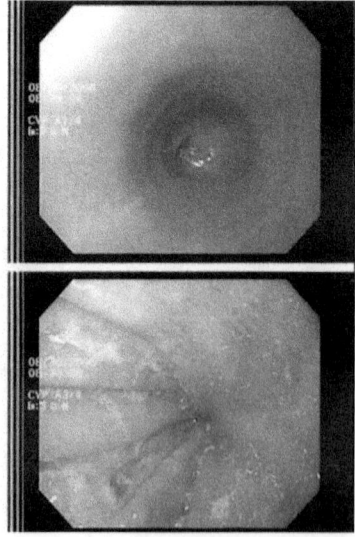

Environmental Multifocal Atrophic Gastritis (EMAG)
- 85% of EMAG caused by *H. pylori*
- Body
  - Atrophic gastritis
  - Pseudopyloric metaplasia "stains positive for pepsinogen 1 (PG1)
- Body and antrum
  - Atrophy
  - Intestinal metaplasia

Autoimmune Metaplastic Atrophic Gastritis, Diffuse Corporal Atrophic Gastritis (AMAG or DCAG) **or Type A Gastritis**
- Parietal cell antibodies to H^+, K^+ – ATPase
- Thin fundic or body mucosa
- Flat gastric folds
- ↑ gastrin
  - ↓ HCl
  - Antral G–cells (secrete antibacterial HD-5 [human defensin-5)
  - Progression of metaplasia to dysplasia / GCA: ↑ CDX_2 (type III)

SO YOU WANT TO BE A GASTROENTEROLOGIST!

- AMAG / DMAG (autoimmune metaplastic atrophic gastritis) results in increased antibodies to parietal cell antigens
- The parietal cell antibodies to H^+, K^+ ATPase lead to increased CD_4^+ lymphocytes.

- Give the consequences of the increased CD_4^+ lymphocytes in AMAG/AMAG.

  The increased CD_4^+ lymphocytes in the inflammation of AMAG/DMAG leads to
  - ↑ Th1 cytokines → ↑ secretion of immunoglobulins by B lymphocytes
  - ↑ cytotoxicity mediated by performin
  - ↑ FAS ligand-mediated apoptosis

Phlegmonous Gastritis (PG)
- PG is also known as suppurative gastritis (SG)
- PG or SG may progress to the following conditions:
  - Acute necrotizing gastritis (ANG) representing gangrene of the stomach
  - Emphysematous gastritis due to necrotic gastric wall infected with a gas–forming organism (i.e. *Clostridium welchii*)

➤ Clinical
- Acute bacterial inflammation of the mucosa and submucosa (usually hemolytic *Streptococci*; usually prior debility, rarely prior to ischemic necrosis)

➤ Endoscopy

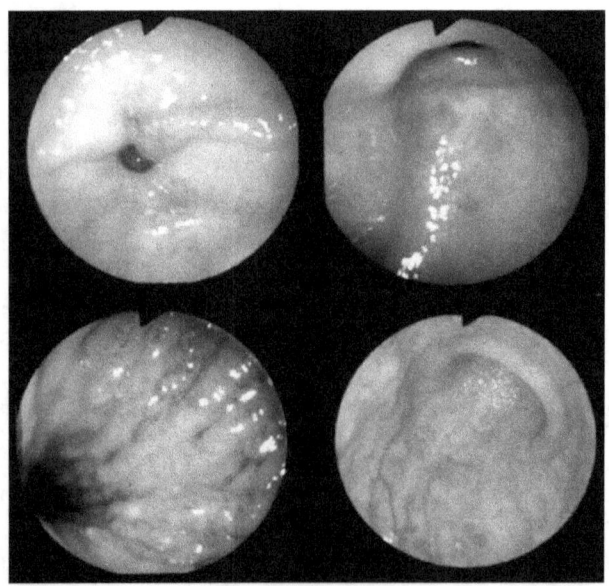

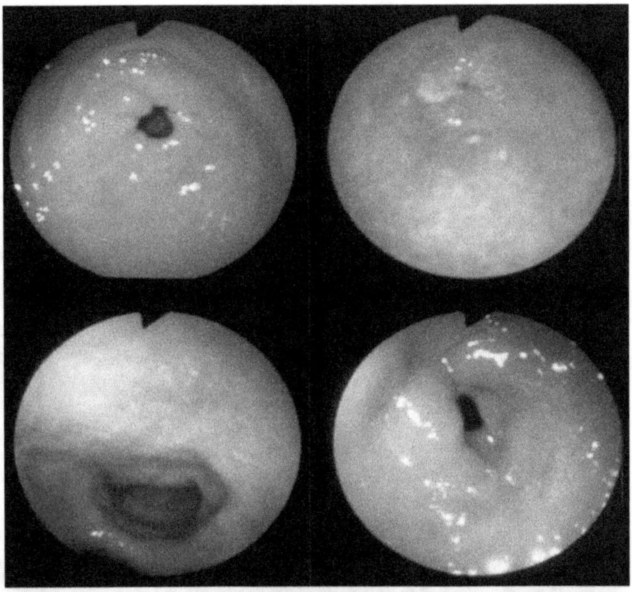

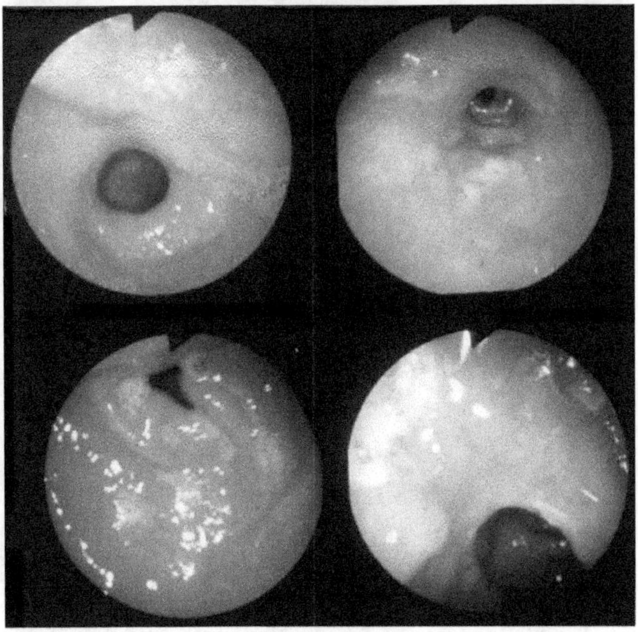

FROM COMPETENCE TO EXCELLENCE
The Stomach

© A.B.R. Thomson

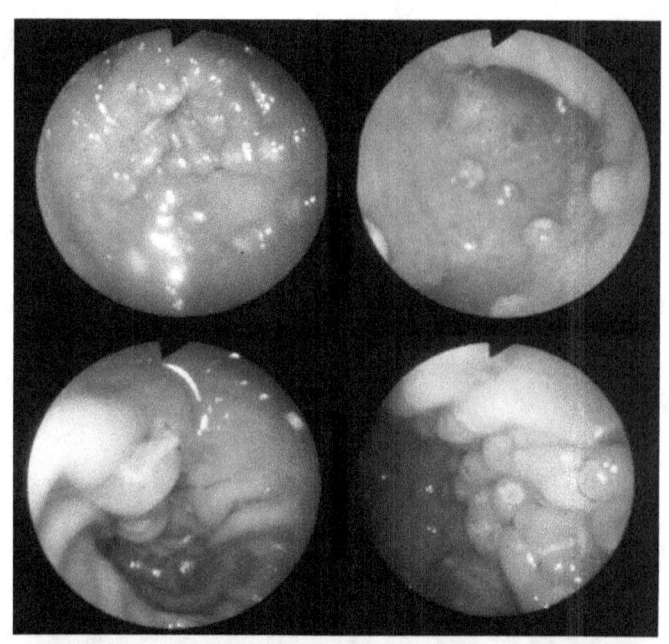
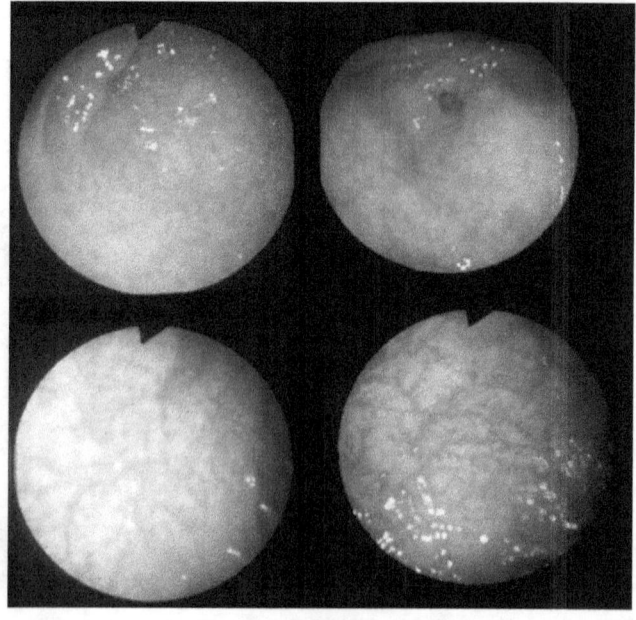

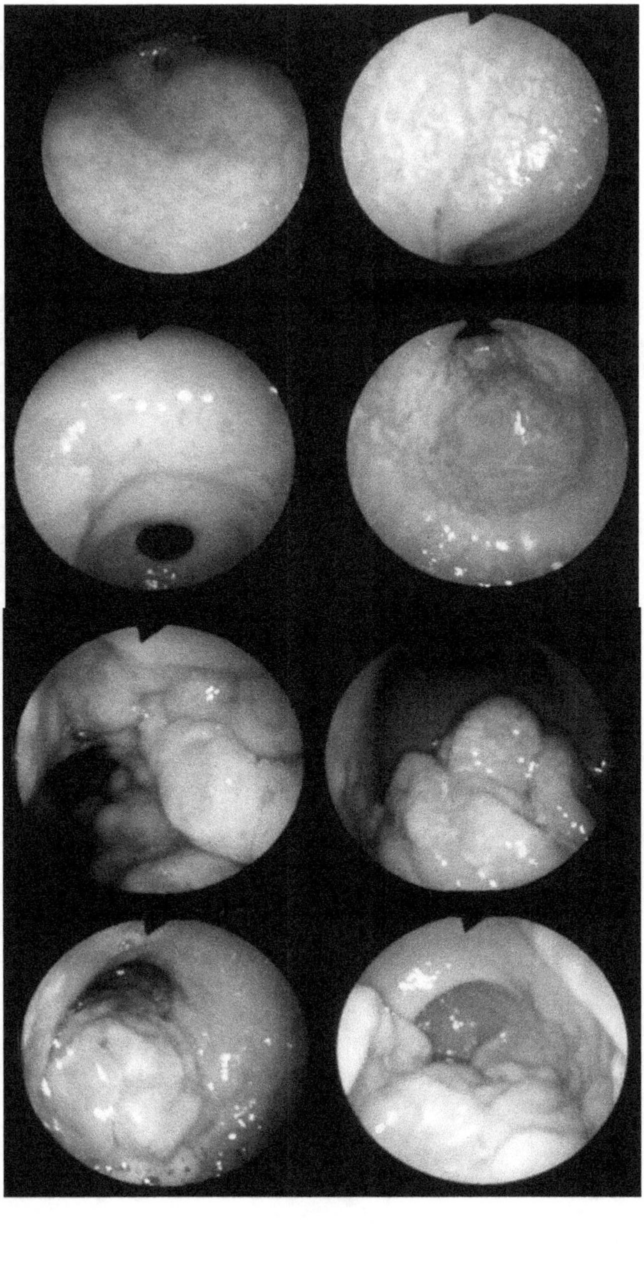

207

FROM COMPETENCE TO EXCELLENCE
The Stomach

© A.B.R. Thomson

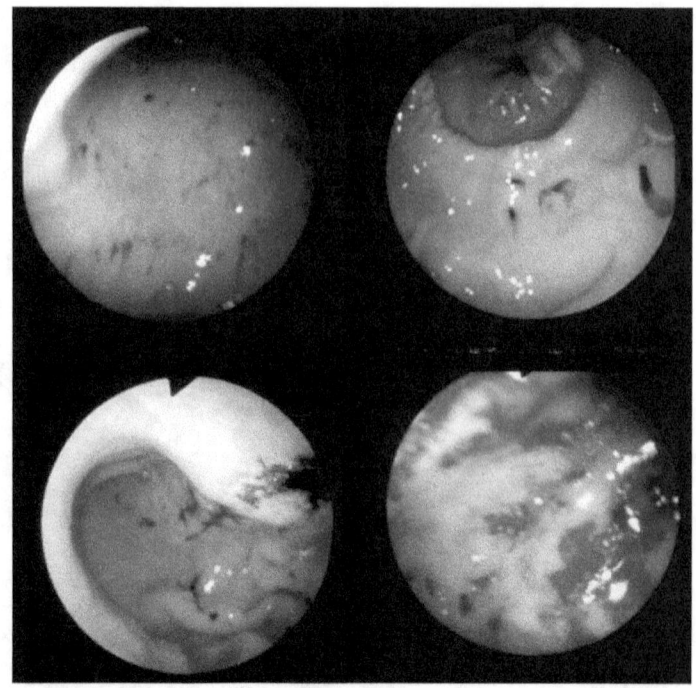

- ➤ Histopathology
    - ○ Severe erythema or exudate or erosive gastritis
    - ○ Severe acute gastritis
    - ○ Severe abdominal pain simulating an acute abdomen
    - ○ Purulent vomiting
    - ○ Broad spectrum antibiotics

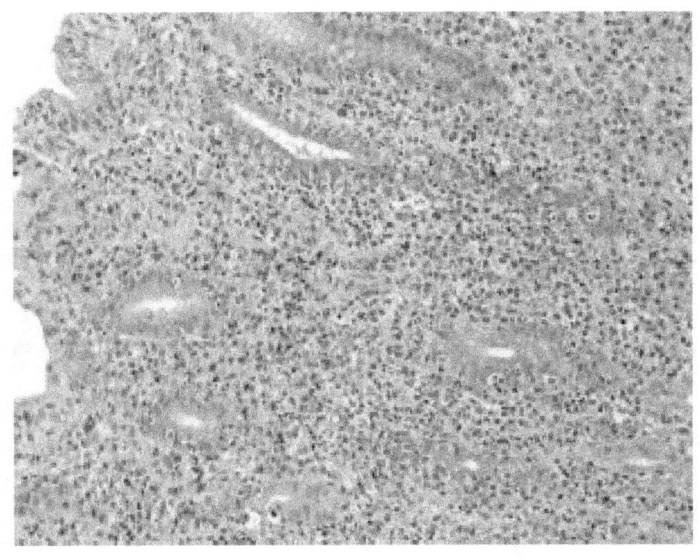

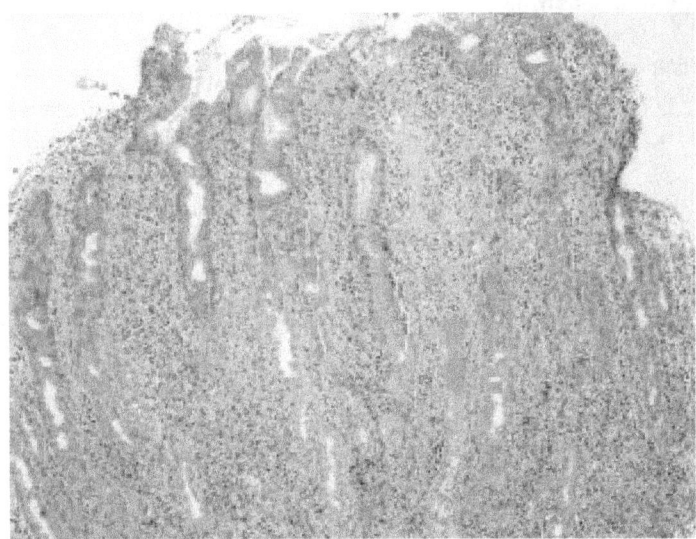

Provided kindly by Dr. Aducio Thiesen, University of Alberta

> **SO YOU WANT TO BE A GASTROENTEROLOGIST!**
> - Give the endoscopic and microscopic appearances of lymphocytic gastritis.
>
>   - Endoscopy (varioliform)
>   - Thick folds
>   - Nodular mucosa
>   - Aphthous "ulcers" (erosions)
>
>   - Lymphocytic gastritis
>   - Antrum, body, or antrum plus body
>   - ↑ lymphocytes and plasma cells in lamina propria
>   - > 5 lymphocytes per 100 cells
>   - Associated with *H. pylori*, celiac disease, Crohn disease in children
>   - Associated with
>   - *H. pylori* infection
>   - Celiac disease

Collagenous Gastritis

- Definition
  - Lymphoplasmacytic infiltration of the lamina propria, with diffuse or patchy band of type I and III collagen > 10 μm in thickness
  - A discontinuous band of collagen > 10 μm in the subepithelial basement membrane layer (normal < 2 μm), with associated damage to the surface epithelium and lymphoplasmacytic inflammation of the lamina propria
  - Degradation of foveolar epithelium
  - No ↑ association with H. pylori

- Demography
  - Very rare
    - About 1 case per year reported worldwide since 1989
    - F > M

- Differential
  - Lymphocytic gastritis
  - H.pylori associated gastritis

- o Amyloidosis (use amyloid attains eg, Congo Red [curiously, shows up as green birefringenee] or thioflavin T, as is negative on trichome stain)
- o Lymphoma (polyclonal CD3, Cd20, K and λ T lymphocytes)
- o Lamina propria fibrosis
  - Scleroderma
  - Ischemia
  - Radiation damage

➢ Clinical
- o Non–specific
  - Upper GI symptoms
- o Other GI symptoms depending upon associated disorders
- o Associations
  - Lymphocytic gastritis
  - Celiac disease
  - Collagenous colitis
  - Lymphocytic colitis
  - Other autoimmune disorders

➢ Diagnosis
- o Gastric mucosal biopsy
- o Biopsy small bowel and colonic mucosa to exclude possible associated conditions

➢ Differential diagnosis

SO YOU WANT TO BE A GASTROENTEROLOGIST!

- What are the pathological features distinguishing collagenous gastritis from amyloidosis, infiltration and scleroderma of the stomach, or radiation gastritis?

Features	Collagenous gastritis	Gastritis amyloidosis	Sclero- derma	Radiation gastritis
o Deposit				
- Mucosa	+	+		
- Submucosa	-	+		
- Vessel walls	-	+		
o Fibrosis				
- Subepithelium	+		+	
- Diffuse or patchy			+	
- Deeper than subepithelioid	-	-		+
- Mucosal necrosis	-	-		+
- Lamina propria hyaline in blood vessels	-	-		+
- Reactive glandular changes	-	-		+
o Special stains				
- Congo red	-	+		
- Thioflavin T	-	+		
- Trichrome	+	-		

➢ Endoscopy
  o Redness, nodularity or erosions in the gastric body or antrum
  o Gastric biopsy or antrum
  o Range of findings
    - Normal
    - Patchy – diffuse redness, nodularity, erosions, ulcers

- Histopathology
    - Diffuse or patchy collagen band under the epithelium
    - ↑ thickness of subepithelial band (normal; 2-3 µm; collagenous gastritis
        - \> 10 µm
        - Average 30-40 µm
    - Collagen band has irregular lower edge which traps WBC and capillaries
    - Surface epithelium
        - Degeneration of foveolar epithelium
            - Flat / cuboid
            - ↓↓ mucin
            - Stripping
    - Lamina propria
        - ↑ lymphocytes (T-cells)
        - ↑ plasma cells
        - Mild, patchy fibrosis
    - Chronic gastritis
        - Superficial
        - Patchy
    - Atrophy
        - Focal
    - Collagen
        - Focal deposits
        - Subepithelial thickening of the collagen band (20 to 75 mm thick)
    - Quantitative (> 2 µm, subepithelial layers of collagen: usually > 10 µm best seen with Masson's trichrome stain for collagen type I and IV and qualitative abnormality with
        - Surface damage: foveolar epithelial degeneration with cuboidal or goblet cells, ↓ mucin, loss of epithelium
        - Ragged border of collagen
        - Lymphoplasmacytosis in lamina propria
        - Trapping of capillaries

- Special studies
  - Positive stain for collagen (Masson trichrome)
  - Polyclonal T lymphocytes CD3, CD20, κ, λ
  - Subepithelial collagen I and III (negative for IV and laminin)

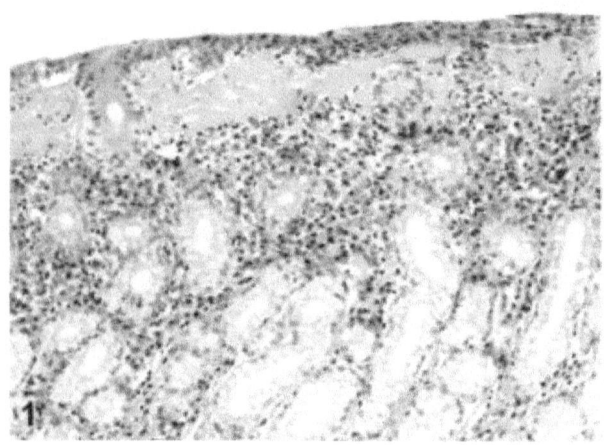

Hematoxylin-eosin x200

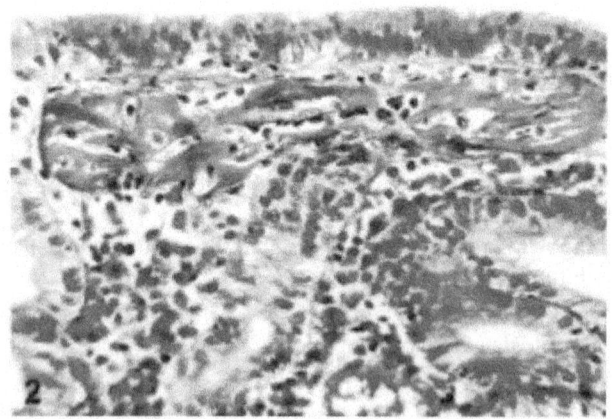

Trichrome x400

http://www.archivesofpathology.org/doi/pdf/10.1043/1543-2165(2004)128%3C229%3ACGAUAW%3E2.0.CO%3B2

> **Pathology Tips**
> - Histopathological features of lymphocytic gastritis (> 20 lymphocytes per 100 epithelial cells) may co-occur with collagenous gastritis.
> - Lymphocystic gastritis associated with collagenous gastritis is not coinfected with H. pylori, as is usual when lymphocystic gastritis occurs by itself

- Treatment
    - Symptomatic
    - Corticosteroids → immnosuppressants
    - If associated
        - Celiac disease
        - Collagenous colitis
            - 5-ASA (aminosalicylic acid) preparation po / pr

- **Gastritis cystica profunda** (GCP)
    - Rare and unknown cause
    - May be associated with
        - Gastric surgery (Bilroth II)
        - Atrophic gastritis
        - Inverted hyperplastic gastric polyp
    - Histology
        - Foveolar hyperplasia
        - Cystic glands extending into muscularis mucosae, submucosa, muscularis propria

- For such a rare and innocuous conditionas GCP, give the reason why do we need to know about it?
    - GCP may be associated with
        - Synchronous or metachronous gastric adenocarcinoma (GCa)
        - GCa of postoperative gastric stump

- **Reactive gastropathies** (aka acute erosive gastritis)

- Diagnostic imaging
    - Erosion surrounded by (halo edema)
    - Central erosion along the crest of in a rugal fold
    - Usually multiple

- Single
  - Artifact
  - Pancraeatic rest
  - GIST
  - Metastases

➤ Endoscopy

- Necrosis of superficial lamina propria in area of erosion
- Foveolar hyperplasia
- Gastric pits
  - Elongated
  - Corkscrew
- Hemorrhage
  - From > 25% of biopsy samples
  - Atypical nuclei

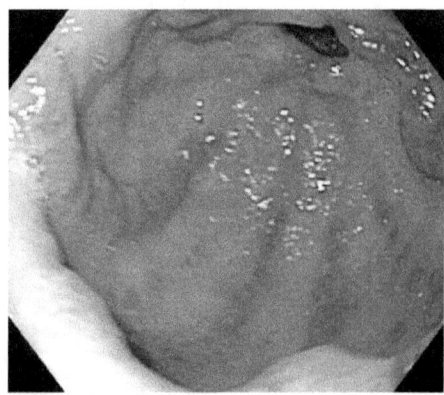

Reactive changes in foveolar eptihelial cells; loss of mucus, enlarged nuclei

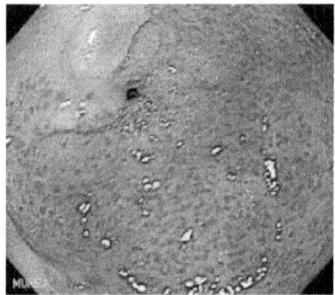

Corkscrew appearance of foveolae

NSAID–Induced Mucosal Damage

➢ Pathophysiology
  o Topical irritant effect on the epithelium (ion trapping; depletion of ATP via uncoupling of oxidative phosphorylation)
  o ↓ hydrophobicity of the mucus gel layer
  o ↓ barrier properties — acid back diffusion
  o ↓ prostaglandin synthesis
  o ↓ gastric mucosal blood flow
  o ↓ repair of superficial injury
  o ↓ hemostasis
  o ↓ growth factors

➢ Endoscopy
  o Redness, erosions, ulcers, polyp

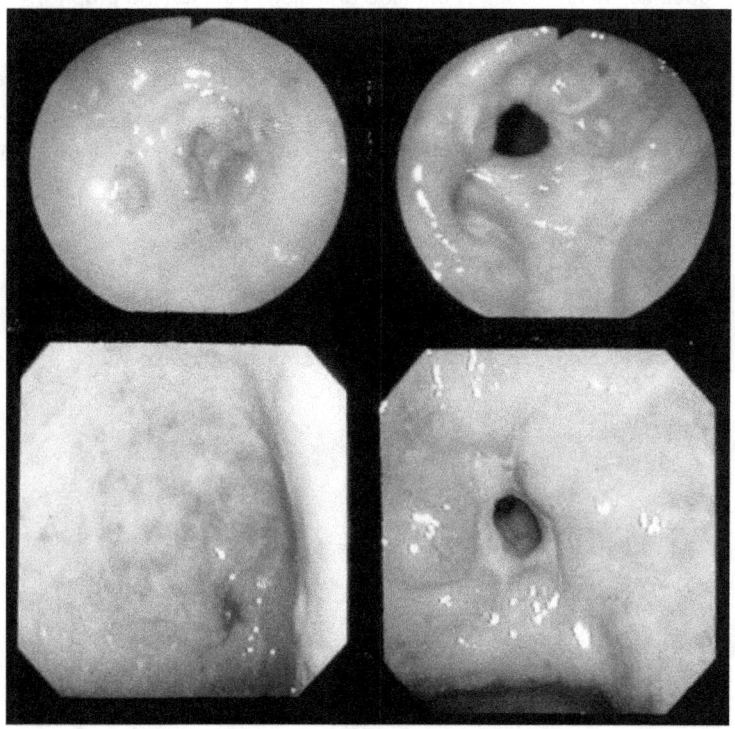

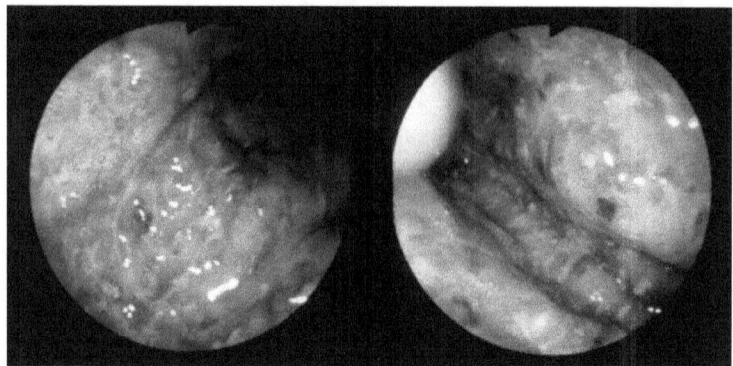

- ➢ Histopathology
  - o Foveolar hyperplasia in the absence of significant inflammation
  - o Capillaries, venules, and lymphatics are congested but not ecstatic
  - o Foveolar hyperplasia, inflammation at edge or base of erosion (in gastritis, inflammation is diffused and also in the lamina propria)
  - o Epithelial regenerative changes include loss of foveolar cell mucin
  - o Marked foveolar elongation results in villous or papillary appearance
  - o Large, round and hyperchromatic nuclei, immature cells rearranging epithelial surface → regeneration + fibrous lamina propria + mucin depletion
  - o These features mimic dysplasia
  - o Cytologic detail and uniformity help in the distinction
  - o Common pattern
    - Marked foveolar hyperplasia
    - Nuclei is enlarged, hyperchromatic, and crowded; mitoses is frequent
    - Empty, pink lamina propria

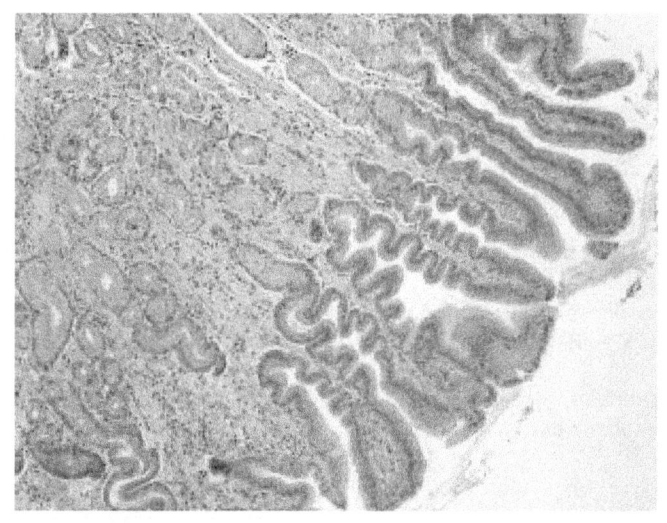

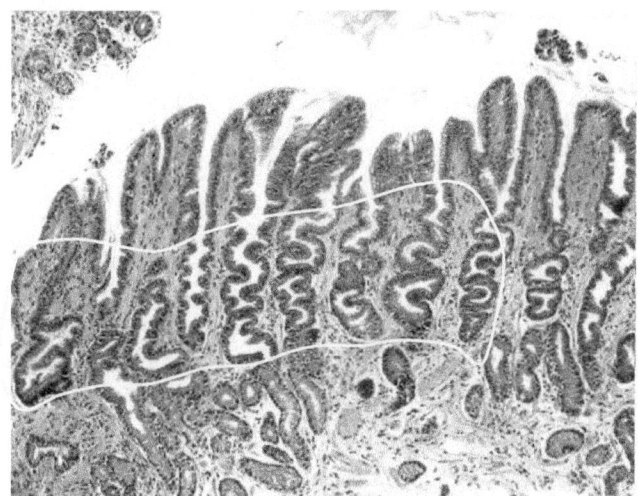

Foveolar Hyperplasia

Provided kindly by Dr. Aducio Thiesen, University of Alberta

Carditis

➢ Definition
- o "Inflammation of the small rim of the cardiac glands at the proximal portion of the stomach" (Feldman, M., et al. *Sleisenger and Fordtran's Gastrointestinal and Liver Disease*. 2010. 9th Edition. Saunders/Elsevier, Philadelphia. page 848).

➢ Causes and associations

SO YOU WANT TO BE A GASTROENTEROLOGIST!

- Differentiate Ménétrier's disease from HHG, both show foveolar hyperplasia and cystic dilation on mucosal biopsy.

	Ménétrier's disease	HHG
o Protein–losing gastropathy	+	+/-
o Acid secretion	↓	N/↑
o Parietal and chief cells	N/↓	↑
o Inflammation	+/-	-
o Mucus secretion	N/↑	-
o Associated with lymphocytic gastritis	+	-
o Carcinoid–like syndrome (↑ PGE$_2$)	+	-

Even in the absence of decreased parietal cells in Ménétrier's disease, there is reduced acid secretion (hypochlorhydria) or achlorhydria.

- Explain the changes in acid secretion in Ménétrier's disease.

Acid secretion may be reduced or absent in Ménétrier's disease even in the absence of a reduction in parietal cells, because of the following:
- o ↑ TGF–α
- o ↑ TGF–α → ↑ EGFR
- o EGFR is a receptor of TK
- o ↑ EGFR and ↑ TK → ↓ HCl

FROM COMPETENCE TO EXCELLENCE
The Stomach

© A.B.R. Thomson

- Name the common causes and associations of **carditis**.
    - GERD
    - *H. pylori*
    - EMAG
    - AMAG

Note: Hyperplastic gastropathies may be confused with or miscalled Ménétrier's disease (hyperplastic hypersecretory gastropathy)

Gastric Epithelial Dysplasia (GED)

➢ Definition
   - Localized growth of dysplastic gastric epithelium appearing normal (flat) on endoscopy (EGD), and has the risk of developing into gastric adenocarcinoma

➢ Demography
   - M > F
   - Age > 50 years
   - Prevalence
     - USA ~ 3%
     - Japan ~ 20%

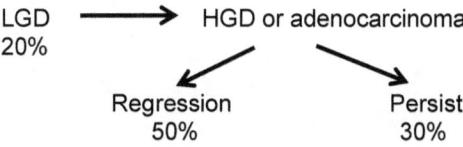

   - GED is more common in the following conditions:
     - Familial adenomatous polyposis (FAP)
     - Early gastric cancer (EGC)
     - Adenomas are polypoid (AA)
   - Flat (adenomas are polypoid)

➢ Risk factors
   - Age, gender, geography
   - Pernicious anemia
   - FAP

- Endoscopy
    - Flat areas of endoscopically (white light) normal antral mucosa
- Histopathology
    - About 50% of GED is associated with the following conditions:
        - Early gastric cancer
        - Advanced cancer
        - Regression of low grade dysplasia (LGD)
    - ~ 15% of low grade GED → high grade dysplasia
    - 80% of high grade GED → carcinoma (infiltrating), in weeks to years
    - Vienna classification of gastrointestinal epithelial neoplasia
        - Negative for dysplasia
        - Indefinite for dysplasia
        - Low grade dysplasia (LGD), non–invasive
        - High grade dysplasia (HGD), non–invasive (carcinoma *in situ*)
        - Invasive carcinoma (intramucosal or submucosal carcinoma)
    - Cytology
        - Nuclear crowding
        - ↑ chromatin
        - Nuclei
            - Basal
        - Nucleoli
            - Elongated
            - Prominent
        - ↓ mucin
        - Lumen
    - Classification of dysplasia
        - Negative
        - Indefinite
        - Non–invasive low grade dysplasia (LGD)
        - Non–invasive high grade (HGD; *in situ* carcinoma)
        - Invasive carcinoma
            - Intramucosal
            - Submucosal

	GED	Reactive and regenerative change
➢ Architecture		
o Gastric glands		
- Crowded	+	Immature cuboidal cells
- Branched	+	↑ basophilic cytoplasm (↑ mucus retention)
- Budding	+	
- Dilated	+	
o ↓ stroma between glands		
o Back–to–back glands		
- Intraluminal folding	+	
➢ Cells		
o Nuclei		
- Enlarged	+	+
- At the base of the cell	-	+
- ↓ polarity	+	-
- Stratification of luminal side of gland	+	-
- Round	+	-
- ↑ chromatin	+	-
- Mitosis	↑ (bottom and top of gland)	+/- (of present, only at bottom of gland)
- N:C ratio	↑	
o Intraluminal necrotic material	+	No

➢ Differential diagnosis
   o Gastric adenoma (please see below)
   o Pyloric gland adenoma
   o Regenerative changes
      - Cytological
          ▪ Cuboidal
          ▪ Immature
          ▪ Basophilic cytoplasm
          ▪ ↓ mucus secretion
          ▪ Nuclei
              - Large
              - Vesicular
              - Pleomorphic
              - Mitotic figures in the basal but not in the surface glands
              - Basal nuclei
              - Minimal pseudostratification

Allergic Gastroenteropathy

- Demography
  - Mainly in the first and second decades

- Pathophysiology
  - Manifestations of allergy (i.e. asthma, eczema, allergic rhinitis)
  - Definite history of allergy to milk, proteins or meat

- Clinical
  - Growth retardation, edema

- Laboratory
  - ↓ albumin, ↓ globulin, protein–losing
  - Anemia, blood eosinophilia

- Histopathology
  - Small bowel eosinophilic infiltration in the mucosa and submucosa

- Treatment
  - Favorable response to elimination diet or corticosteroids

Disseminated Eosinophilic Collagen Disease

- Demography
  - Middle age, mainly male patients

- Histopathology
  - Persistent eosinophilia in the blood
  - Diffused organ infiltration by eosinophils (hepatosplenomegaly, heart disease, nervous system abnormalities, pulmonary disease)
  - No other cause for eosinophilia (infectious or parasitic disease, neoplasia)

- Clinical
  - Fever, anorexia, and weight loss, recurrent abdominal pain, persistent non–productive cough with chest pain, various neurologic abnormalities, pruritic rash, congestive heart failure, hepatosplenomegaly, lymphadenopathy
- Prognosis
  - Significant morbidity and mortality (average survival)

Hypereosinophilic Syndrome (HES)

- Demography
  - Middle age, mainly male patients
- Histopathology
  - Persistent hypereosinophilia — > 1500 eos/mm3
  - Diffuse organ infiltration by eosinophils (hepatosplenomegaly, heart disease, nervous system abnormalities, pulmonary disease, fever, weight loss, anemia)
- Cause
  - No other causes of eosinophilia (infectious or parasitic disease, neoplasia)

Active Chronic Antral Gastritis With Lymphoid Hyperplasia

- Histopathology
  - Lymphoid nodule in chronic gastritis beneath the groove on the edge of areae gastricae
  - Endoscopy showing normal or red mucosa, friable nodules with erosions
  - Varioliform gastritis, mucosal hemorrhage; lymphoid hyperplasia
  - Sites: *H. pylori* — body or antrum; autoimmune — body; Crohn's disease — antrum; (may be associated granulomatous reaction)
  - Mononuclear cell infiltration in lamina propria and few intraepithelial neutrophils
  - Neutrophils associated with reactive or regenerative antral epithelium

ffuse Antral Gastritis
- Often *H. pylori* associated
- Most patients are asymptomatic (#1 indication for EGD is dyspepsia)
- Pathology
  - Diffuse, antral predominant
  - Chronic inflammation (lymphocytes and plasma cells) +/- polymorphonuclear cells (PMNs)
    - vs. Acute *H. pylori*: PMNs only
  - Erosions
  - Lymphoid follicles w/ germinal centers
  - *H. pylori* organisms in the mucus layer of the surface, usually seen best with silver stain

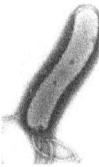
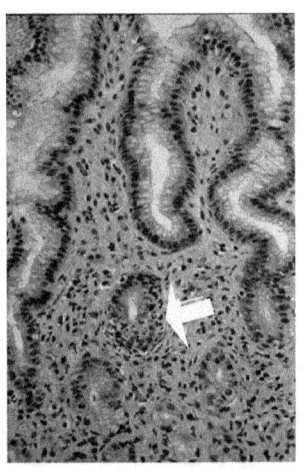
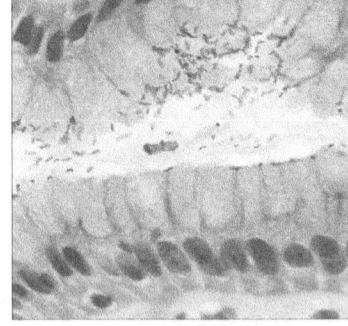

PMNs infiltrating the epithelium

Acute Erosive or Hemorrhagic Gastritis

- ➢ Definition
  - o A pathological diagnosis of gastric erosions associated with patchy, small, multiple mucosal defects, superficial necrosis, and petechial hemorrhage

- ➢ Causes
  - o Drugs, toxins, radiochemotherapy
  - o Low flow states (i.e. heart failure, sepsis, hypotension, head injury, severe burns or "stress")

- ➢ Clinical
  - o Asymptomatic
  - o Sudden onset of dyspepsia
  - o Upper GI bleeding

- ➢ Endoscopy
  - o Multiple, small erosions with petechial hemorrhage
  - o Site
    - Fundus
      - Body
      - Stress
    - Antrum
  - NSAIDs

- ➢ Histopathology
  - o Mucosal necrosis and sloughing
  - o Neutrophilic (fibropurulent) exudate
  - o Reactive (healing) changes
    - Glands
  - Syncytial architecture
    - Epithelial cell nuclei
  - ↑ size or darkness
  - ↑ nucleoli
  - ↑ mitosis
    - Cytoplasm
  - Amphophilic

- Hemorrhage
  - Hemorrhage in the lamina propria without degenerative or regenerative epithelial changes
- Acute erosive gastropathy
  - Punctate areas of redness and friability from mucosal hemorrhage or vascular ectasia, erosions, ulcers
  - Hemorrhage, congestion, necrosis, with minimal inflammation or regenerative changes (foveolar hyperplasia)
  - Fibrosis within lamina propria
  - Immature surface gastric cells with mucin depletion
  - Cork screen architecture (crowded pits, ducts attempted regeneration)

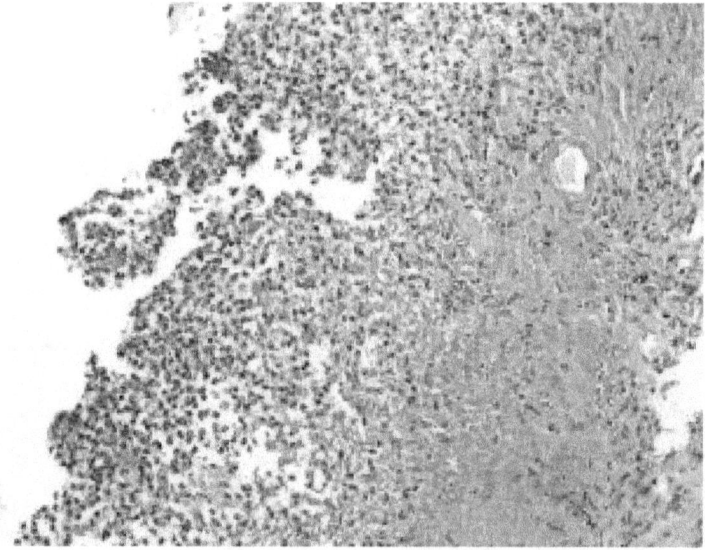

ovided kindly by Dr. Aducio Thiesen, University of Alberta

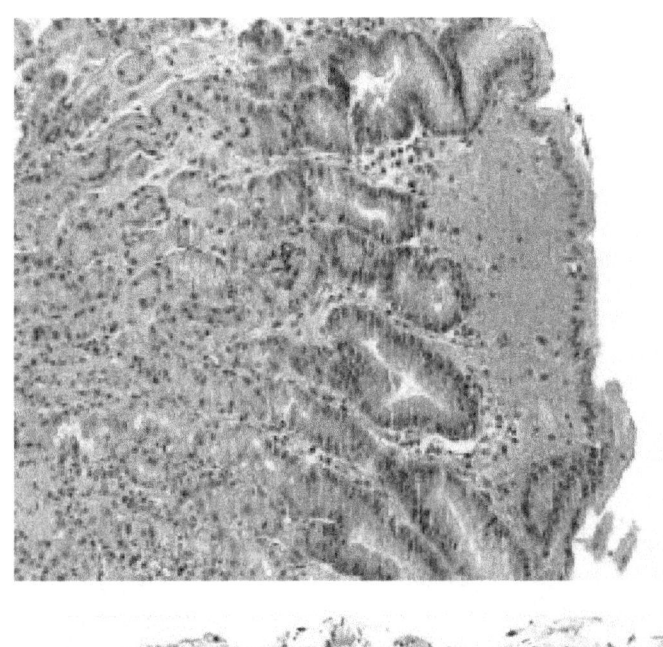

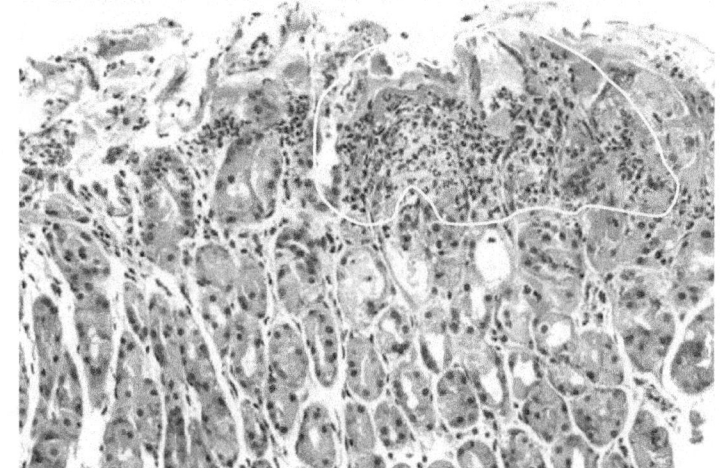

ovided kindly by Dr. Aducio Thiesen, University of Alberta

- ➤ Treatment
  - ○ Correct the associated deficiencies
  - ○ Carcinoid tumors
    - Polypectomy
    - Antrectomy
  - ○ Beware of ↑ risk of adenocarcinoma
    - No screening or surveillance recommendations

Both acute erosive gastropathy (AEG) and chemical gastropathy (CG; type C gastritis) may be caused by NSAIDs, and associated with regenerative changes.

- What are the histopathological changes distinguishing AEG from CG?

	CG	AEG
○ Architecture	ncytial	veolar hyperplasia
○ Mucosal gastric pits		long, tortuous (corkscrew) gastric pits)
○ Smooth muscle, lamina propria		
○ Chronicity, WBC	acute, PMN exudate and eosinophils in pockets)	chronic lymphocytes or plasma cells)
○ Metaplasia	)	:s

"Teaching is the art of acting. I don't teach Gastro', I teach about myself."

Grandad

CHRONIC GASTRITIS

- Endoscopy

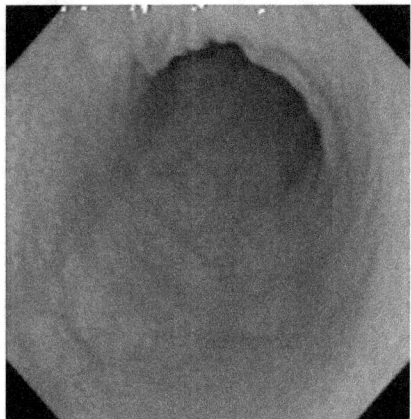

- Histopathology
  - Intestinal metaplasia
  - Goblet and intestinal absorptive cells partially replace the foveolar epithelium
  - Loss of rugal folds, prominent submucosal vesicles
  - Focal or multifocal areas of intestinal metaplasia appearing as white or pearly nodules, surrounded by red mucosa and prominent vessels

Chronic Non–Specific Gastritis

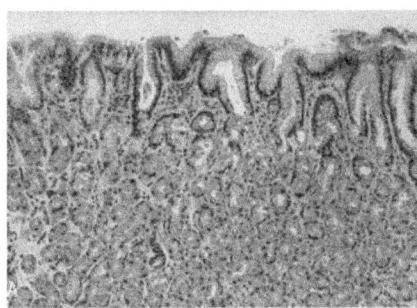

Normal gastric body   Normal gastric antrum

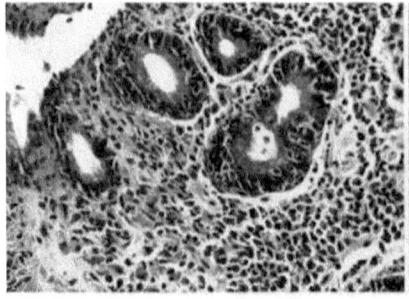
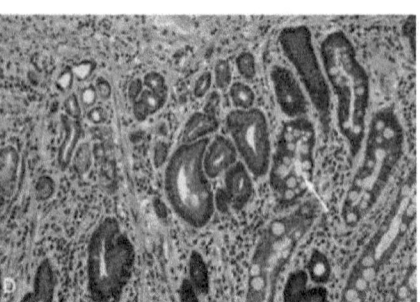

'fuse antral gastritis (DAG)
- Glands show infiltrate of neutrophils and inflammatory cells in the lamina propria

ıltifocal atrophic gastritis (MAG) with intestinal metaplasia (IM)
- Diffuse corporal atrophic gastritis i a man with pernicious anemia

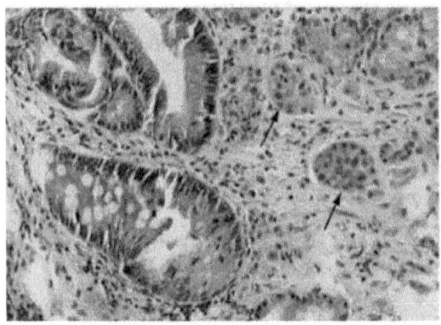

'fuse atrophic gastritis of the body of the stomach
- Gland in the lower left is lined by goblet cells
- Nests of enterochromaffin–like cells are also visible (arrow)

p://clinicalgate.com/gastritis-and-gastropathies/

Chronic Atrophic Gastritis of Body

- Histopathology
  - Body mucosa is chronically inflamed and completely replaced by thin, intestinalized mucosa with lymphoid hyperplasia
  - Site of biopsy to be confirmed by endoscopy, otherwise pathologist may think as the antrum
  - Loss of gastric glands by intestinal metaplasia, with body glands replaced by antral or pyloric glands
  - Residual inflamed body–type mucosa (left); extensive intestinal and focal pyloric metaplasia (right)
    - Chronic Gastritis, Intestinal Metaplasia
    - Goblet and intestinal absorptive cells partially replace foveolar epithelium
    - Loss of gastric glands by intestinal metaplasia, with body glands replaced by antral or pyloric glands
    - Residual inflamed body–type mucosa
    - Extensive intestinal and focal pyloric metaplasia
  - Chronic Atrophic Gastritis
    - Body mucosa replaced by intestinalized epithelium with goblet, absorptive, and Paneth cells.
    - Residual body–type glands (left)

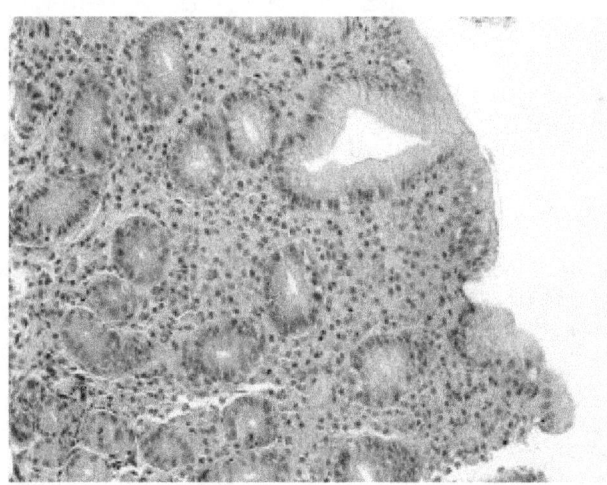

Provided kindly by Dr. Aducio Thiesen, University of Alberta

> Multifocal atrophic gastritis

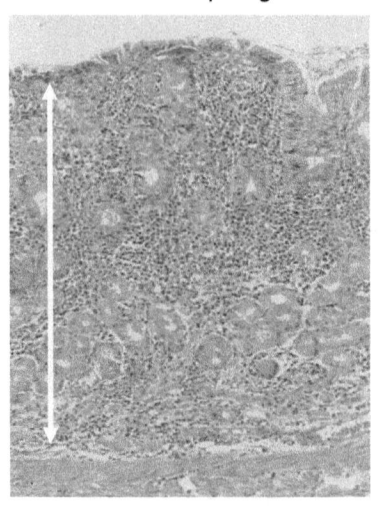

H. pylori with full thickness mucosal inflammation

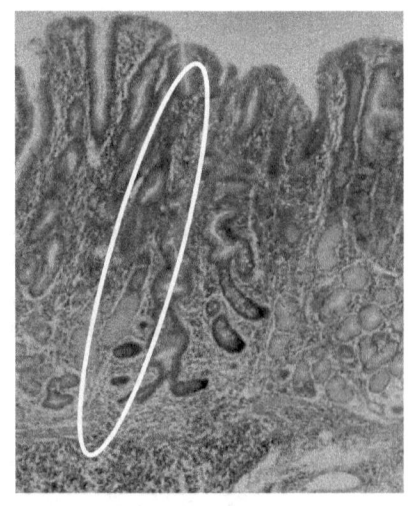

Focus of intestinal metaplasia

Diffuse Corporal Atrophic Gastritis

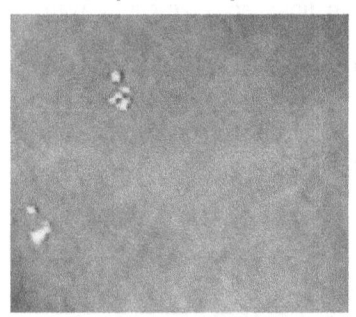

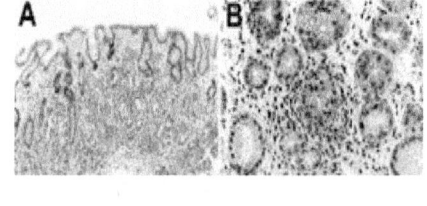

Thinning of the corpus mucosa: loss of folds and increased visibility of the submucosal vessels

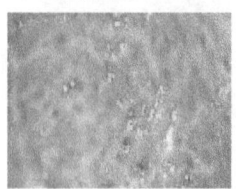

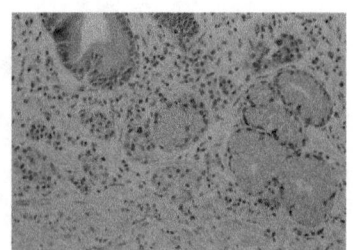

Enterogastric Reflux Gastritis

- Pathophysioloyg
  - Reflux of biliary and pancreatic juice
  - Conversion of lecithin into lysolecithin through pancreatic and possibly H.py phospholipase A2
  - ↑ lysolecithin lowers mucus layer hydrophobicity
  - ↓ of hydrophobicity reduces mucosal defense against acid

- Diagnosis

EGD, why biopsy when the mucosa appears to be endoscopically normal?

  - To contribute in unravelling the cause of symptoms, justifying the endoscopy
  - To detect and grade histologic gastritis
  - To detect uncommon causes of gastritis (eg. infections, granulomatous, eosinophilic, vasculitis)
  - To detect atrophy and intestinal metaplasia
  - To detect (early) dysplasia

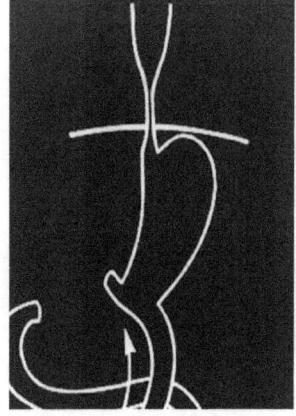

➢ Endoscopy

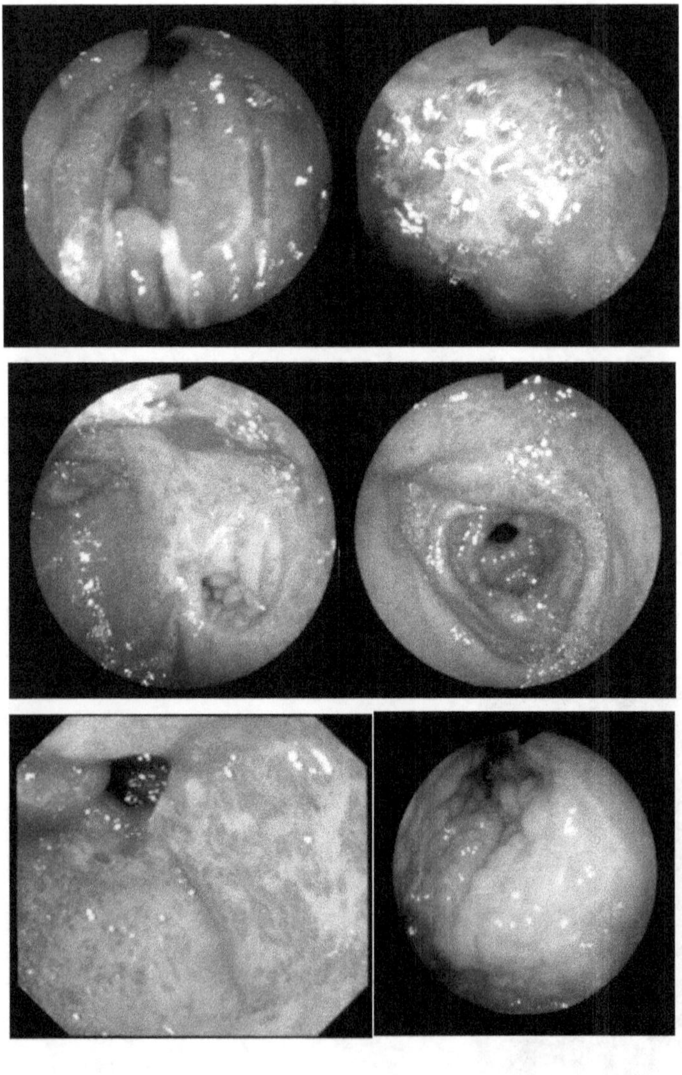

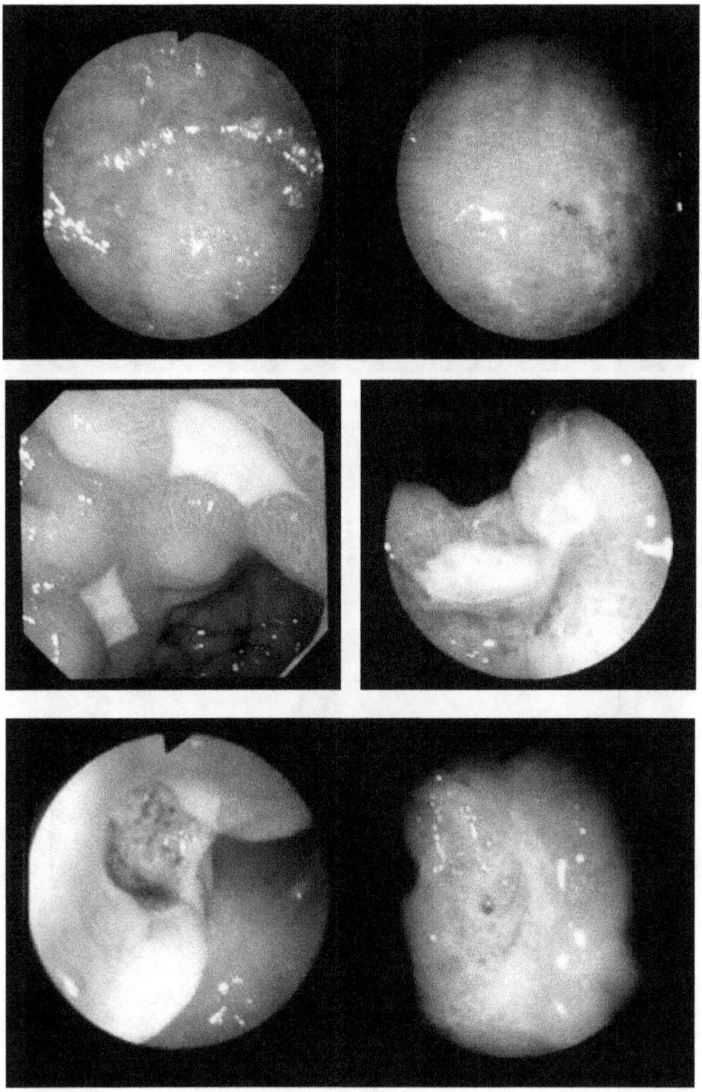

FROM COMPETENCE TO EXCELLENCE
The Stomach

© A.B.R. Thomson

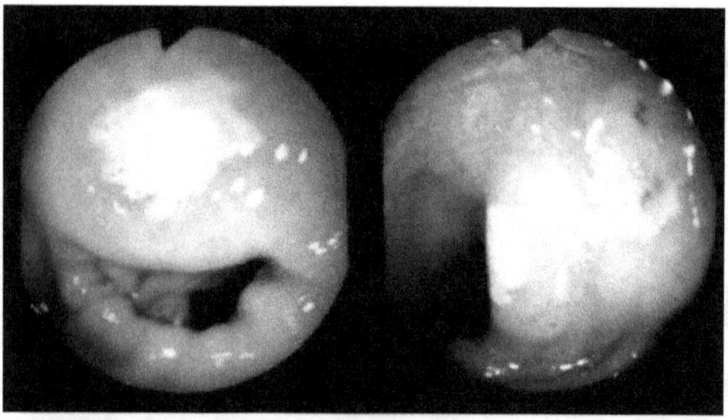

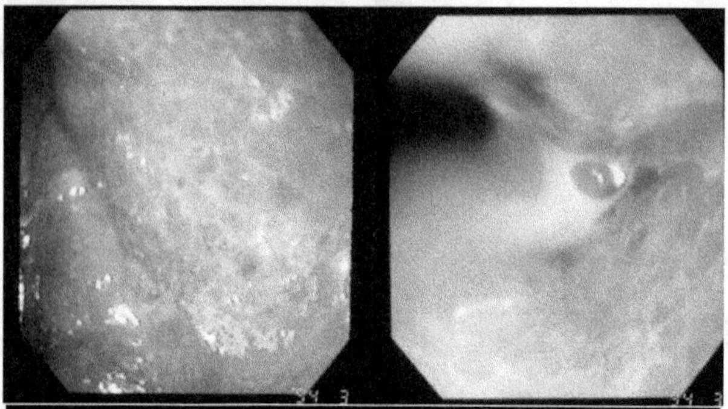

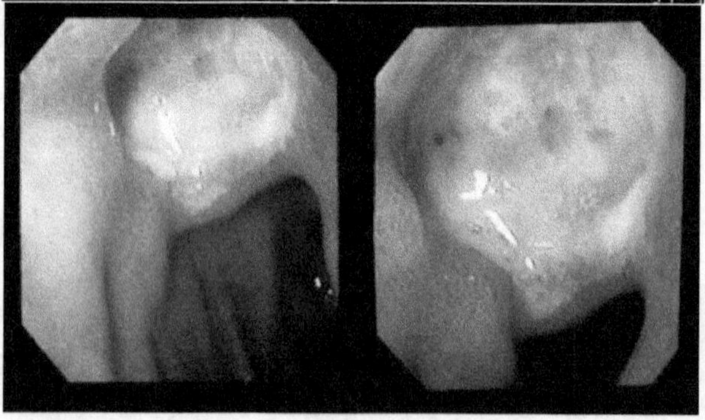

FROM COMPETENCE TO EXCELLENCE
The Stomach

© A.B.R. Thomson

238

***Helicobacter pylori*–Associated Gastritis**

- Definition
  - Chronic active gastritis — neutrophils, lymphocytes and plasma cells, mostly in the luminal side of the mucosa, due to infection with curved, flagellated, microaerophilic, gram negative *Bacillus* (rods) seagull wing–shaped (S–shaped)

- Demography
  - Prevalence of infection is high in developing countries (~ 80% of population), and in certain groups of patients in developed countries, where the prevalence may be < 20%
  - Only a small portion of patients with *H. pylori* infection develop an *H. pylori*–associated disease
  - *H. pylori* infection in ~ 25% of Canadians
  - More common in some "New Canadians" or "First Nation Canadians"
  - *H. pylori*–associated GI and non–GI diseases or disorders
  - Most common cause of chronic active gastritis (> 95%)

- Pathogenesis
  - Depends on
    - Adhesions
      - Bab A, Sab A, urease
    - Virulence factors
      - Cag A, Vac A, urease
    - Production of cytokines
      - IL–8, attracts neutrophils

- Clinical
  - Depends on disease which develops as of the H. pylori infection
  - H. pylori-associated disease
    - Peptic ulcer disease (GU and DU)
    - Dyspepsia
    - Gastric adenocarcinoma
    - MALT lymphoma
    - Fundic gland polyps
    - Idiopathic urticarial

SO YOU WANT TO BE A GASTROENTEROLOGIST!

Gastric MALT lymphoma is a complication of *H. pylori* infection associated with gastric lymphoid hyperplasia, which is difficult to distinguish from gastric marginal zone B–cell lymphoma (low–grade MALT lymphoma).

- Give the histopathological features distinguishing *H. pylori*–associated gastric lymphoid hyperplasia and gastric MALT lymphoma.

Histopathological findings	*H. pylori*–associated lymphoid hyperplasia	MALT lymphoma
o Germinal center and mantle B–cells		CD20 positive
o Peripheral T–cells		CD3 positive
o Intraepithelial lymphocytes	CD3 positive T–cells	CD20 positive neoplastic B–cells
o Destructive lymph epithelial lesions	-	+
o Monomorphic B–cells below the muscularis mucosae	Only superficial changes	+ (deeper changer)
o Clonal lymphocytes	+	+

Both lymphocytic gastritis and MALT lymphoma are associated with *H. pylori* infection of the stomach.

- Differentiate thee two complications of *H. pylori*.

    o Lymphocytic gastritis
    - > 25 lymphocytes per 100 epithelial cells
    - CD8–positive T lymphocytes
    - Reactive lymphoid follicles
    - Lymphoepithelial lesions of the glands
    - Associated with celiac disease

    o MALT
    - Diffuse population of B–cells in the lamina propria

➢ Differential diagnosis
  o *Helicobacter heilmannii* (larger than *H. pylori*, and usually intracellular)
  o MALT lymphoma — CD3–positive T–lymphocytes in the periphery or CD20 positive B–lymphocytes in the germinal centers
  o Crohn's disease, chemical gastropathy (may have active gastritis)

Curiosity

  o Autoantibobodies to gastric parietal cells target H^+ / K^+ ATPase, and are present in 60 – 85% of patients with autoimmune gastritis.
  o Autoantibodies against H^+ / K^+ ATPase are also present in some patients with *H. pylori* infection, and explain why gastric HCl inhibitory effects of PPIs may be less in patients with *H. pylori* infection, even when there is no associated pangastritis leading to reduced gastric body parietal cells.

➢ Performance characteristics for the tests for *Helicobacter pylori*.

Tests	Sensitivity	Specificity	Comments
❖ Non–biopsy tests			
o Blood serology	88 – 92%	86 – 95%	- Useful if positive - Not useful in follow–up re–eradication - ↑ false negative (↓ sensitivity with HIV infection
o Stool antigen test	89%	94%	- Useful in proving eradication
o Urea breath test (UBT)	90 – 100%	98 – 100%	- Acid–lowering therapy (i.e. PPIs) will ↓ sensitivity unless stopped for 2 weeks - Useful in proving eradication

Tests	Sensitivity	Specificity	Comments
❖ Gastric mucosal biopsies (G)			
o Warthin–Starry modified Giemsa	84 – 99%	90 – 99%	- May be falsely negative in presence of fresh blood, i.e. from upper GI bleeding
o Rapid urease tests	89 – 98%	93 – 98%	
o Culture	77 – 92%	100%	- Possibly useful in patient not eradicated by useful treatment

Modified from: Bhattacharya, B. 2010. *Gastrointestinal and Liver Pathology*. Chapter 3. Elsevier, 2nd Edition. page 78.

- Endoscopy

Acute gastritis → chronic → EMAG → MAG → dysplasia → gastric adenocarcinoma

- o Mucosa is red, granular or nodular (lymphoid hyperplasia), erosions, ulcers, tumor (adenocarcinoma, MALT lymphoma)
- o Antral redness, granularity, nodularity, erosions, ulcer

- Histopathology
    - o Superficial mucosa
        - PMNs
        - Lymphoplasmacytic infiltration
    - o Gastric pits
    - o Pititis (crypt abscesses)
    - o Foveolar hyperplasia
    - o Erosion, ulcers
    - o Lymphoid follicles
    - o *H. pylori* organism
        - Giemsa stain
        - Silver stain
            - Warthin–Starry
            - Genta
        - Immunohistochemistry

- Spectrum of changes
  - Acute gastritis
  - Chronic active gastritis
  - Few PMNs, cluster of plasma cells
  - Lymphocytic gastritis
  - Marked intraepithelial lymphocytes (differentiated from MALT [T/B cell lymphoma])
  - Follicular gastritis
  - Marked lymphoid follicles
  - Granulomatous gastritis
  - Hyperplastic polyp
  - Fundic gland polyp
  - Ulcer (extension through the muscularis mucosae)
  - Fibrinoid necrosis
  - Inflammation
  - Granulation
  - Tissue fibrosis, scarring
  - Type B gastritis (multifocal atrophic gastritis, or EMAG)
  - Multifocal intestinal metaplasia
  - Atrophic gastritis
  - Dysplasia
  - Gastric adenocarcinoma
- *H. pylori* identified
  - Curved rods
  - Mucus
  - Surface foveolar epithelium
  - Pits
  - Special stains: Gemsa, Warthin–Starry, immunohistochemistry (with PPI treatment, *H. pylori* migrates proximally into the gastric body, and immunostains may be useful to detect in parietal cells)
- Superficial epithelium – inflammation:
  - PMNs plus lymphoplasmacytic cells
  - Lymphoid follicles
- Foveolar epithelium – hyperplasia
- Pits
  - Active inflammation ("pititis")
  - Crypt abscesses
- Degenerative changes

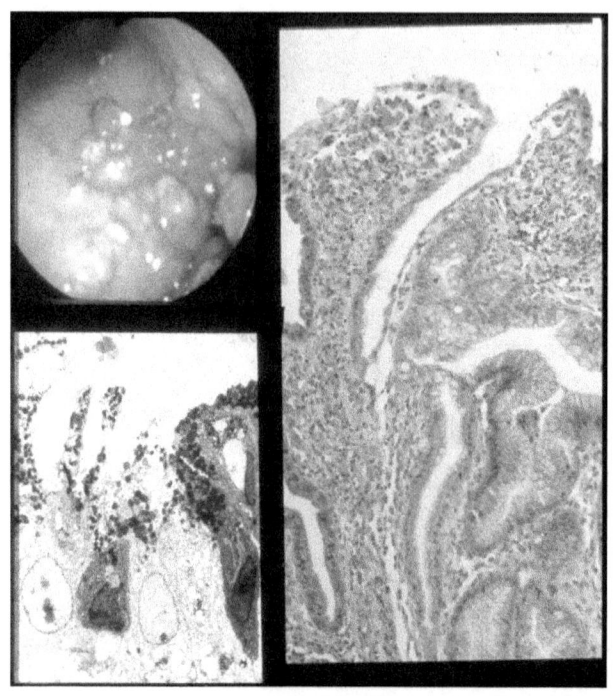

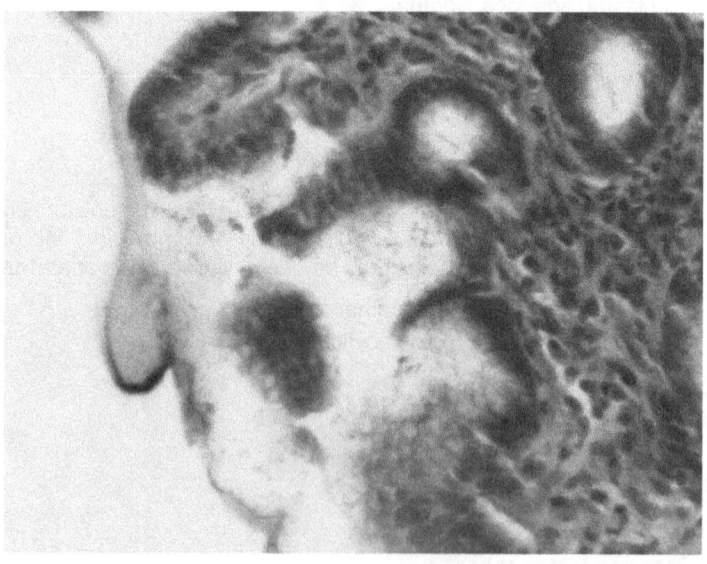

Gastric tissue, Giemsa stain for *Helicobacter pylori*

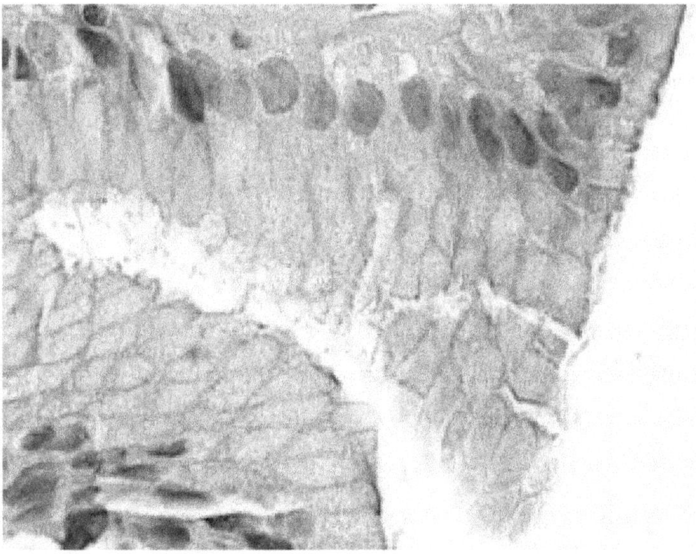

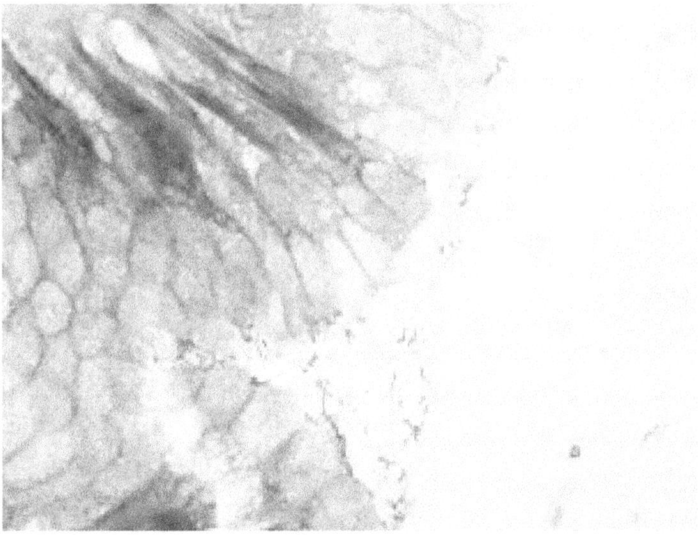

Provided kindly by Dr. Aducio Thiesen, University of Alberta

FROM COMPETENCE TO EXCELLENCE
The Stomach

© A.B.R. Thomson

Autoimmune Gastritis (Autoimmune Metaplastic Atrophic Gastritis)

- Definition
  - An immune–mediated chronic inflammation directed against the parietal cells of the gastric body
  - Aka type A gastritis
- Demography
  - F >> M = 3:1
  - Caucasians = F > 50 years
  - Affects 2% of people > 60 years
  - ↑ risk of gastric carcinoma
    - Adenocarcinoma
      - 2 – 3x
    - Carcinoids
      - ~ 5%
- Pathogenesis
  - HLA haplotype HLA–B8, DR–3
- Clinical
  - ↓ parietal cells → ↓ H⁺ / ↓ intrinsic factors
  → absorption of Fe^{3+} / cobalamin (vitamin B12)
  → iron deficiency, megaloblastic anemia, degeneration of posterior columns
- Laboratory
  - Stomach   — Parietal cells
    - Parietal cell antibodies 60 – 85%
    - Intrinsic factor antibodies 30 – 50%
    — Chief cells
    - ↓ HCL secretion
    - ↓ serum secretion
  - Gastrin   — G–cell
    - ↑ gastrin (secondary to loss of H⁺ feedback)
  - Cobalamin concentrations   — ↓ (lack of intrinsic factor)
  - Schilling test   — Investigation of vitamin B12

- Iron deficiency — Anemia
- Vitamin B12 deficiency — Anemia
  — Posterior column defects

> Differential diagnosis
  - Environmental metaplastic atrophic gastritis (EMAG)
  - Diffuse or multifocal atrophic gastritis
  - Atrophic gastritis associated with autoimmune polyglandular syndrome (APS)

- Differentiate AMAG and EMAG.

		AMAG	EMAG
o	Synonyms	Type A gastritis Diffuse corporal gastritis	Type B gastritis Diffuse antral gastritis Multifocal atrophic gastritis
o	Population affected	Northern European and Scandinavian descent	Worldwide
o	Sex	Female predominance	No sex predilection
o	Etiology	Immune mediated	H. pylori infection
o	H. pylori colonization	< 20%	90 – 100%
o	Location	Body and fundus	Antrum predominantly with extension to body, multifocal
o	Anti–parietal cell antibody	Positive	Negative
o	Anti–intrinsic factor antibody	Positive	Negative
o	Vitamin B_{12} level	Low	Normal
o	Serum gastrin	Very high	Normal or low

Source: Iacobuzio-Donahue, C. A. and Montgomery, E. A. 2011. Gastrointestinal and Liver Pathology. 2nd Edition. Table 3-4. page 86.

> **SO YOU WANT TO BE A GASTROENTEROLOGIST!**
> Autoimmune gastritis (AIG, from metaplastic atrophic gastritis) and autoimmune polyglandular syndrome (APS) have no of gastric body parietal cells on biopsy.
>
> - What are the laboratory tests that help distinguish the two?
>
> | | | AIG | APS |
> |---|---|---|---|
> | o Lab | Parietal cell antibodies | + | - |
> | | Gastrin | ↑↑ | N / ↓ |
> | o Biopsy | Antral metaplastic gastritis | No | Yes |

- Endoscopy
    - Loss of rugal folds of the gastric body and fundus
    - Reddened mucosa
    - Visible blood vessels (atrophy of mucosa)
    - Polypoid lesions
        - Hyperplastic
        - Pseudoplastic
        - Carcinoids
        - Adenocarcinoids
        - Adenocarcinoma

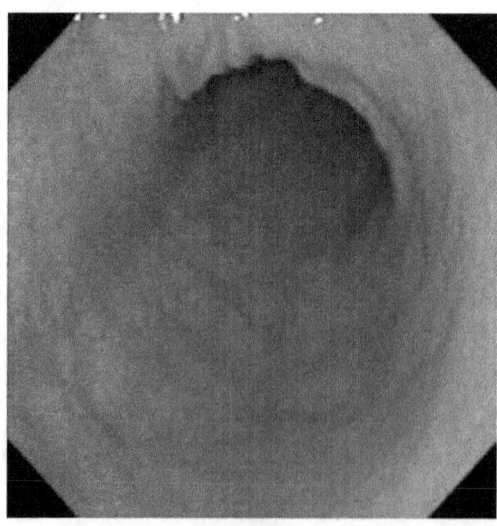

- Histopathology
  - Body and fundus
    - ↑ lymphocytic and plasma cell infiltration in submucosa
    - ↓ parietal cell
    - ↓ chief cell
    - Metaplasia
      - Pseudopyloric (mucosa–like glands, but no G–cells)
        - Linear nodular ECL
        - Hyperplasia
      - Intestinal metaplasia (goblet cells and Paneth cells)
      - Pancreatic acinar metaplasia
  - Antrum
    - Gastropathy
    - Chronic gastritis (mild)
    - G–cell hyperplasia

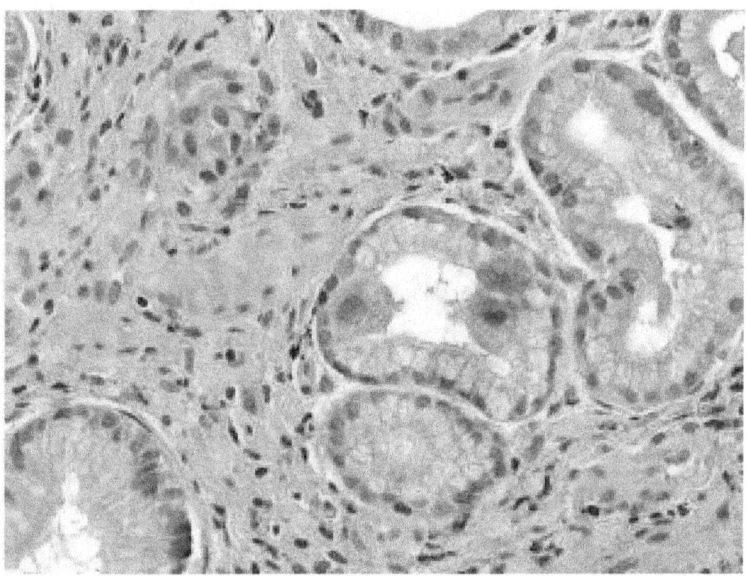

Provided kindly by Dr. Aducio Thiesen, University of Alberta

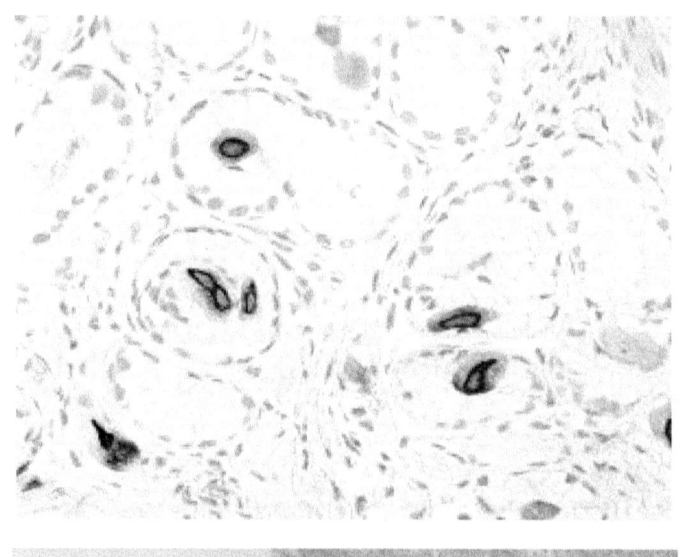

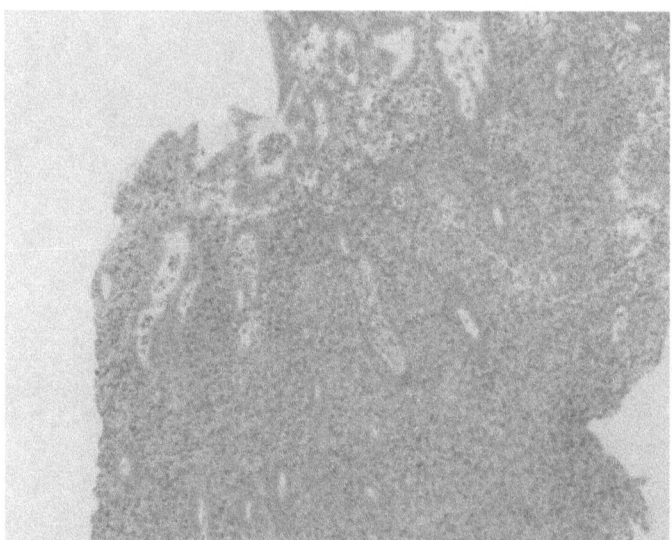

Provided kindly by Dr. Aducio Thiesen, University of Alberta

- Special stains
  - G–cell hyperplasia (antrum)
  - Pseudopyloric metaplasia (body), negative for gastrin
  - Gastrin–stain positive with intestinal metaplasia (rare)

Gastritis Cystica Polyposa

- Definition
    - Dilated cystic gland in the mucosa and submucosa causing sessile polyp near the gastric stoma
    - Breaks the record for synonyms: gastritis cystica profunda, gastritis cystica superficialis, gastric cystic polyposis, stromal polypoid hypertrophic gastritis, polypoid cystic gastritis

- Differentials
    - Invasive adenocarcinoma
        - Does have pleomorphism and desmoplastic stroma
        - Does not have thick, splayed smooth muscle bundles

- Endoscopy
    - Single or multiple polyp near the gastric stoma
    - Sessile, 1 – 3 cm polyps
    - Multiple polyps may become confluent and forms a peristomal mass

- Histopathology
    - Dilated cystic glands in the mucosa, submucosa and muscularis propria
    - Lamina propria
        - Splaying of muscles
        - Fibrosis
        - Thickening
    - Surface epithelium has regenerative change and may show atrophy
    - Foveolar hyperplasia
    - No pleomorphism or desmoplastic stroma
        - Chronic inflammation
    - Gastric remnants (away from the stoma)
        - ↓ parietal and chief cells
        - Intestinal metaplasia, dysplasia, adenocarcinoma ("stump carcinoma")

Infectious Gastritis

- ❖ CMV
  - Viral inclusions
    - Nuclear and cytoplasm
      - Glandular epithelium
      - Mesenchymal cells
        - Endothelial
        - Fibroblasts
- ❖ HSV
  - Viral inclusions
    - Nuclear
      - Glandular epithelium
      - Mesenchymal cells
        - Endothelial
        - Fibroblasts
    - Necrosis
- ❖ Other causes of infections:
  - Anisakiasis
  - *Aspergillus*
  - Cryptosporidiosis
  - Giardiasis
  - *Histoplasma*
  - *Schistosoma mansoni*
  - *Strongyloides stercoralis*
  - Whipple's disease

Candidiasis

- ➤ Definition: immune–mediated chronic gastritis leading to loss of oxyntic (chief and parietal) cells
- ➤ Demography
  - F > M, 3%
- ➤ Differentials
  - May be associated with autoimmune polyglandular syndrome, type I
  - Distinguish AMAG from EMAG

- ➢ Endoscopy
  - ○ Contamination from GI tract is common
  - ○ May aggravate and perpetuate ulceration
  - ○ Usually, treatment is not necessary
  - ○ Body and fundal involvement
  - ○ Atrophic, pale shiny mucosa with prominent vascular pattern
  - ○ Loss of rugal folds
  - ○ Tumors
    - Fundic gland polyps
    - Hyperplastic polyps
    - Carcinoid (may be multiple)
    - Adenocarcinoma

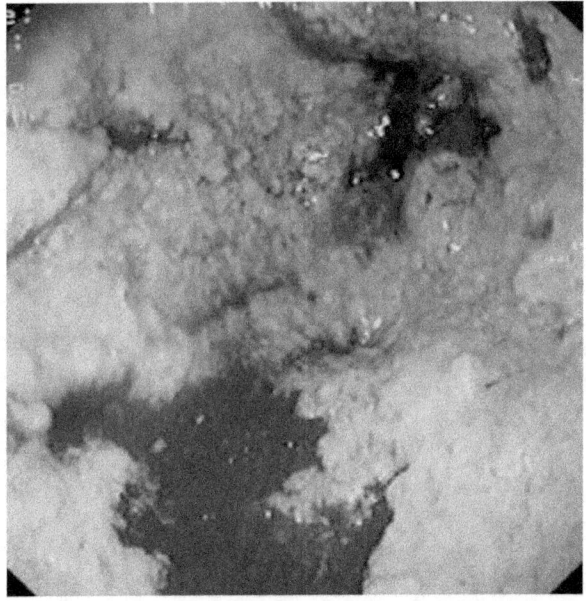

- Histopathology
    - Different changes in the gastric body or fundus versus antrum (yes: unlike the endoscopic changes seen only in the body or fundus, histological changes occur in the antrum [please see below])
        - Body or fundus
            - Lymphoplasmacytic infiltration of the body or fundus, particularly in the deeper layers
            - Loss of the parietal and chief cells (reflected by the lymphoplasmacytic)
            - Pseudopyloric metaplasia – mucous glands in the antrum, like the pyloric glands, but is called "pseudo" because there are no G–cells (gastrin–containing cells)
                - Intestinal metaplasia (goblet cells and Paneth cells)
                - Pancreatic acinar metaplasia
                - Cells in the foveolar epithelium may become megaloblastic when severe B_{12} deficiency develops
                - Fundic gland polyps
                - Gastric carcinoids (prevalence is ~ 5%)
                - Adenocarcinoma (↑ RR 2 – 3x)
        - Antral mucosa
            - Mild chronic gastritis, or reactive (chemical) gastropathy
            - G–cell hyperplasia (nodular or linear, 5 or more ECL cells in a line)

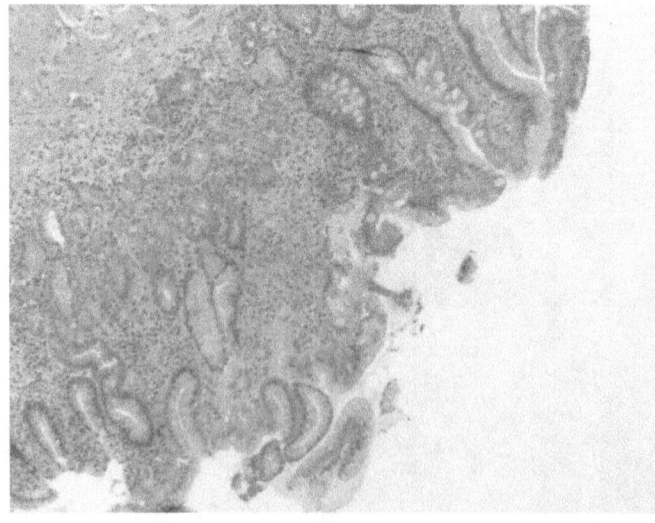

Cytomegalovirus *(CMV)*

- ➤ Definition
  - o CMV infection of the epithelial and endothelial cells, and of the fibroblasts of the gastric glands
- ➤ Demography
  - o Seen in patients with immunosuppression
- ➤ Clinical
  - o Ulceration
  - o Symptoms and signs of associated disease(s)
- ➤ Differential diagnosis
  - o Take biopsies from the edge as well as the base of ulcer (if ulcer is present)
  - o Viral inclusions of enlarged epithelial cells of the gastric glands and vascular endothelial cells
  - o Eosinophilic nuclear inclusions, perinuclear halo, cytoplasmic red granules
  - o May mimic ischemic gastritis, if there is marked CMV involvement of the vascular endothelial cells
  - o May cause thickened gastric folds resembling Ménétrier's disease in children
  - o Distinguish from gastric mucosal calcinosis (aluminum calcinosis), which has large, extracellular, basophilic depots under the foveolar tips

SO YOU WANT TO BE A GASTROENTEROLOGIST!

- Differentiate the nuclear inclusions in CMV and HSV infections.

	CMV	HSV
o Optimal site of mucosal biopsy from ulcer	Margin	Base
o Eosinophilic	+	-
o Perinuclear halo	+	-
o Ground glass		+
o Necrosis		+
o Multinucleated		+
o Marginated		+
o Molding		+

- Endoscopy
    - Ulcers (often single, and deep)
    - Polyps
    - Thick folds
    - May look like adenocarcinoma

- Histopathology
    - Inclusions in the nuclei and cytoplasm of enlarged epithelial cells and fibroblasts
        - Eosinophilic
        - Perinuclear halo
    - Cytoplasm with red granules
    - Lamina propria
        - Condensed
    - Glands
        - Loss or drop out

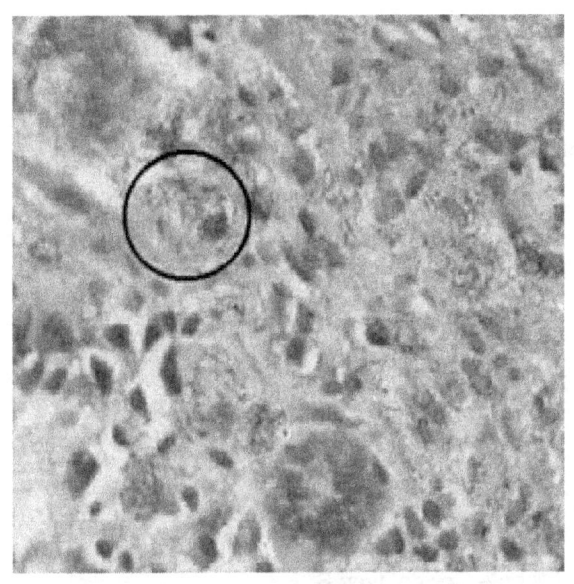

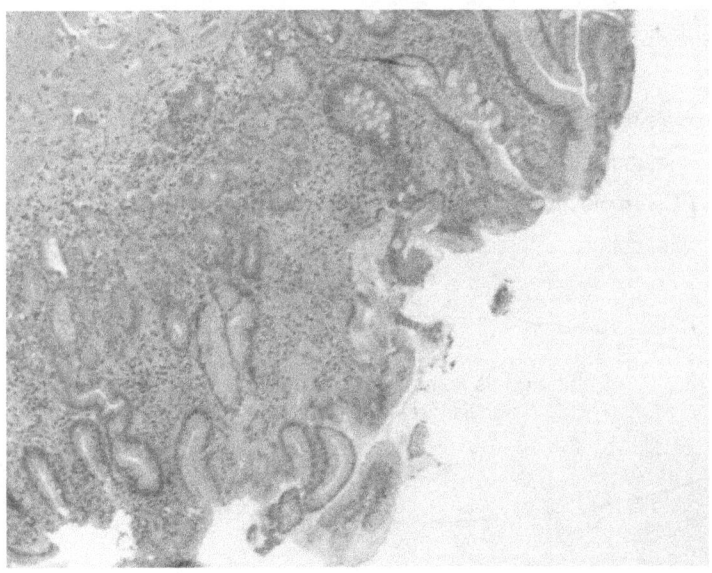

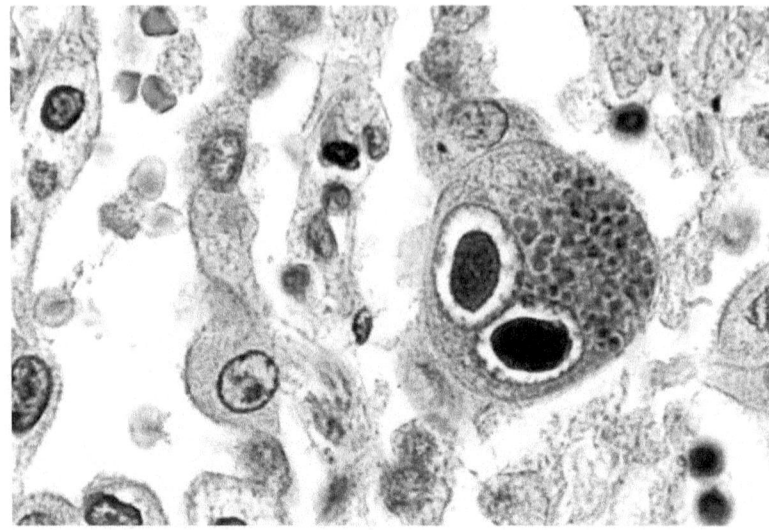

Owl's eye inclusion – Cowdry type B

http://emedicine.medscape.com/article/215702-overview#a6

- Specials studies
    - Immunohistochemistry (immunostains)
    - PCR (molecular studies)
    - Viral culture

"Setting goals is the first step in turning the invisible into visible.

Tony Robbins

Mycobacterial Gastritis

➢ Pathology

Histopathology	TB	MAI
o Foamy histiocytes with acid–fast bacilli	+	+
o Granulomas caseation		

➢ Treatment

A 70–year old immunocompetent patient develops benign gastric ulcer after a 4–week course of standard dose of ibuprofen for osteoarthritis. Six mucosal biopsies confirm the lesion is benign, but show an admixture of *Candida*–like fungal yeast and pseudohyphae.

- What is the treatment for gastric ulcer?
  - PPI in standard dose *po od* ½ hour before breakfast for 12 weeks
  - Repeat endoscopy to confirm ulcer healing
  - Stop NSAID, if NSAID cannot be stopped (Some conditions apply)
  - Do not treat Candida infection (fluconazole) unless the ulcer does not heal with 12 wk PPI, since ~1/5 of benign gastric ulcers are colonized with this fungus.

Suppurative (Phlegmonous) **Gastritis**

- Culture of the slough of necrosis, infected phlegmonous gastritis may reveal the following organisms:
  - *Streptococci*
  - *Staphylococcus*
  - *E. coli*
  - *Proteus*
- On endoscopy, the surrounding area is soft, easily compressed, and crepitus is suspected

Granulomatous Gastritis

- Definition
    - Granulomatous infiltration and inflammation in the stomach
    - Circumscribed, nodular collection of epithelioid histiocytes, lymphocytes, eosinophils, giant cells (occasional PMNs)
    - May be a lymphoid cuff, or central necrosis
- Causes
    - Infection
        - TB
        - Histoplasmosis
        - Whipple's disease
        - Schistosomiasis
    - Inflammation
        - Crohn's disease (50%)
            - Granulomatous gastritis affects ~ ¼ of Crohn's disease patients
            - Endoscopically, may have the appearance of linitis plastica
            - Granulomas are caseating with a cuff of lymphocytes
        - Sarcoidosis (10%)
            - 10% of patients with multisystem granulomatous disease have gastric involvement
        - Vasculitis (Churge–Strauss Disease plus granulomas)
    - Infiltration
        - Tumor
    - Idiopathic (25%)
    - Foreign body
        - Suture material
        - Food (10%)

- Endoscopy
  - Nodules
  - Erosions
  - Ulceration
  - Strictures
  - Thick folds
  - Gastric outlet obstruction
  - Erythema
  - Erosions (aphthous) and ulcers
  - Nodules
  - Thick gastric folds
  - Narrowing
- Histopathology
  - Nodular, circumscribed lesion
  - Collection of the following:
    - Epithelioid histocytes
    - Giant cells
    - Lymphocytes
    - Eosinophils
  - Lymphoid cuff
  - Central necrosis may be present
  - Focal mixtures of PMNs plus lymphohistiocytic clusters
  - Characteristic granulomas (please see above)
  - Special stains for possible etiology, i.e. *H. pylori*, TB, histoplasmosis, Whipple's (rarely syphilis, leprosy)
  - Chronic gastritis with epithelial granuloma
  - Presence of necrosis suggests an infectious cause (i.e. TB, fungal)
  - Patchy, focal, active chronic inflammation and an epithelioid granuloma

- Special considerations
  - Crohn's disease
  - Sarcoidosis
  - Foreign body granulomas (i.e. sutures, barium) endoscopy may show ulcers, nodularity, thick folds, segmental linitis plastica
  - Appearance: microscopy may show non–caseating granulomas with a cuff of lymphocytes
- Granulomatous Gastritis (Crohn's disease)
  - Crohn's — sharply punched–out aphthous erosion
  - Active chronic inflammation and an epithelioid granuloma
  - Full thickness section with (1) transmural fissure (2) and transmural inflammation characteristic of Crohn's disease
- Antrum, Granulomatous Gastritis
  - Caseous granuloma and active chronic inflammation rich in eosinophils
  - Necrosis favors infection

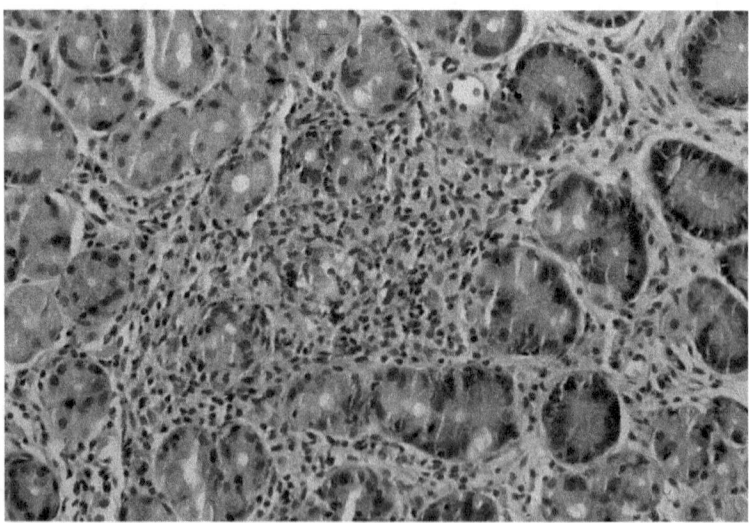

Mixed inflammatory cell infiltrate in the stomach

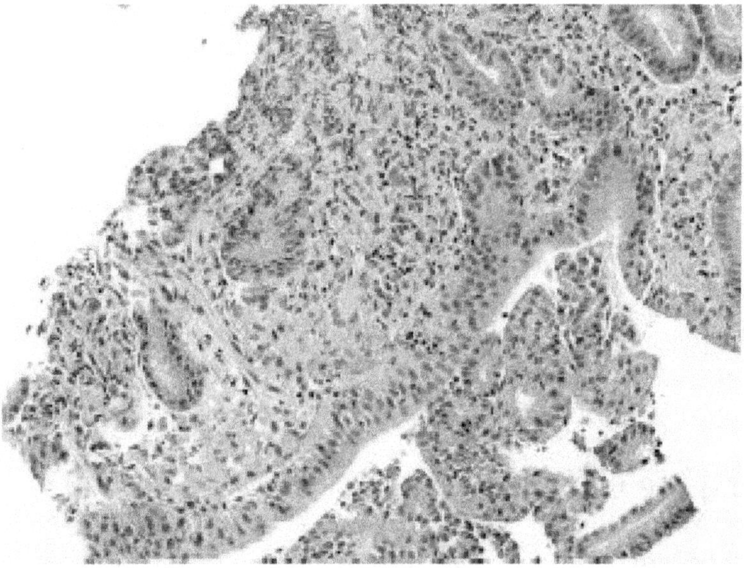

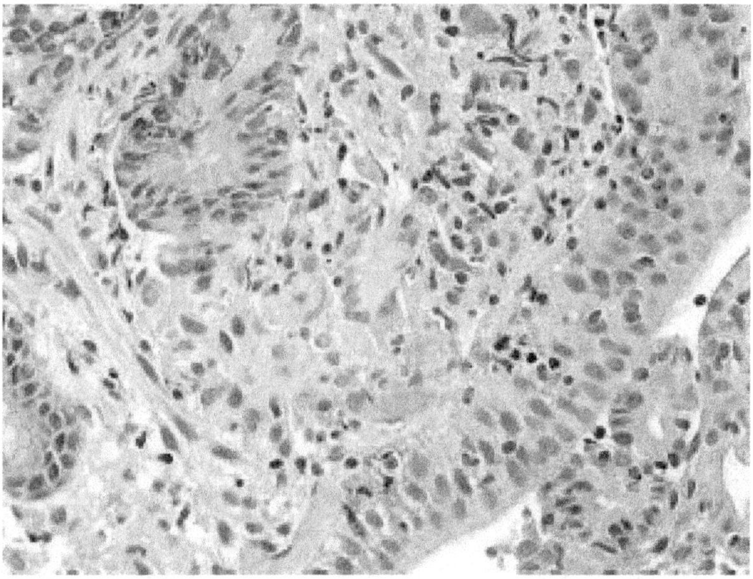

Provided kindly by Dr. Aducio Thiesen, University of Alberta

Lymphocytic Gastritis

- Definition
  - ↑ lymphocytes in the epithelium of gastric surface and pits
- Demography
  - Diagnosed in ~ 2% of esophagogastroduodenoscopy (EGDs)
- Clinical
  - May be associated with dyspepsia
  - Associated with the following diseases in ~ 1/3 of patients:
    - Celiac disease
    - *H. pylori* infection
    - Lymphocytic colitis, when patient has associated celiac disease
- Diagnostic imaging (barium study)
  - Nodule with central erosion ("volcano"; halo central barium flick)

o Single contrast	- Erosion
o Double contrast	- Central spot of barium with surrounding "halo" (volcano–like)

- Differentials
  - Gastric MALT lymphoma
    - CD20– and CD43–positive malignant B lymphocytes
    - Destruction of the epithelium and lamina propria
  - Chronic active gastritis from *H. pylori*
    - Superficial infiltration of PMNs and plasma cells, but not the prominent lymphocytosis
    - Positive identification of *H. pylori*

SO YOU WANT TO BE A GASTROENTEROLOGIST!

- Explain why gastric mucosal biopsies, though to be due to lymphocytic gastritis, need to be stained for gastrin and/or chromogranin, as well as for *H. pylori*.
  - Gastric, gastrin and chromogranin staining would be positive in hyperplasia of the endocrine cells, which may be confused with lymphocytic gastritis.

- Endoscopy
    - Normal
    - Nodules
    - Erosions
    - Thick folds (varioliform)
    - Nodule with central erosion ("volcano"; halo central barium flick)
- Histopathology
    - Eroded nodule on the crest of large fold in the body (varioliform gastritis)
    - Nodule consists of localized lymphocytic gastritis
    - Increased intraepithelial lymphocytes without evidence of epithelial damage in contrast to lymphoepithelial lesions of MALT lymphoma
    - Lymphocytes have twisted nuclei, a characteristic of T–cells
    - Lymphocytic gastritis (varioliform gastritis, chronic erosive verrucous gastritis)
        - Prominent intraepithelial CD3 and CD8 cytotoxic or suppressor T–lymphocytes (> 25 lymphocytes per 100 epithelial cells in the epithelium of the lamina propria of the gastric body and the antrum)
        - H. pylori gastritis has ~ 5 lymphocytes per 100 epithelial cells, with no lymph in deep layers
    - Site   - Body
            - When associated with *H. pylori* infection
        - Antrum
            - When associated with celiac disease
    - Nuclei   - Dark (condensed)
        - Surrounding clear halo

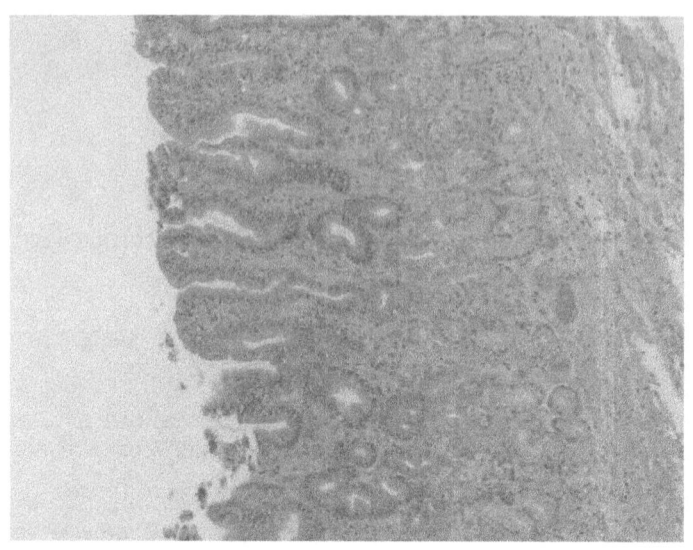

Provided kindly by Dr. Aducio Thiesen, University of Alberta

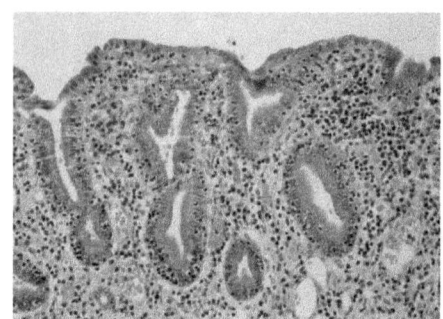

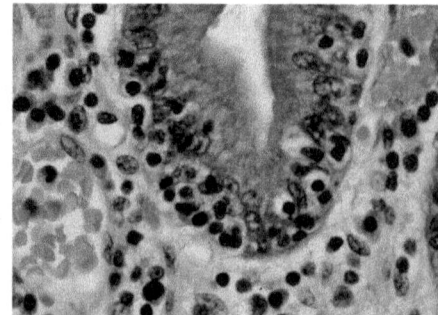

MAC w/in LP macrophages

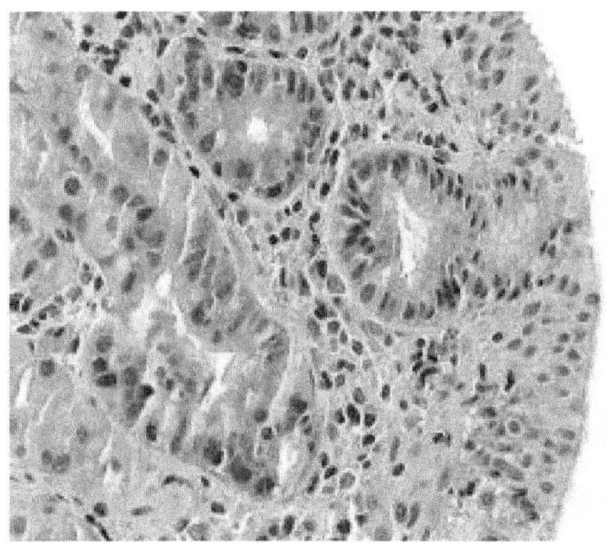

Provided kindly by Dr. Aducio Thiesen, University of Alberta

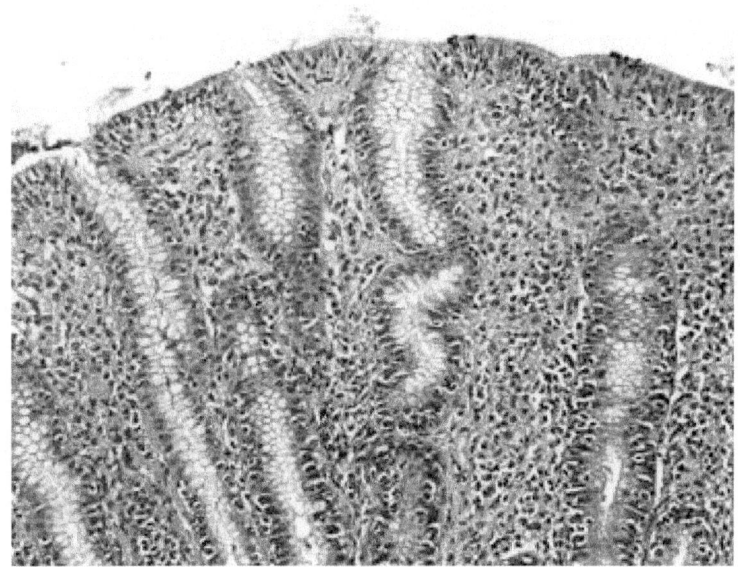

Printed with permission: McKenna, B. J. and Appelman, H. D. 2006. *Nat Clin Pract Gastroenterol Hepatol*. Primer: histopathology for the clinician—how to interpret biopsy information for gastritis. 3: 165–171.

- Special strains

	Lymphocytic Gastritis	MALT Lymphoma
o B–lymphocytes	–	CD20– / CD43–positive
o T–lymphocytes	CD3– / CD8–positive	–

> **Endoscopic Alert**
>
> o Thick gastric folds confused with gastric polyps

> **SO YOU WANT TO BE A GASTROENTEROLOGIST!**
>
> - What are the endoscopic and histological changes in lymphocytic gastritis?
>
>   o Endoscopy (varioliform)
>   - Thick folds
>   - Nodular mucosa
>   - Aphthous "ulcers" (erosions)
>
>   o Histopathology
>   - Antrum, body, or antrum plus body
>   - ↑ lymphocytes and plasma cells in the lamina propria
>   - > 5 lymphocytes per 100 cells
>   - Associated with the following conditions:
>   - *H. pylori* infection
>   - Celiac disease
>   - Crohn's disease in children

Gastropathies causing Thickening of Gastric Folds

- ❖ Ménétrier's disease (MD)
  - ○ ↓ oxyntic glands
    - Replaced by mucous glands
  - ○ Deep body mucous glands
    - Long
    - Tortuous
    - Foveolar epithelium (foveolar hyperplasia)
    - Mucous cells
    - Cystic dilation
  - ○ Superficial submucosa
  - ○ May be associated with lymphocytic gastritis
  - ○ Usually, have the following condition:
    - Little inflammatory infiltrate
      - May be associated with lymphocytic gastritis
    - Little regenerative changes

- ❖ Zollinger–Ellison Syndrome (ZES)
  - ○ Hyperplasia
    - Oxyntic mucosa
    - Enterochromafin–like (ECL) cells
  - ○ No foveolar hyperplasia

- ❖ Hyperplastic hypersecretory gastropathy (HHG)
  - ○ Hyperplasia of the parietal and chief cells

- ❖ Hyperplastic polyps (inflammatory [chronic inflammation, mucosal proliferation, dilation of the cystic glands], or regenerative fundic gland polyps)
  - ○ Multiple
  - ○ Small (< 1 cm)
  - ○ Fundus
  - ○ Associated with FAP (fundic gland polyposis syndrome, multiple hyperplastic polyps despite FAP elsewhere being adenomas)
  - ○ Regenerative changes
  - ○ Inflammatory infiltration

- Non–involved (non–*H. pylori* tissue)
  - Atrophy
  - Intestinal metaplasia

➤ Diagnostic imaging

60–year old woman with history of vague dyspepsia, mild microcytic anemia and hypoalbuminemia

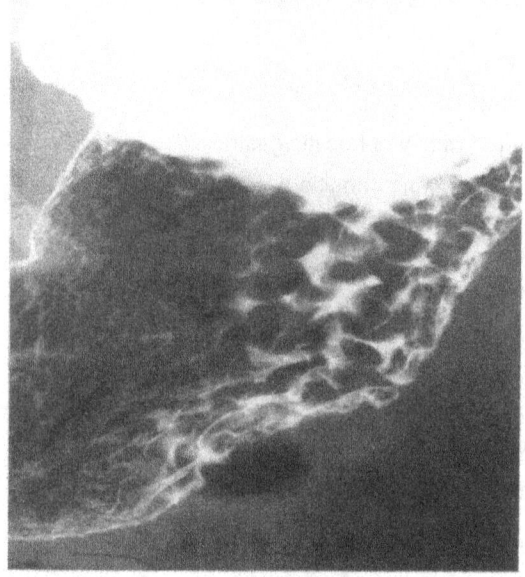

➤ Differentials
  - Lymphoma
  - Nodular, irregular, thick folds in variable size
  - Mass due to an adenocarcinoma
  - Ménétrier's disease
    - Proximal stomach
    - Thick gastric folds
    - Usually in the proximal half of the stomach
    - Common in the greater curve
    - Pliable (stomach cannula is distended)

- Histopathology

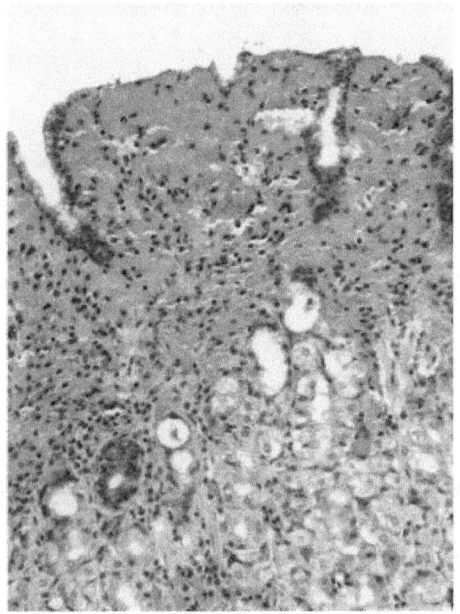

    - Hemorrhage is confined to the superficial portion of the mucosa
    - Paucity of the inflammatory cells

Ménétrier's Disease (MD)

- Definition
    - Rare, idiopathic giant gastric mucosal rugae, hypertrophy of the rugae of the gastric body, protein–losing gastropathy, and hypochlorhydria
- Demography
    - M > F, 3:1
    - Age 40 – 60 years
- Causes and associations
    - Children with CMV or other infections
    - Carcinoma in the adults

- Pathophysiology
  - Possibly due to ↑ production of TGF–α
- Clinical
  - Non–specific upper GI symptoms
  - Hypoproteinemia, edema
- Laboratory
  - ↓ serum
    - Albumin
    - Transferrin
    - Immunoglobulins

- The **risk factors** associated with the development of gastric adenocarcinoma.
  - Genetic—First degree relative with gastric cancer (hereditary diffuse gastric cancer) (2 – 3 fold increased risk): with mutations in E–cadherin CDH1 gene
  - HNPCC >> APC
  - Polyps—adenomatous gastric polyps (HNPCC, APC), Peutz-Jeghers syndrome, hamartomas, Ménétrier disease
  - Gastric atrophy—H.pylori infection, pernicious anemia, chronic atrophic gastritis, subtotal surgical resection with vagotomy for benign gastric ulcer disease
  - Diet—salted, pickled or smoked foods, low intake of fruits and vegetables
  - Life Style—Smoking (EtOH is not an independent risk factor)
  - Esophageal—Barrett's esophagus (cancer of cardia)
  - Late onset hypogammaglobulinemia
  - Intestinal metaplasia, type III

Abbreviation: HNPCC, hereditary nonpolyposis colon cancer

Adapted from: Abrahms, J. A. and Quante, M. 2016. *Sleisenger & Fordtran's Gastrointestinal and Liver Disease: Pathophysiology/ Diagnosis/Management*. 10th Edition. *Saunders/Elsevier*, Philadelphia, Box. 54-1, page 902.

- Differential diagnosis
  - Benign
    - Gastritis
      - *H. pylori*
      - CMV
    - Peptic ulcer disease
    - Zollinger–Ellison syndrome
    - Gastric varices
    - Ménétrier's Disease
  - Crohn's disease
  - Collagenous gastritis
  - Cetuximab (anti–epidermal protease inhibitor)
  - Malignant
    - Carcinoma
    - Lymphoma
    - Metastases
  - Site
    - Antrum
      - *H. pylori* gastritis
      - Collagenous gastritis
    - Cardia and fundus
      - Varices
      - Ménétrier's disease

> "The decisions of our own past are the architects of our present" [and future]
> Dan Brown, Infornd

SO YOU WANT TO BE A GASTROENTEROLOGIST OR GI PATHOLOGIST!

- Pathology
    - Foveolar hyperplasia
        - Gastric ulcers
        - Hyperplastic polyps
        - Chemical gastroenteropathy
        - Stoma site after gastroenterostomy
    - Hyperplastic polyps

	Ménétrier's disease (MD)	Hyperplastic Polyps (HP)
o Sites	Body	Antrum
o Inflammatory infiltrates	-	+
o Regenerative changes	-	+
o Uninvolved mucosa		
- Chronic atrophy	-	+
- Intestinal metaplasia	-	+

- Physiology
    - Thick gastric folds, hyperplasia of the parietal and chief cells

	Ménétrier's disease (MD)	ZES	Hyperplastic Hypersecretory Gastropathy (HHG)
o Acid (HCl) secretion	↓	↑↑	N / ↑
o Serum gastrin	Normal	↑↑	Normal
o Protein–losing gastropathy	+	No	No
o Foveolar hyperplasia	+	No	No

> Diagnostic imaging (barium)
>   - Gastric
>   - Wall
>   - Thick (1 – 3 cm)
>   - Folds
>   - Thick
>   - ↑ mucus secretion
>   - Reticular pattern of barium

- Endoscopy
  - Thick (1 – 3 cm) polypoid folds in the gastric body
  - Cerebriform appearance
  - Site
    - Children
      - Antrum
    - Adult
      - Body

A 64–year old woman with a long history of recurrent, severe dyspepsia, presented with dyspepsia and diarrhea while on PPI. Her fasting gastrin concentration was 750 pg/ml. Describe the endoscopic findings and management.

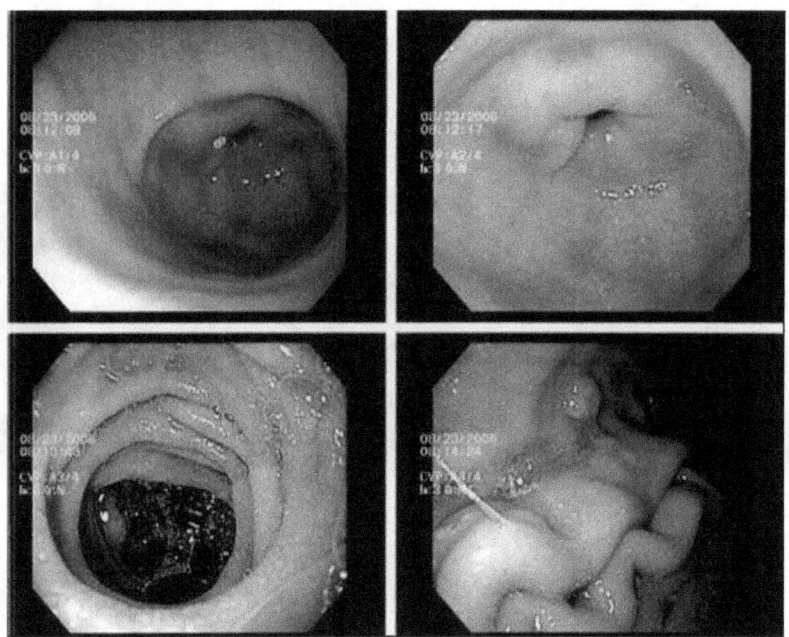

- Histopathology
    - ↑↑ foveolar hyperplasia
        - Tortuous
        - Elongated
        - ↑ mucous cells

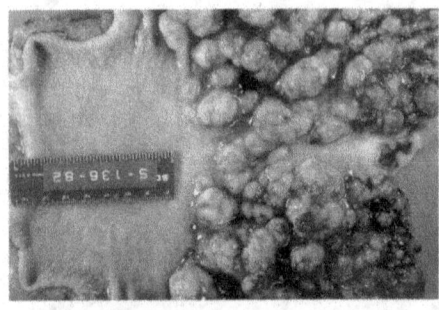
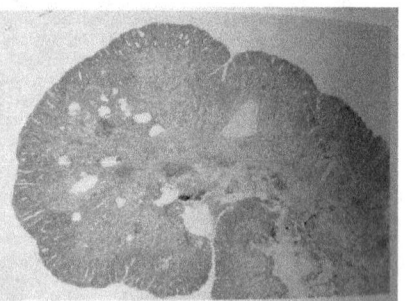

- Special studies
    - ↑ TGF–α
    - May be associated with CMV–positive immunostains in children
    - Rule out incidentally associated *H. pylori* infection

Congestive Gastropathy

- Endoscopic appearances of congestive gastropathy

    - Mild   – Scarlatina (fine pink speckling)
    - Moderate   – More pronounced patchy reddening – striped appearance
    - Severe   – Snake skin (quite specific) – white reticulated pattern
        - Cherry red spots – diffuse hemorrhagic

Hypertrophic Gastropathy (from Zollinger–Ellison syndrome)

- Definition
    - Fasting hypergastrinemia, gastrinoma, gastric acid (HCl) hypersecretion, and severe peptic ulcer disease
- Define end genetics of MEN–1 syndrome.
    - Autosomal dominant condition
    - Mutation in MEN–1 gene on chromosome 11q13 which encodes for MENIN (a protein with 610 amino acid)
    - 3Ps
        - Adenomas in pituitary
        - Hyperplasia of parathyroid
        - Adenomas less frequent in other endocrine glands
- Demography
    - Incidence ~ $1/10^6$ population
    - Mean age is 50 years
    - M = F
- Clinical
    - Multiple peptic ulcers including ulcers in the unusual sites with aggressive ulcer disease
    - Diarrhea, steatorrhea
    - 20% have associated MEN–1
    - Reduced healing response to acid inhibitory agents

- Laboratory
  - ↑ fasting and fed serum concentrations of gastrin
  - ↑ fasting gastrin concentration (> 200 pg/ml) after weight–based injection, or ↑↑ serum gastrin concentration in response to standard dose of IV calcium, sufficient to cause hypercalcemia
  - ↑↑ BAO > 10 mEq/hour, ↑ MAO with ratio of BAO / MAO > 60%
- Diagnostic imaging
  - Abdominal ultrasound, CT, MRI, octreotide scan, EUS
- Endoscopy
  - Thick gastric rugal folds in the body
  - Large multiple ulcers in unusual sites
  - Tumors
    - Linear nodular formation in the fundus and body (ECL hyperplasia)
    - In MEN–1 associated ZES, 1/3 have gastric carcinoid tumors

A 64–year old woman with a long history of recurrent, severe dyspepsia, presented with dyspepsia and diarrhea while on PPI. Her fasting gastrin concentration was 750 pg/ml. Describe your endoscopic findings and management.

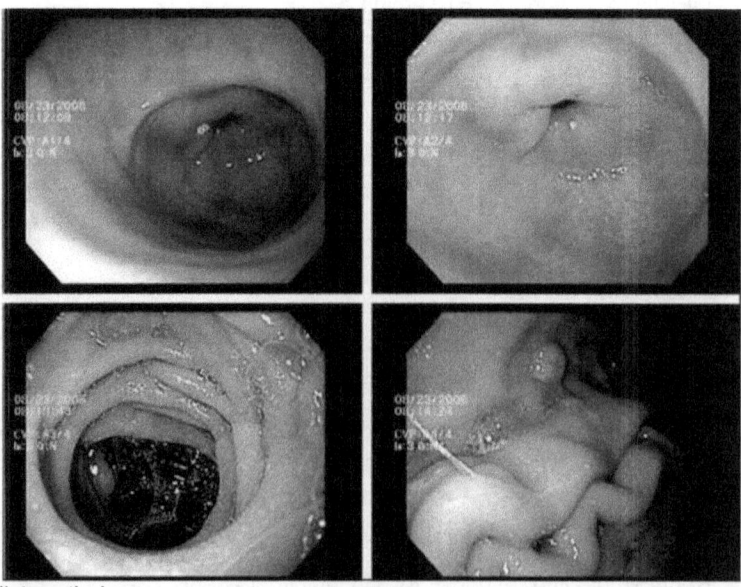

- Histopathology

- Gastrinoma
  - Site
    - 80% sporadic (gastrinoma triangle)
  - Usually multifocal
  - > ½ are malignant
- Thick gastric wall
- Hyperplasia of the parietal and chief cells, ECL cells
- Gastric foveolar epithelium
  - Long, tortuous (foveolar hyperplasia)
  - Lined by mucous cells
- Mucous glands
  - Cystic (dilated) mucous glands
- Parietal and chief cells are reduced (replaced by mucous glands)
- Inflammation – spectrum from none to ↑ intraepithelial lymphocytes
- No dysplasia

- Special studies (immunohistochemistry positive)

  - Gastrinoma
    - Gastrin
    - Chromogranin
    - Synaptophysin

  - Carcinoids
    - Chromogranin
    - vMAT–2

  - ECL cells
    - Chromogranin
    - vMAT–2
    - Gastrin, somatostatin and serotonin-negative

Abbreviation: vMAT–2, vesicular monoamine transporter isoform–2

GASTRIC MUCOSAL CALCINOSIS (GMC; aka aluminocalcinosis)

- ➤ Definition
    - o Extracellular deposition of calcium under the tips of the foveola or slightly deeper in the lamina propria of any part of the stomach

- ➤ Demography
    - o Occurs 0.1% of all gastric mucosal biopsies
    - o Adult females

- ➤ Clinical
    - o Asymptomatic
    - o Non-specific dyspepsia
    - o Associated conditions
        - Hypercalcemia and hyperphosphatemia (especially chronic renal failure, dialysis, and solid organ transplantation)
        - Gastric
            * Adenocarcinoma
            * Ulcer
            * CMV
        - Chemical gastropathy

- ➤ Endoscopy
    - o White plaques in any part of the stomach

- ➤ Histopathology
    - o Small (50–500 µm) extracellular, deposits of calcium
    - o Deposits at the tips of the foveola, or deeper in the lamina propria
    - o Basophilic refractile
    - o Hyperplasia of the foveola
        - Mucin deposits
    - o Reactive changes of the epithelium

- • Special studies
    - o Positive on calcium stains
        - von Kossa
        - Alizarin red

GASTRIC NEOPLASM

Gastric Polyps

> Demography

Types of polyps	% distribution
o Neoplasias	34
– Tublular Adenoma	17
– Tubulopapilliary adenoma	2
– Papillary adenoma	0.2
– Pyloric gland adenoma	0.4
– Adenocarcinoma	12
– Carcinoid tumor	3
– Tumor–like lesions	66
o Hyperplastic polyp	57
o Inflammatory fibroid polyp	5
o Heterotopia	3
o Peutz–jeghers polyp	0.6
o Juvenile polyp	0.3
o Cronkhite–Canada polyp	0.1
o Sites of polyps	
– Cardia	4
– Fundus	3
– Corpus	49
– Antrum	38
– Pylorus	2
– Anastomosis	4

> Classification

- o Epithelial polyp
  - Fundic gland polyp
  - Hyperplastic polyp
  - Adenomatous polyp
  - Hamartomatous polyp
    - Juvenile polyp
    - Peutz–Jegher syndrome
    - Cowden syndrome

- Polyposis syndrome (non–hamartomatous)
  - Juvenile polyp
  - Familial adenomatous polyposis
- Non–mucosal intramural polyps
  - Gastrointestinal stromal tumor (GIST)
  - Leiomyoma
  - Inflammatory fibroid polyp
  - Fibroma and fibromyoma
  - Lipoma
  - Ectopic pancreas
  - Neurogenic and vascular tumors
  - Neuroendocrine tumors (carcinoids)

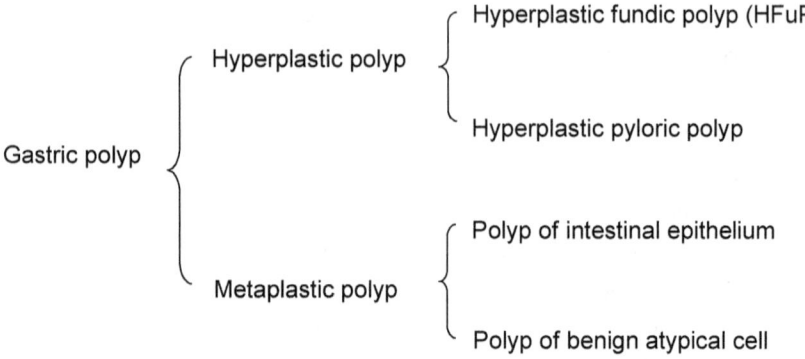

- Neuroendocrine tumors
  - Neuroma, neurofibroma
  - Granular cell tumor
  - Lipoma
  - Sarcoma
    - Neurosarcoma, fibrosarcoma
- Lymphatic
  - Mucosa associated lymphoid tissue (MALT) lymphoma

Hyperplastic Fundic Polyp (HFuP)
- Frequent in middle–aged female
- Originate from the fundic gland region without atrophy
- Hemispheric in shape
- Multiple
- Almost the same color as the surrounding mucosa
- No elongation of the foveolar epithelium
- Hyperplasia and cystic dilation of the fundic gland

Hyperplastic foveolar polyp (HFoP)
- Severe atrophy of fundic gland
- Pyloric antral region
- With stalk
- Single
- Red on the surface
- Marked hyperplasia of the foveolar epithelium
- Formation of the gland is seldom seen
- Edematous interstice
- Infiltration of inflammatory cells is sometimes seen

Tumor–like Lesion
- Fundic gland polyp
- Hyperplastic polyp
- Inflammatory fibroid polyp
- Brunner's gland heterotopia
- Pancreatic heterotopia
- Peutz–Jeghers polyp
- Cronkhite–Canada polyp
- Juvenile polyp
- Metaplastic polyp
  - Polyp of the intestinal epithelium
  - Polyp of benign atypical cell

- Causes and associations

- What are the causes of thick gastric folds seen on an upper GI series or EGD?
    - Folds are not actually thickened (i.e. barium study is wrong for varices)
    - Malignant — adenocarcinoma, lymphoma
    - Benign infiltration — granulomas, i.e. sarcoidosis, TB, Crohn's disease, severe gastritis (ethanol, *H. pylori*), Ménétrier's disease (hyperplasia) eosinophilic gastritis
    - Multiple gastric polyps (HNPCC, FAP, fundic gland polyps)
    - Hypersecretion (Zollinger–Ellison Syndrome)
    - Fundic varices
    - Worms

Abbreviations: EGD, esophagogastroduodenoscopy; FAP, familial adenomatous polyposis; GI, gastrointestinal; TB, tuberculosis

- Clinical

- Clinical situations or syndromes associated with fundic gland polyps.
    - *H. pylori* infection
    - PPI use
    - Hypergastrinemia
    - Familial adenomatous polyposis (FAP; Attenuated FAP, 0.5 – 1.0% lifetime risk of gastric cancer)
    - Cowden syndrome
    - Idiopathic

➤ Diagnostic imaging of gastric cancer

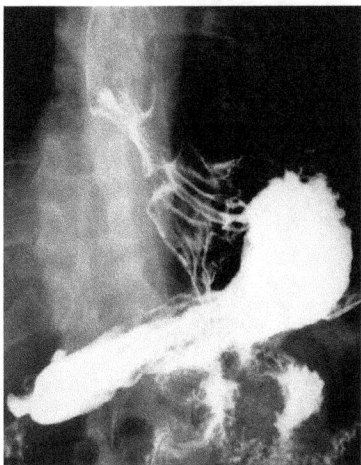

72-year old female presents with dysphagia and weight loss

Diffuse infiltration of the distal stomach, compatible with linitis plastica

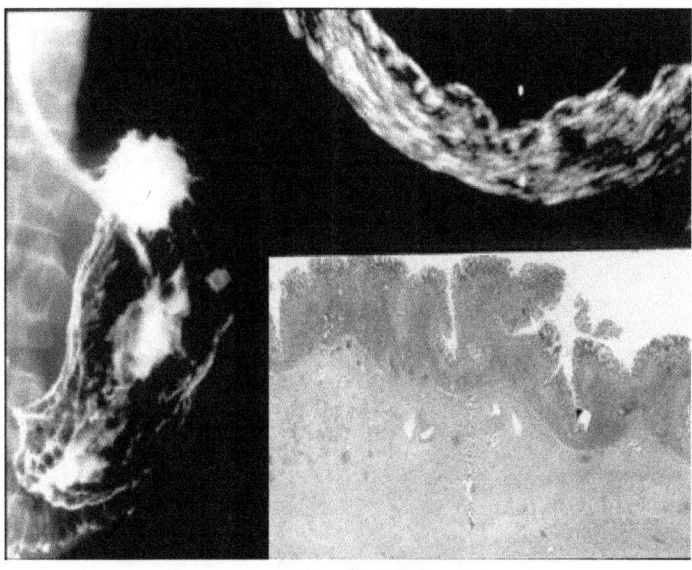

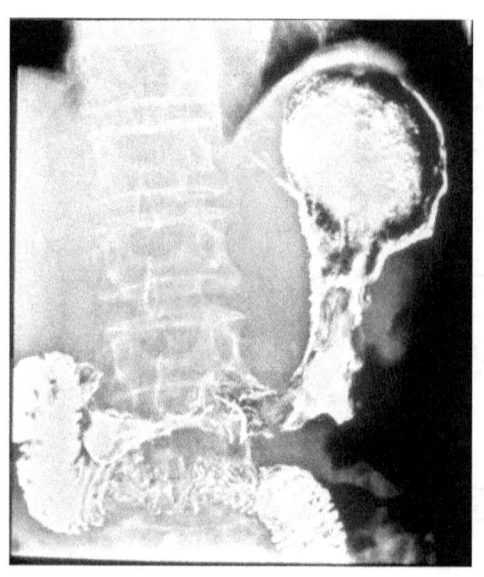

72–year old male presents with weight loss and early satiety

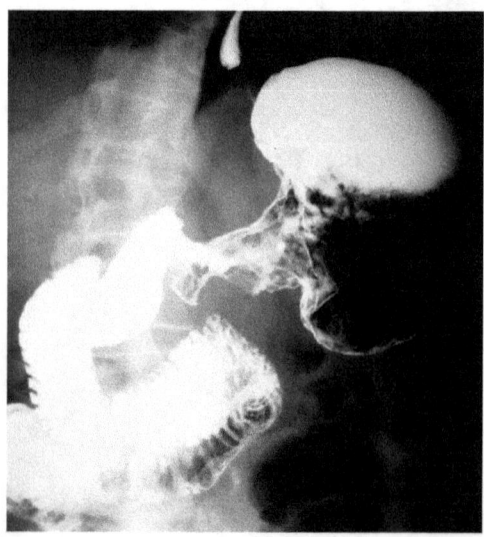

- Ulcer
  - Ulcerating mass
  - Lobulated contour of the mass
  - Irregular surface (mucosa–based lesions)
  - Nodular orifice and floor of ulcer
  - Tissues around the ulcer is nodular
  - Tissues around the ulcer stops suddenly with an acute angle to the normal gastric tissue
  - Ulcer crater does not project beyond the expected location of the gastric wall
  - Ulcer is placed asymmetrically in the surrounding tissue
  - Ulcer is wider than deep (width > depth)
- Converging folds
  - Clubbed
  - Fused
  - Tapered
  - Amputated
  - Stop before the ulcer crater
  - Lack of mucosal markings (gastric folds) usually indicates ulceration
- Carman meniscus sign
  - Lesser curve malignant ulcer
  - Nodular tissue around ulcer
  - Compression of both sides of the nodular surrounding tumor produces a half moon, crescent–shape (pathognomic for adenocarcinoma)
  - Usually single
- Infiltrative scirrhous tumor
  - Narrowing of the stomach ("leather bottle")
    - Mucosa nodular
    - Ulceration
  - Thick walls of fundus or body
  - Contour of stomach is irregular, scalloped
  - Stomach is not distensible
  - Long segment, with intact folds

- Metastatic gastric cancer
  - Serosal contours of the gastric wall are irregular and fuzzy
  - CT shows thickened wall
  - Lymphadenopathy
    - Parapancreatic
    - Para–aortic
    - Para–middle colic artery
  - Soft tissue masses
    - Spread to perigastric, omentum, peritoneum
  - Below renal pedicles:
    - Ovary (Krukenberg tumor)
    - Pancreas
    - Liver
- Lymphoma
  - May be solitary, or multiple masses
  - Mass
    - Ulcerative
    - Infiltration
    - Polypoid
    - Intraluminal fungating
  - May narrow stomach by infiltration
  - May be localized or extensive
  - Nodules (stomach; duodenum [crosses the pylorus])
  - Infiltration of the submucosa
  - Body of the stomach
    - Remains distendable (compliant)
    - No narrowing of the lumen
  - Thickened folds
  - CT shows lymphadenopathy of the perigastric and not below the renal pedicles

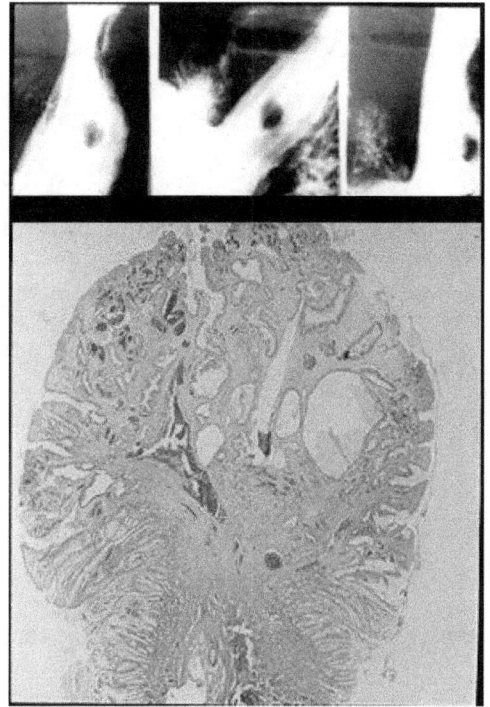

- ➢ Differential Diagnosis
  - o Focal foveolar hyperplasia
  - o Lymphatic follicles
  - o Giant folds
  - o Varioliform gastritis
  - o Extensive resection for cure
  - o If extensive resection is not possible (incomplete resection, locally or systemically advanced [metastatic] disease) → palliation
  - o Chemoradiation
  - o Endoscopic stents

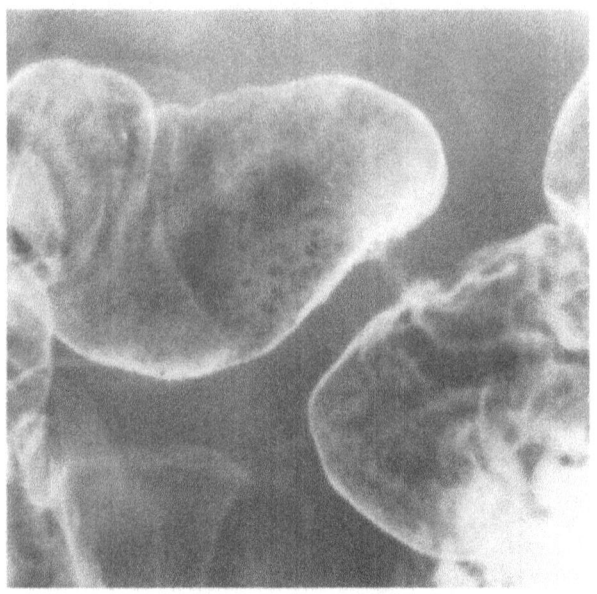

Dyspeptic 51–year old man, worried about having gastric cancer

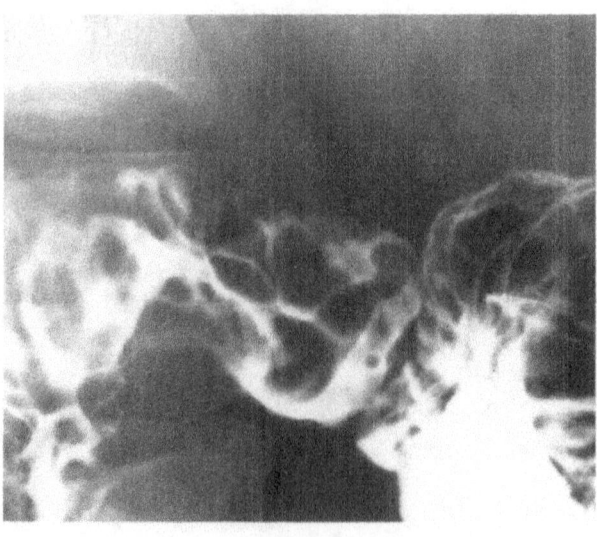

Nausea, indigestion, but no bleeding or weight loss in 60–year old woman

- Filling Defects
  - Benign tumors
    - Polyps
      - Fundic gland polyp
      - Hyperplastic
      - Hyperplastic, FAP
      - Adenoma
    - GIST
    - Lipoma
    - Other submucosal tumors
    - Ectopic pancreatic rest
  - Malignant tumors
    - Adenocarcinoma
    - Lymphoma
    - GIST
    - Metastases
  - Non–neoplastic
    - Fundus
      - Varices
      - Post–fundoplication
    - Antrum
      - Ectopic pancreatic rest
    - Anywhere
      - Bezoar
      - Acute erosive gastritis
- Pathology

Benign Gastric Ulcer

- Round or oval ulcer crater
- Hampton line (thin line of the normal mucosa around the ulcer crater)
- Multiple in ~ 15% (multiple ulcers are likely benign)
- Giant ulcer (> 3 cm) is not more likely to be malignant
- Ulcer collar (wider, submucosa around the ulcer, smooth, symmetrical collar of edematous)
- Sump ulcer (edema around the ulcer may form a mass effect around the ulcer, with sharp definition of edge with normal gastric wall, and shape that does not change with peristalsis)
  - Smooth, symmetrical folds running to edge of ulcer crater (i.e. cross the mound of surrounding, tapered edema)
  - No nodularity or clubbing of folds

- o Ulcer extends beyond the normal gastric contour
- o Usually in the lesser curve
- o Benign ulcer may penetrate or fistulizes forming abscess or perforates the pneumoperitonium
    - posterior wall, body or antrum
    - when on lower greater curve
        - ASA or NSAIDs
        - Carcinoma of the upper greater curve

- What are the causes of **thick gastric folds** seen on an upper GI series or EGD?
    - o Folds are not actually thickened (i.e. barium study is wrong in varices)
    - o Malignant — adenocarcinoma, lymphoma
    - o Benign infiltration — granulomas, i.e. sarcoidosis, TB, Crohn's disease, severe gastritis (ethanol, *H. pylori*), Ménétrier's disease (hyperplasia) eosinophilic gastritis
    - o Multiple gastric polyps (HNPCC, FAP, fundic gland polyps)
    - o Hypersecretion (Zollinger–Ellison Syndrome)
    - o Fundic varices
    - o Worms

- What are the EGD characteristics and pathological features of the 8 types of benign gastric polyps?

Polyp types	Location	Size	EGD	Pathological features	Comments
❖ Fundic gland (75%)	Fundus and upper body	< 1 cm	Smooth, glassy, transparent; usually multiple polyps are found	*Helicobacter pylori*-associated gastritis is rare	o Associated with PPI use, may regress o Dysplasia found in patients with FAP o Fundic gland polyp: distorted glands and microcysts lined by parietal and chief cells; no or minimal inflammation

Polyp type	Location	Size	EGD	Pathological features	Comments
❖ Hyper-plastic (20%)	Random, adjacent to the ulcers or stoma sites, or in the cardia if related to acid reflux	Generally, < 1 cm	Small polyps have smooth dome Large polyps are lobulated, and erosions are common	o Atrophic gastritis with intestinal metaplasia o *Helicobacter pylori-* associated gastritis (25%) o Dysplasia is rare (< 3%) and found in polyps < 2 cm	o *Hyperplastic* elongated, cystic, and distorted foveolar epithelium o Marked regeneration o Stroma with inflammation, edema, and smooth muscle hyperplasia
❖ Adenoma	*Incisura angularis*, found in the antrum than in the fundus	< 2 cm	Velvety, lobular surface; exophytic, sessile or pedunculated; usually solitary (82%)	o Atrophic gastritis with intestinal metaplasia o May be accompanied by coexistent carcinoma	o Dysplastic intestinal- or gastric-type epithelium o Variable architecture
❖ Inflammatory fibroid	Submucosal, found near the pyloric sphincter	Median 1.5 cm; generally < 3 cm	Single, firm, sessile Well-circumscribe Ulceration is common	o Pernicious anemia is commonly found; atrophic gastritis o Genetic mutations are common	o CD34⁺ spindled stromal cells, o Inflammatory cells o Thin-walled vessels in a myxoid stroma
❖ Peutz-Jeghers	Random	< 1 cm	Pedunculated with a velvety or papillary surface	o Risk of adenocarcinoma is rare in gastric polyps	
❖ Juvenile	Found more in the body than in the antrum	Variable	More rounded than hyperplastic polyps Superficial erosion Multiple	o Polyps may exclusively involve the stomach o Risk of adenocarcinoma is rare in gastric polyps	

FROM COMPETENCE TO EXCELLENCE
The Stomach

© A.B.R. Thomson

Polyp type	Location	Size	EGD	Pathological features	Comments
❖ Xanthoma	Antrum, lesser curvature, prepyloric	< 3 mm	o Can be multiple in group o Sessile o Pale-yellow o Nodule or plaque	o Chronic gastritis o No association with hyperlipidemia	o Xanthoma aggregates of lipid-laden macrophages in the lamina propria
❖ Pancreatic heterotopias	Antrum, prepyloric	0.2-4.0 cm	o Solitary o Dome-shaped with central dimple o Smooth surface	o Normal o Very rare instances of associated pancreatitis, islet-cell tumors, adenocarcinoma	o Normal components of the pancreatic parenchyma
❖ Gastrointestinal stromal tumor	Random, submucosal	Variable (median 6 cm)	o Well-circumscribed o Overlying mucosa may be ulcerated	o Normal o 25% are malignant o Risk of aggressive behaviour depends on size and mitotic count	o CD117+, CD34+ spindle cell or epithelioid cell tumor o Variable pattern mitoses, and stroma
❖ Carcinoid	Body and fundus	< 2 cm, larger if sporadic	o Hypergastrinemic lesions o Firm o Yellow, broad-based o Multiple o Sporadic lesions: large and single	o Autoimmune atrophic gastritis with intestinal metaplasia o Parietal cell hyperplasia in ZES o Normal mucosa if lesion is sporadic o Associated with - Hypergastrinemia - Autoimmune - Atrophic gastritis - ZES or MEN I	o Nodular proliferation of neuroendocrine cells > 500 μm in diameter

Abbreviations: EGD, esophagogastroduodenoscopy; FAP, familial adenomatous polyposis; MEN, multiple endocrine neoplasia; ZES, Zollinger-Ellison syndrome

Adapted from: Carmack, S. W., et al. Am J Gastroenterol. 2009.104(6): 524-532.; and Carmack, S. W., et al. Nat Rev Gastroenterol Hepatol. 2009.6(6): 331-341.

A 54–year old obese woman with "gas" and bloating following a fundoplication. Describe the endoscopic findings, give the most likely causes, and provide your management.

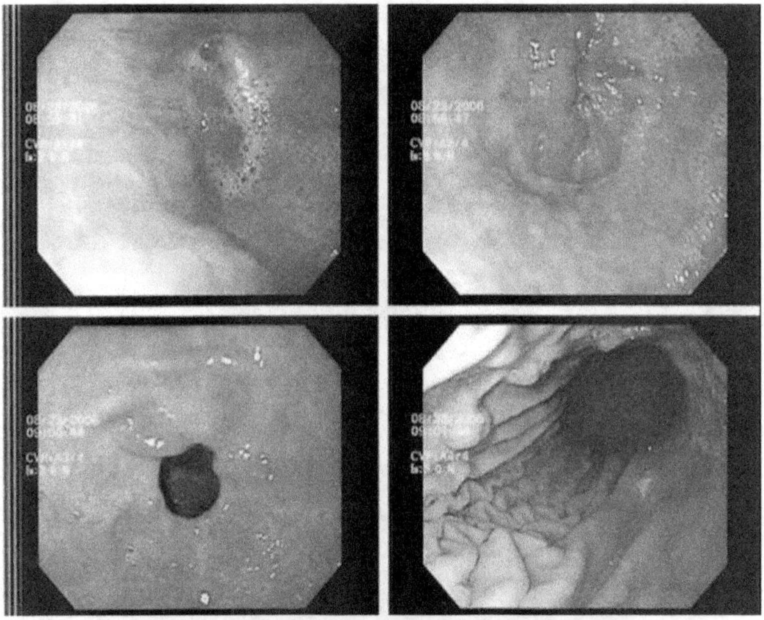

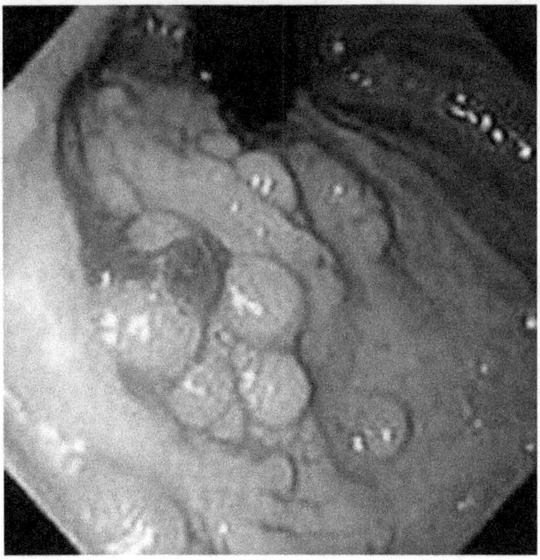

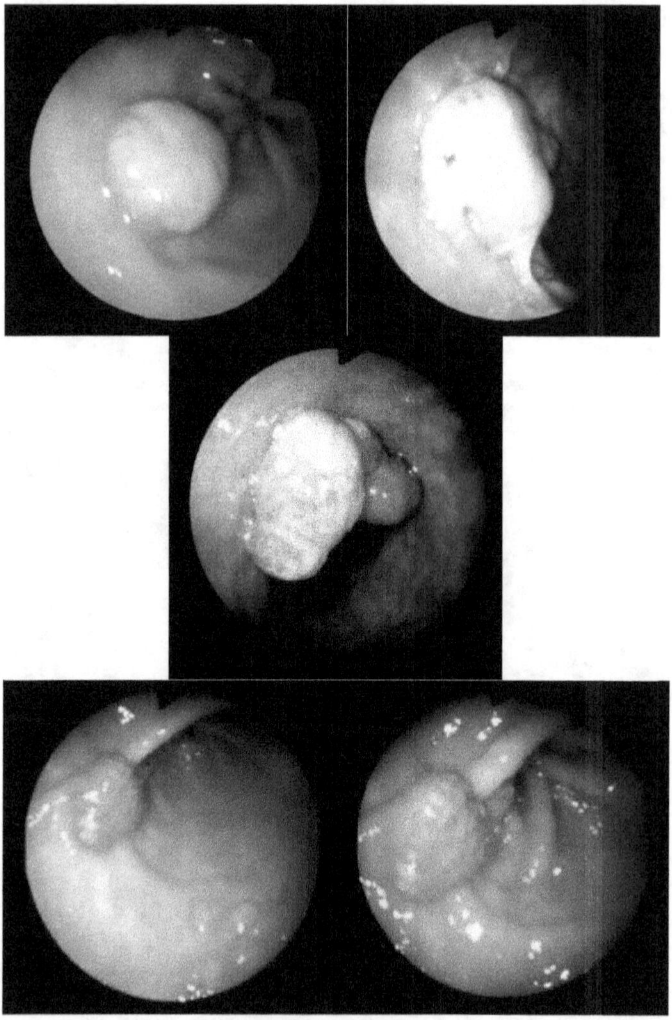

FROM COMPETENCE TO EXCELLENCE
The Stomach

© A.B.R. Thomson

296

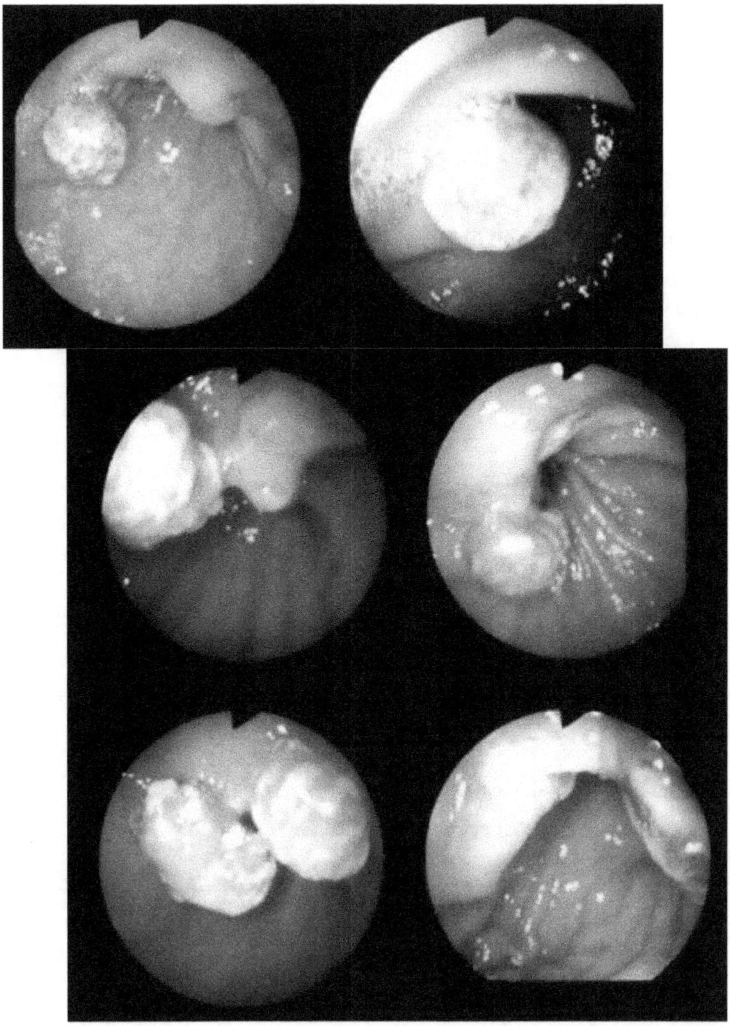

Fundic Gland Polyps

➢ Definition
   o "Fundic gland polyp" needs to be understood in its context: when the endoscopist reports fundic gland polyps, strictly speaking this means that there are polyps in the fundus or fundic gland area of the stomach. However, the term "fundic gland polyps" is sometimes used interchangeably with the term "fundic gland polyposis".
   o Hyperplasia of the oxyntic glands in the gastric body and fundus, as well as in the dilated fundic cysts
   o Oxyntic gland mucosa shows cystic dilation
   o Other gastric cells (parietal, ↓ chief, mucous neck cells)

➢ Demography
   o May now be the most common type of benign gastric polyps
   o Occurs in ~ 3% of EGDs
   o F > M, 1:3
   o Average age is 57 years
   o When associated with familial adenomatous polyposis (FAP)
      - Seen in ¼ to ¾ FAP patients
      - Usual age 20 – 30 years, rather than 40 – 70s
      - Risks
         ▪ Small risk of dysplasia (~ 25%)
         ▪ Large risk of colonic FAP

➢ Pathogenesis of non–FAP FGPs
   o Not associated with *H. pylori* infection or use of PPIs is controversial, since non–FAP FGP may disappear with stopping the use of PPIs

➢ Clinical
   o Asymptomatic

- Associations
- What are the clinical situations or syndromes associated with fundic gland polyps?
  - Hypergastrinemia
  - *H. pylori* infection
  - PPI use
  - FAP, attenuated FAP, 0.5 – 1.0% lifetime risk of gastric cancer
  - Cowden syndrome
  - Idiopathic

- Types

There are two types of fundic gland polyposis, sporadic or familial.

- Name the distinguishing features between sporadic versus familial fundic gland polyposis as defined by the above histopathology.

Features	Sporadic	Familial
Associated mutations		
– β–catenin gene	+	–
– APC gene (chromosome)	–	+
Dysplasia	3%	25%

  - Familial polyposis syndrome affecting the stomach
    - Autosomal dominant germline mutation of the APC gene on chromosome 5q21
    - Gastric polyps occur in ~ 30% of FAP cases
      - With no diclectin, 50 mg – 10 FGP (fundic gland polyps, 95%)
      - Adenoma of the stomach (5%) and duodenum
    - EGD *q* 1 – 2 years with age 50, then EGD *q* 5 years
  - Juvenile polyposis
    - Mutations in BMPRIA, 10q22.3, SMAD4, 18q21.1

- Differential diagnosis

> **SO YOU WANT TO BE A GASTROENTEROLOGIST!**
>
> Both fundic gland polyps without the associated long term use of PPIs as well as PPIs themselves may develop hyperplastic parietal cells and fundic cysts. What are the histological features determining the PPI–effect on the gastric mucosa?
> - Fundic gland polyps
>   - Parietal cells are hypertrophic and have cytoplasmic protrusions ("snouts")
> - PPI effects
>   - Parietal cells are flattened

- Progression to dysplasia and cancer
    - Fundic gland polyp (FGP) (~ 50%)
        - FGP > 1 cm, progression to GCa ~ 1% per year
        - FGP in FAP, dysplasia in 40%
    - Adenomas (10%)
        - Progress to GCa (*in situ*), 11% in 4 years
    - Ménétrier's disease
        - Progress to GCa in 15%
    - Previous partial gastrectomy
        - Especially Billroth II
        - Low risk of the development of stromal (marginal) ulcer > 25 years after surgery
    - Hyperplastic
        - Rare progression to GCa

- Endoscopy
    - Clusters of multiple, small (1 – 7 mm), sessile, shiny polyps in gastric fundus or body
    - Color of the surface looks like the same as surrounding mucosa
    - Body or fundus
    - May be single, or multiple in clusters, hundreds of FGPs covering the mucosa ("syndromic" may show LGD)
    - Small (< 7mm) sessile, hemispheric

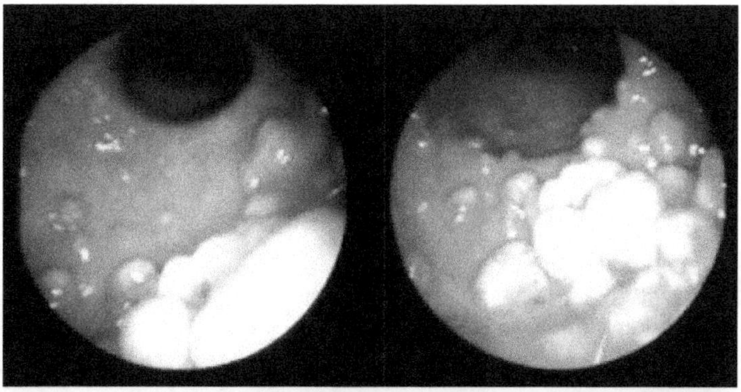

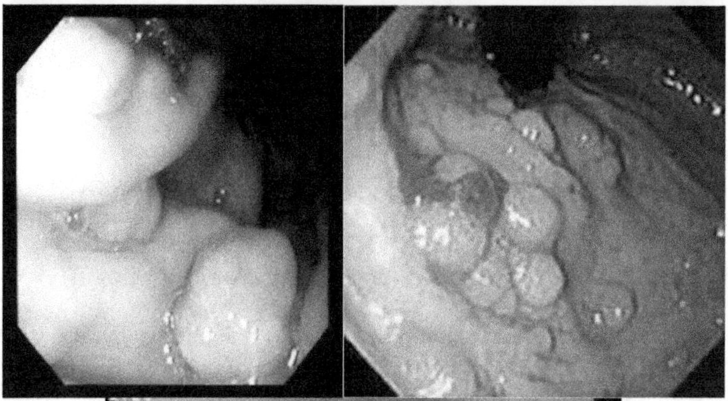

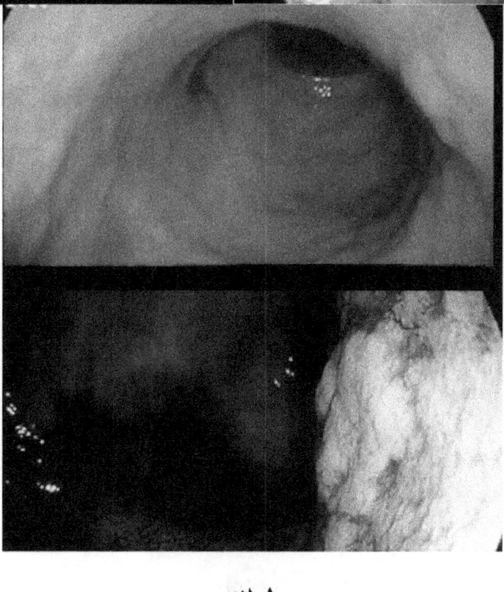

FROM COMPETENCE TO EXCELLENCE
The Stomach

© A.B.R. Thomson

- Histopathology
  - Dilated cystic glands lined by parietal cells and chief cells
  - Hypertrophic parietal cells
  - Dilated glands
  - Protrusions of the apical cytoplasm
  - Surrounding mucosa si normal
  - Hyperplasia of the oxyntic mucosa
    - Dilated fundic glands, or microcysts
    - Budding of the glands
  - Cysts in the fundus
  - Lined by flattened cells:
    - Parietal and chief cells
    - Mucus neck cells
  - Microcysts lined by flattened parietal cells
  - Dilated cysts lined by parietal and chief cells
  - Microcysts lined by flattened parietal cells
  - Minimal inflammation
  - Normal surrounding mucosa (unlike hyperplastic polyposis)

  - Small, sessile, epithelial polyp with a mixture of fundic and foveolar glands, many of which are cystic
  - Normal and dilated oxyntic (fundic or body) glands
  - No nuclear enlargement or other signs of cellular atypia
  - Small, round, sessile lesions in the gastric fundus, made up of fundic and foveolar cystically dilated glands

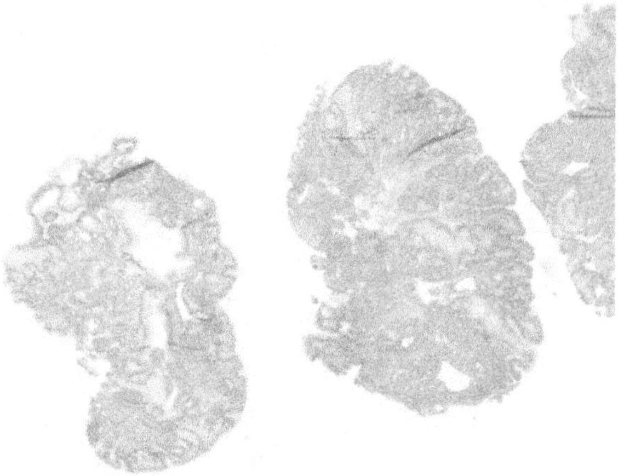

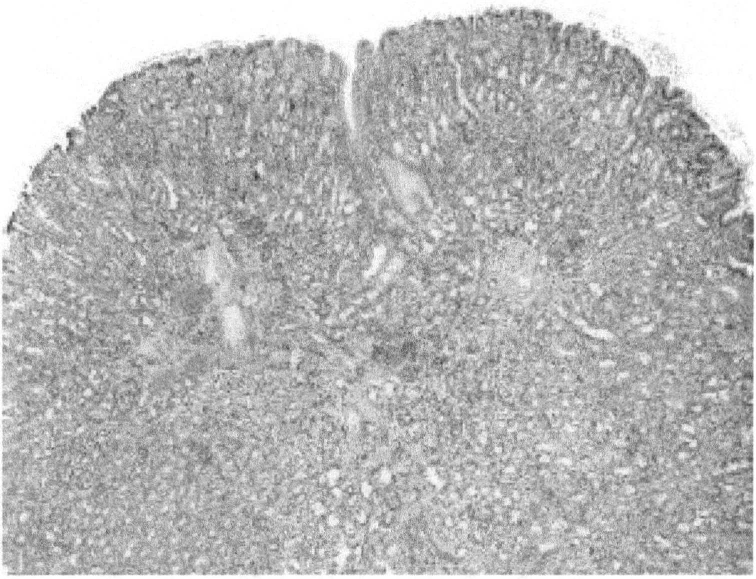

Provided kindly by Dr. Aducio Thiesen, University of Alberta

FROM COMPETENCE TO EXCELLENCE
The Stomach

© A.B.R. Thomson

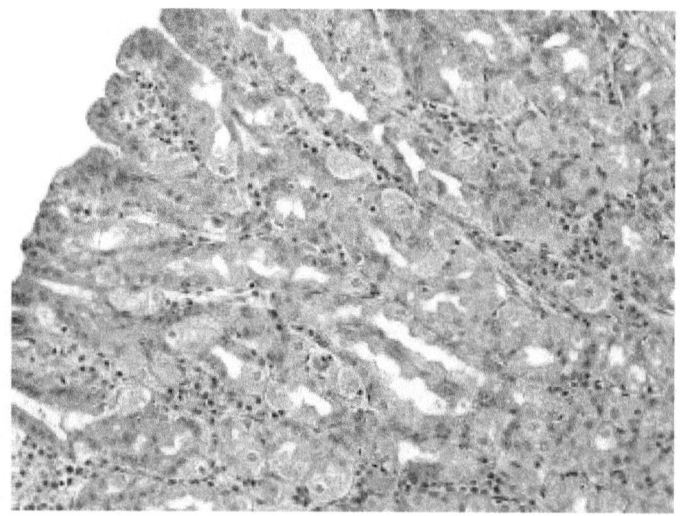

Provided kindly by Dr. Aducio Thiesen, University of Alberta

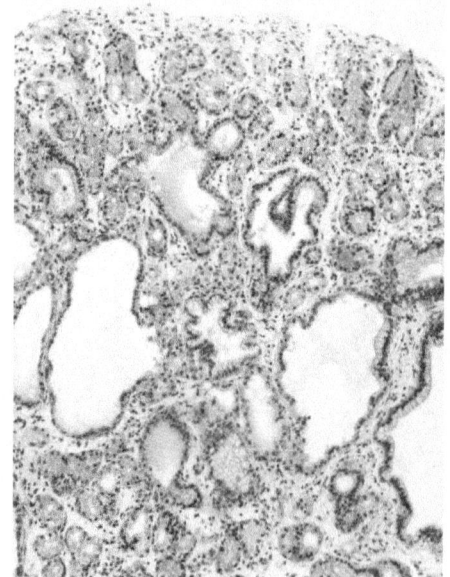

- o Shortening of the gastric pits
- o Cystic dilation

- Special studies (molecular)
  - Sporadic FGP
    - β–catenin mutation (90%)
  - FAP–associated
    - APC somatic gene mutation (50%)

Look towards the future:
- Some studies have shown as many as half of the patients with non–syndromic FAP may have APC gene mutations.
- Dysplasia may be found in FGP: sporadic (not associated with FAP), < 1%; associated with FAP, ~ 25%.
- What is the risk of FGP becoming malignant? In the words of B. Bhattacharya, in Gastrointestinal and Liver Pathology (Elsevier), edited by Iacobuzio-Donahue, C. A., et al, 2012, page 115, "....FGP with low grade dysplasia carry virtually no risk of developing carcinoma [FGP]."

Gastric Neuroendocrine Tumors (NET)

➤ Definition
  - Neoplasm of the neuroendocrine syndrome (no longer called "carcinoid" tumors)

➤ Demography
  - Incidence is $1/10^5$
  - Represents ~ 1% of gastric neoplasms (adenocarcinoma, ~ 95%)
  - Gastric carcinoid represents ~ 1/3 of all GI NET and ~ 6% of all NETs
  - Age and gender

	Gender	Mean age at diagnosis
WHO		
- Type I	F > M	60s
- Type II	M = F	40s
- Type III	M > F	50s

WHO Type

Demography	I	II	III
o Gender	F > M	M = F	M > F
o Mean age at diagnosis	60s	40s	50s

- Classification
  - Well–differentiated tumors
    - Carcinoid tumors of the gastrointestinal tract
    - Endocrine pancreatic tumors
  - Poorly differentiated neuroendocrine carcinomas (based on):
    - Tumor localization
    - Tumor size
    - Angioinvasion
    - Hormone production
    - Histological grade
    - Proliferative index

Stomach: Clinicopathologic Classification of Neuroendocrine Tumors

- ❖ Well–differentiated tumor (carcinoid)
  Benign behavior: non–functioning, confined to the mucosa, submucosa, non–angioinvasive, ≤ 1 cm in size
  - o ECL cell tumors of the corpus, fundus–associated with hypergastrinemia, chronic atrophic gastritis (CAG, often with pernicious anemia) or MEN–1 syndrome
  - o Serotonin–producing tumor
  - o Gastrin–producing tumor
  - o Uncertain behavior: confined to the mucosa–submucosa, > 1cm in size or angioinvasive
  - o ECL cell tumors with/without CAG or MEN1 syndrome or sporadic gastrin, somatostatin or serotonin-producing tumors (rare)

- ❖ Well–differentiated endocrine carcinoma (malignant carcinoid)
  Low grade malignant: extending beyond submucosa, angioinvasive or metastasis
  - o Non–functioning
    - ECL cell carcinoma, usually sporadic, rarely in CAG or MEN–1 syndrome
    - Gastrin, somatostatin or serotonin–producing tumors (rare)

- Functioning
    - Gastrinoma
    - Serotonin–producing carcinoma with carcinoid syndrome
    - ECL cell carcinoma with atypical carcinoid syndrome
    - ACTH–producing carcinoma with Cushing syndrome

❖ Poorly differentiated endocrine carcinoma
  High grade malignant (small to intermediate cell) carcinoma
    - Usually non–functioning, occasionally with Cushing syndrome

➤ Clinical
  - Asymptomatic (30%)
  - Aggressive peptic ulcer disease
  - Diarrhea
  - Carcinoid syndrome (~ 10%, especially type III [sporadic])

- Give the clinical features of neuroendocrine tumors suggesting "carcinoid syndrome".

    - Hormones
        - Serotonin
        - Histamine
        - Substance P
    - Clinical
        - Head
            - Headache
        - Face
            - Flushing
            - Edema
        - Lung
            - Bronchospasm (asthma)
        - GI
            - Diarrhea

➤ Differential diagnosis
  - Glomus tumor of the stomach is the major differential for gastric carcinoid, since both shows certain uniform round cells with centrally placed hyperchromatic nuclei

- What are the features distinguishing gastric NETs from glomus tumor?

	NET	Glomus tumor
o Nuclear chromatin	- Fine - Granules	- Course - Lumps
o Cytoplasmic color	- Pale pink (eosinophilic)	- Amphophilic
o Immunohistochemistry		
- Chromogranin	+	-
- Synaptophysin	+	-
- Actin	-	+

- ➤ WHO types

	WHO types of NET		
	I	II	III
o Size	< 1 cm	> 1 cm	> 2 cm
o Multiple	+	-	-
o ↑ gastrin	+	+	+
o Gastric H+	↓	↑	↑
o Aggressive nature	+	++	+++
o Carcinoid syndrome	-	+	++

- ➤ Endoscopy
  - o Small to large submucosal tumors in the body (type I) or fundus and body (type II) and prepyloric (type III)
  - o Central dimple ("umbilication") in the larger tumors with focal erosion
  - o Peptic ulcer disease, if there is hypergastrinemia plus hypersecretion

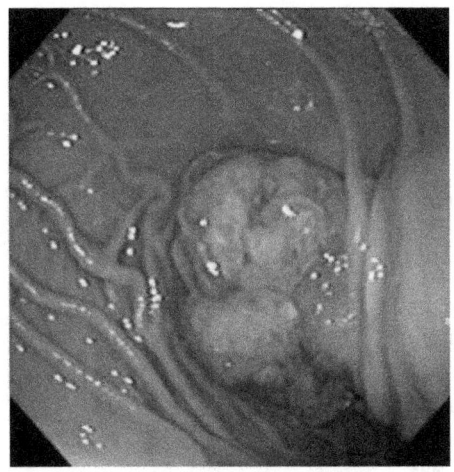

Metastatic tumor (often from the breast, not prostate)

- Histopathology
  - Cords or nests of NE cells
  - Surrounding mucosa shows autoimmune gastritis

- ❖ Neuroendocrine tumors (NETs)
  - Monomorphic roots, ribbons, trabecular collections of round cells
  - Nuclei
    - Central
    - Fine chromatin ("salt and pepper")
  - Cytoplasm
    - Clear

- ❖ Glomus tumors
  - Small round cells
  - Nuclei
    - Central
    - Hyperchromatic
    - Lumpy, course chromatin
  - Cytoplasm
    - Pale, eosinophilic

- o Mucosal clusters ("nests") of small, round cells
- o Organization of clusters
  - Solid
  - Trabecular
  - Ribbon–like
- o Morphometric
- o Centrally placed nuclei
- o Chromatin
  - Fine granules
  - Hyperchromatic
  - Speckled ("salt and pepper") appearance
- o Mitotic figures are rare
- o Cytoplasm
  - Amphophilic
- o Mass lesion
- o Distinguish from type IV endocrine heterotopia
- o Tinge nests of endocrine cells in the submucosa and muscularis
- o Stromal response
- o Neuroendocrine tumor cells seen as trabeculae, tubules, rosettes

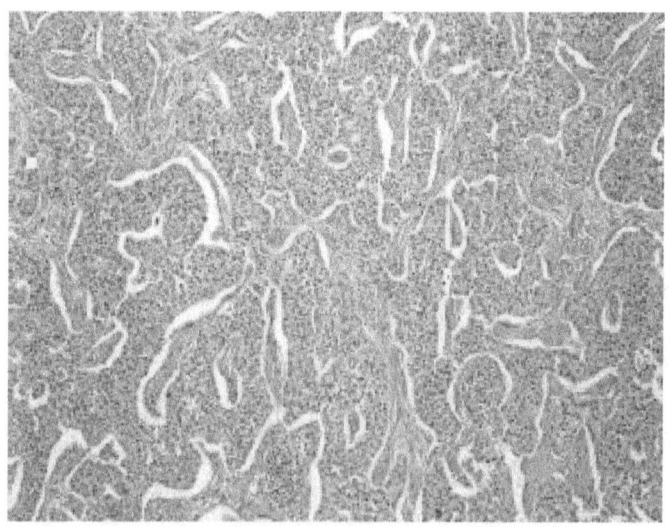

Provided kindly by Dr. Aducio Thiesen, University of Alberta

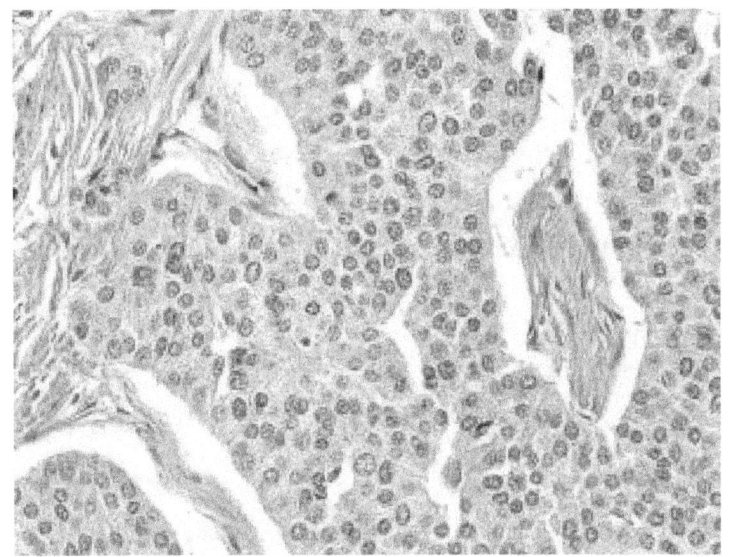

Provided kindly by Dr. Aducio Thiesen, University of Alberta

- Special studies (immunostains)
    - To diagnose NET
        - Chromogranin A
        - Synaptophysin
        - Neuron-specific enolase (NSE)
        - Pancytokeratin markers
    - To determine primary site of origin
        - Gastroduodenal
            - PDX1-positve
            - CDX2- / TTF-negative
    - Specific hormones, i.e. gastrin

- Give the special immunostains to diagnose benign mesenchymal tumors.

Tumors	Marker
o KIT-negative GISTs	- PDGFRA
o Schwannoma	- S-100
o Leiomyoma	- Desmin
o Solitary fibrous tumor	- BCI-2
o Perineuroma	- EMA
	- Glut-1
	- Claudin

Abbreviations: PDGFRA, platelet-derived growth receptor alpha; EMA, endomysial antibody

- Pharmacodynamic action of synthetic somatostatin and octreotide in the human GI tract
    o Inhibition of neuroendocrine secretion
        - Gut peptides
        - Pancreatic peptides
    o Inhibition of exocrine secretion
        - Salivary gland (amylase)
        - Stomach (acid, pepsin, intrinsic factor)
        - Pancreas (enzymes, bicarbonate)
        - Liver (bile flow)
        - Inhibition of intestinal transport
        - Absorption of glucose, fat, amino acids
    o Inhibition of motility
        - Stimulated intestinal secretion
        - Stomach (late phase of gastric emptying)
        - Gallbladder contraction
        - Small intestinal transit time
        - Early gastric emptying
        - Migrating motor complex

- Stimulation of motility
  - Wedged hepatic venous pressure
  - Portal pressure
- Inhibition of splanchnic hemodynamics
  - Splanchnic blood flow

➢ Prognosis

			5–year survival rate
o Type	I		> 90%
	II		~ 50%
	III		Intermediate
o Extent	Local		~ 70%
	Regional		~ 65%
	Distant (metastatic)		~ 25%
o Size	> 2 cm		
o Mitosis	↑		

Gastric Adenomas

➢ Definition
  - Localized polypoid growth of dysplastic gastric epithelium, which has the developing into gastric adenocarcinoma

➢ Demography
  - ~ 10% of gastric polyps
  - M > F, 2:1
  - Peak incidence
    - 70 years
  - Single usually (but may be multiple)
  - Larger (> 1 cm)
  - Antrum

- Pathogenesis
  - Molecular changes
    - APC, kRas and Tp53 genes
  - However
    - Gastric adenomas are not common precursors to adenocarcinoma
    - Sequence of gastric adenoma → adenocarcinoma is not well proven for stomach
  - May be associated with the following conditions:
    - FAP
    - Intestinal metaplasia
    - Atrophic gastritis

- Types
  - Intestinal type
  - Pyloric gland
  - Foveolar gland type

- Differential diagnosis
  - Hyperplastic polyps
  - Pyloric gland adenoma (especially difficult to distinguish from gastric foveolar type adenoma)
  - Reactive epithelial change

- Endoscopy
  - Polypoid mass in the antrum or body
  - Pedunculated, or polypoid

http://www.pathologyatlas.com

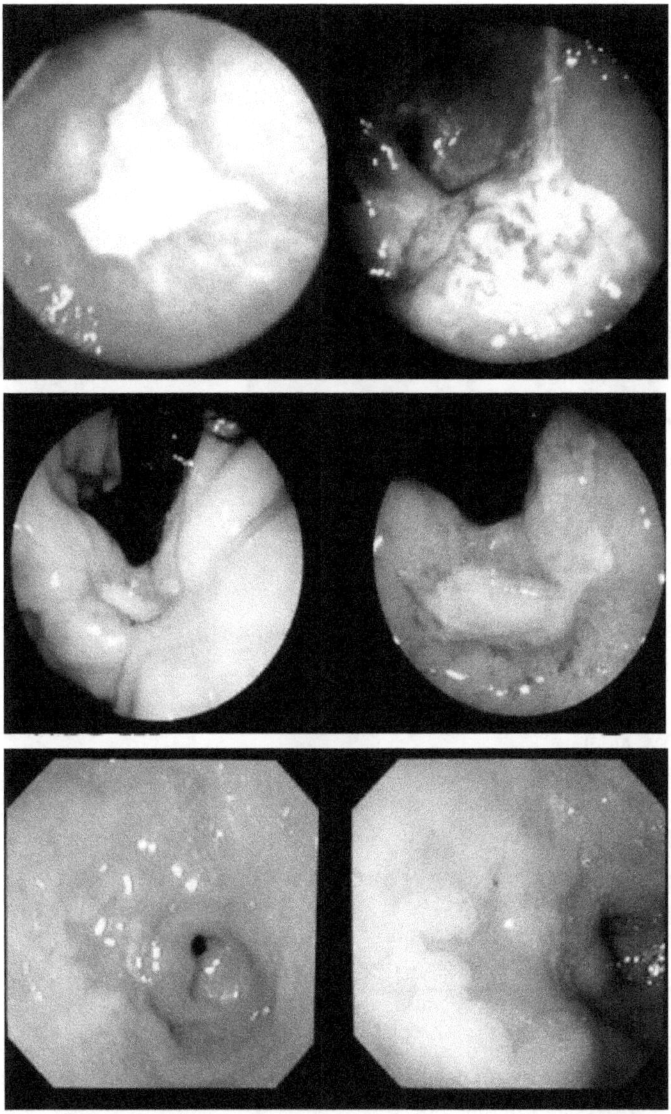

FROM COMPETENCE TO EXCELLENCE
The Stomach

© A.B.R. Thomson

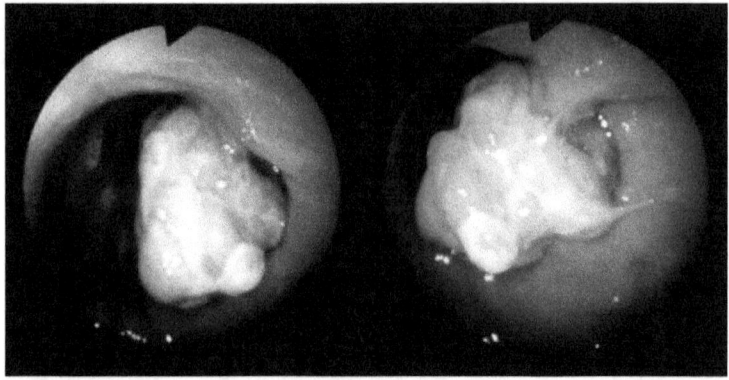

- ➢ Histopathology
    - Gastric type — gastric foveolar epithelial cells
    - Intestinal type — goblet cells
        - Paneth cells
    - Intervening mucosa
        - Atrophic intestinal metaplasia
    - High grade dysplasia
        - Glands
            - Crowded
            - Cribriform
        - Nuclei
            - Stratification
            - Loss of polarity
    - Mucin cap
    - Risk of development of adenocarcinoma from
        - Adenoma, > 30%
        - Surrounding non–adenomatous mucosa, ~ 30%

	Types	Intestinal	Foveolar
o	Commonality	More	Less
o	Glands		
	- Goblet, Paneth cells	+	-
	- Foveolar epithelial cells	-	+
o	Neutral mucin		
	- MUC 5AC	-	+
	- MUC 6	-	-
o	Associated intestinal metaplasia, or atrophy	+	-
o	High risk of HGD or adenocarcinoma	+++	+

Pyloric Gland Adenomas

- Definition
  - Localized polypoid growth of dysplastic gastric epithelium, with differentiation of the pyloric glands, which have the risk of developing into gastric adenocarcinoma

- Demography
  - F:M: ~ 5:1
  - Mean age of diagnosis, > 70 years

- Pathogenesis
  - Similar to intestinal–type adenomas
  - Chromosomal gain
    - Gain
      - 8, 9q, 11q, 20
    - Loss
      - 5q, 6, 10, 13

- Differential diagnosis
  - Gastric foveolar adenoma
    - Expresses MUC 5 AC, but not MUC 6
    - Surrounding mucosa is normal (no gastritis as in gastric pyloric gland adenoma)
  - Hyperplastic polyp
    - No cytoplasmic ground glass appearance
  - Reactive epithelial changes
    - No cytoplasmic eosinophilic to amphophilic colon
    - No basal nuclei

- Endoscopy
  - 3/4 in the gastric body
  - Mean size is 16 mm
  - Pedunculated

- Histopathology
  - Tubular glands lined by cuboidal or columnar epithelial cells
  - Cytoplasm
    - Ground glass
    - Eosinophilic
    - Amphophilic

- Nuclei basally located
- Cells are "ground glass", eosinophilic (red) or amorphic
- No mucin cap
- May be associated low-grade or high grade dysplasia, or adenocarcinoma
- Surrounding area (non-lesional)
  - *H. pylori* gastritis, ~ 40%
  - Autoimmune gastritis, ~ 1/3
  - Chemical gastritis, ~ 1/5

- Special studies
  - Positive immunostains for MUC 5AC and MUC 6

Polyposis Syndromes
- FAP, attenuated FAP, PJS lymphoma, CCS (Cronkhite–Canada syndrome: GI polyposis, pigmented skin, atrophy of nails)
- Gastritis cystica glandularis
- Polyps appear histopathologically similar to hyperplastic polyps

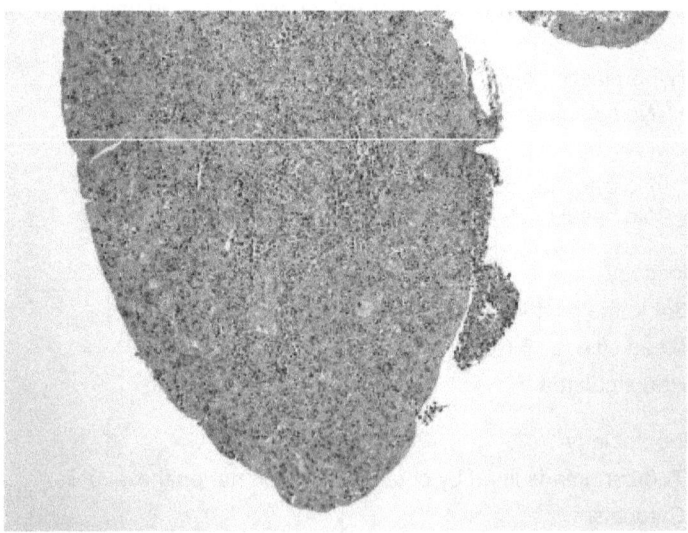

Provided kindly by Dr. Aducio Thiesen, University of Alberta

Gastritis Cytica Polyposa

- Definition
  - "Polypoid gastric lesions occurring near the gastroenteromy stroma, characterized by dilated cystic glands in the mucosa and submucosa" (Bhattacharya, B. In Gastrointestinal and Liver Pathology, Elsevier 2012, page 117)

- Demography
  - Usually men > 70 years and 30 – 40 years after partial gastric resection

- Clinical features
  - Non-specific symptoms after gastric surgery

- Diagnostic imaging
  - Multiple masses near the gastric stoma

- Endoscopy
  - Mass or masses near gastric stroma
  - Mass or masses may slow erosions
  - 1 – 3 cm in size
  - Soft, sessile
  - May surround the stoma

- Histopathology
  - Features of a mucosal prolapse
  - Thick wall of stomach
  - Cystic glands from a dilated pyloric–like glands
  - Present in the mucosa, submucosa, muscularis propria
  - Foveolar hyperplasia with changes in the surface epithelium
    - No pleomorphism
    - No desmoplasia in the stroma
  - Chronic inflammation and fibrosis
    - Lamina propria
    - Submucosa

- o Muscle bundles are characterized by:
  - Thick
  - Splayed
  - Close to surrounding cystic glands
- o Remember the post-surgical stomach
  - ↓ parietal cells (antrectomy → ↓ gastrin → ↓ parietal cells)
  - Chronic gastritis
  - Edema
  - Intestinal metaplasia or dysplasia

Hyperplastic polyps (HP)

➢ Definition
  - o Long, dilated and tortuous gastric foveolar epithelium, associated with lamina propria inflammation and edema, as well as foci of regeneration, intestinal metaplasia, dysplasia or cancer

➢ Demography
  - o ~ 3% of EGDs
  - o Slightly, F > M
  - o Age > 60 years

➢ Pathophysiology
  - o May be related to *H. pylori* infection, and use of PPIs
  - o In some patients associated with genetic changes, point mutation in codon D of the K-Ras oncogene

➢ Clinical
  - o Asymptomatic
  - o Non-specific symptoms
  - o If large and pedunculated, there is obstruction of the pylorus
  - o Symptoms and signs of associations
    - Those listed above
    - Post-transplantation
    - Post-partial gastrectomies for peptic ulcers

> Clinical Tips
> - In patients with suspected gastric hyperplastic polyp, always biopsy the surrounding mucosa, which may contain intestinal metaplasia (37%), dysplasia (2%), or synchronous or metachronous carcinoma (~ 5% in 5 years)

- Differential diagnosis
  - Distinguish hyperplastic foveolar from the following:
    - Goblet cells
    - Signet ring cells
    - Fundic gland
    - Hereditary
      - Peutz–Jeghers (PJ)
      - Juvenile
      - Cronkite–Canada
      - Cowden disease
    - Ménétrier's disease
  - Other types of benign polyps
  - Gastritis cystica glandularis
- Endoscopy
  - Antrum > body (60% vs 30%)
  - Single > multiple (80% vs 20%)
  - Size
    - Mean: 10 mm
  - Sessile > pedunculated
  - Surface
    - Smooth
    - Shining
    - Lobulated
  - Small to large (> 100 cm)
  - Sessile or pedunculated
  - Usually in the antrum (no inflammation in MD)

- Histopathology
  - Foveolar epithelium
    - Long, tortuous
    - Dilated
    - Branched
    - Prominent
  - Inflammatory cells in the lamina propria
  - May contain foci of the intestinal metaplasia (16%), dysplasia (4%), or signet ring carcinoma (< 1%)
  - When hyperplastic polyp is associated with erosion, may show reactive changes of ↓ mucin, hyperchromatic nuclei with prominent nucleoli
  - Pronounced regenerative changes with inflammation (not seen in MD)
  - Bundles of smooth muscles from muscularis mucosa into the lamina propria of the polyps
  - Non–involved mucosa may show chronic atrophy plus intestinal metaplasia (85%); have biopsy appearing mucosa (inflammatory polyp, regenerative polyp, focal or polypoid)
  - Infectious gastritis (*H. pylori*, CMV)
  - Fundic gland polyps (4x more common than hyperplastic polyp)
  - Long, dilated, tortuous foveolar epithelium
  - Contains neutral mucin
  - Lamina propria
    - Inflammation
      - Lymphoplasmacytes
      - Lymphoid aggregates
      - Eosinophils
    - Edema
  - Surrounding foci in non–polypoid mucosa (> 85%)
    - Regeneration
    - Intestinal metaplasia (37%)
    - Dysplasia (2%)
    - Adenocarcinoma is synchronous or metachronous (~ 5% in 5 years)
  - Other associations
    - *H. pylori*
    - Chemical gatropathy
    - Autoimmune gastritis (12%)
    - CMV gastritis
    - Gastric antral vascular ectasia (GAVE)

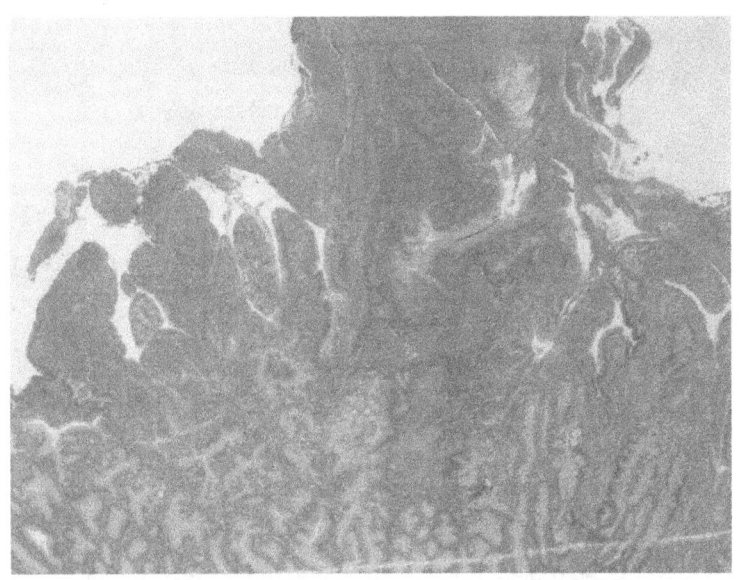

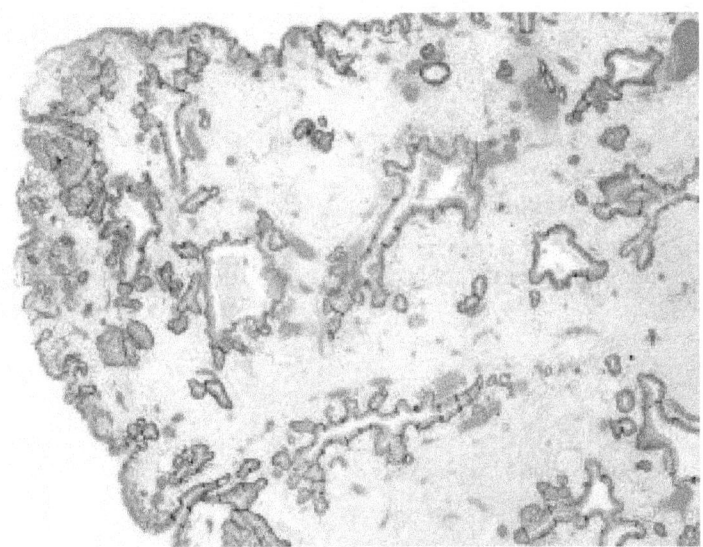

Provided kindly by Dr. Aducio Thiesen, University of Alberta

- Special studies
    - Mucin in the epithelium of foveola
        - Neutral
            - Hyperplastic polyps
        - Acidic
            - Goblet cells
            - Signet ring cells (cancer)
    - Immunohistochemistry
        - ↑ expression of p53 and Ki–67 in dysplasia

Pathology Tips
- Peutz–Jeghers polyps are usually easy to recognize because of their characteristic smooth muscle arborization, but in the stomach, this feature may be absent.
- Gastritis cystica glandular (GCG) contains foveolar hyperplasia, but can be easily distinguished from hyperplasia
    - GCG is usually associated with surgical gastric resections, and mucosal prolapse
    - Dilated glands are often in the submucosa or muscularis propria, rather than in the mucosa
---

➤ Treatment
- Endoscopic resection
- Be certain to biopsy the normal–appearing surrounding non–polypoid mucosa
- Treat the associated *H. pylori* infection (~ 25%)
- Beware of the risk of synchronous or metachronous risk of gastric adenocarcinoma (no guidelines available on surveillance)

Gastric Foveolar Adenoma

➤ Differentials
- Gastric epithelial dysplasia
- Reactive epithelial change
- Pyloric gland adenoma
- Hyperplastic polyp

- Endoscopy
  - Sessile or pedunculated
  - Usually in gastric antrum
- Histopathology
  - Intestinal–type
    - Goblet or Paneth cells (intestinalization)
    - Atrophic intestinal metaplasia
  - Foveolar–type
    - Foveolar epithelial cells containing neutral mucin (mucin cap)
    - Express MUC5AC
    - Less likely than intestinal type to develop dysplasia or adenocarcinoma (in intestinal–type adenomas larger than 2 cm)

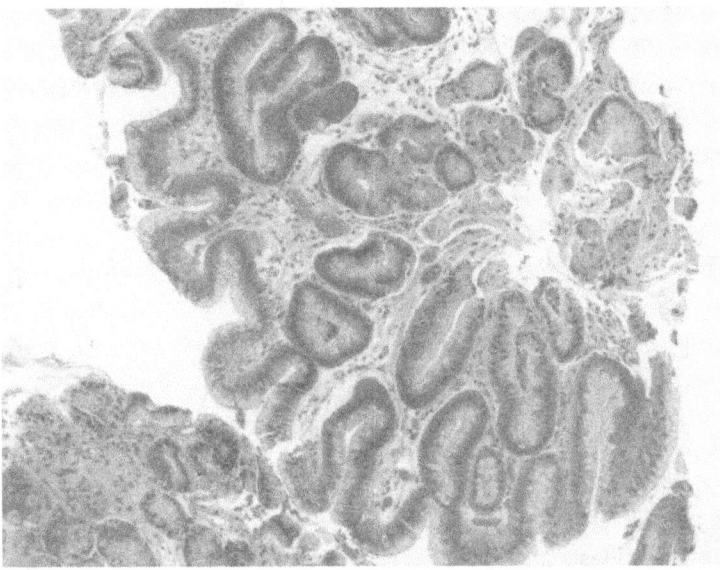

GASTRIC ADENOCARCINOMA

- Demography
  - Common worldwide
  - 2nd most common cancer
  - 1st most common cause of cancer deaths
  - M > F, 2:1
  - Age > 40 years
  - More common in Japan, S. America, parts of Asian mainland
  - $8/10^5$ in North America
  - Higher in Japan, some parts of China, Chile, Peru
  - Lower incidence in Caucasians and in females
  - Cause of more than ¾ million deaths annually
  - 2nd most common fatal malignancy: 14th most common cause of death
  - Changing population structure will result in increased frequency in developing world despite decrease in incidence rate
  - Survival rate less is than 15% in 5 years

- Pathological types (Lauren Classification)

Features	Intestine	Diffuse
Incidence	↓	steady
Low risk areas	-	+
Worse prognosis	-	+
Risk factors diet/environment	+	-
Gland–like tubular structures	+	-
Singly invasive tumor cells	-	+
Linitis plastica	-	+

  - Another classification
    - Proximal cardia, GE junction
    - Distal fundus, body, antrum
    - Incidence
      - Proximal ↑
      - Distal ↓

- Compare and contrast the intestinal– with the diffuse–type of gastric cancer.

Characteristic	Intestinal–type	Diffuse–type
o Clinical	– Comparable	▪ Comparable
o Morphology	– Cohesion, tubular structures	▪ Loss of cohesion ▪ Signet ring cells
o Epidemiology	– High-risk areas	▪ Low-risk areas
o Pathogenesis	– Precursor lesions	
o Molecular Profile	– Depending on the studied population	▪ Type of alteration partly similar

- Pathological conditions associated with gastric cancer
  - Adenomatous gastric polyps (10% focal malignancy)
  - Chronic atrophic gastritis (RR: 18)
  - H. pylori gastritis with atrophy (RR ~ 5)
  - Gastric remnant (RR ~ 1.4)
  - Pernicious anemia (RR ~ 3)
  - Ménétrier's disease
  - Late onset hypogammaglobulinemia
  - Intestinal metaplasia, type III (Incomplete sulphomucin secreting type)
  - HED → GCA in 85%

- Clinical
  - Unusual Presentations of Gastric Cancer
    - Achalasia
    - Silent jaundice
    - Skin metastases
    - Intestinal obstruction
    - Fistula and perforation
    - Duodenal spread
    - Early gastric cancer

- o Infiltration (thick gastric folds seen on an upper GI series or EGD)
    - Folds are not thickened (barium study is wrong for varices)
    - Malignant — adenocarcinoma, lymphoma
    - Benign infiltration — granulomas, i.e. sarcoidosis, TB, Crohn's, severe gastritis (ethanol, *H. pylori*), Ménétrier's disease (hyperplasia) eosinophilic gastritis
    - Multiple gastric polyps (HNPCC, FAP, fundic glands)
    - Hypersecretion (ZES)
    - Fundal varices
    - Worms

- Common sites for metastasis of gastric cancer:
    - o Liver
    - o Lungs
    - o Supraclavicular lymph nodes
    - o Distant abdominal lymph nodes
    - o Peritoneum (ascites)

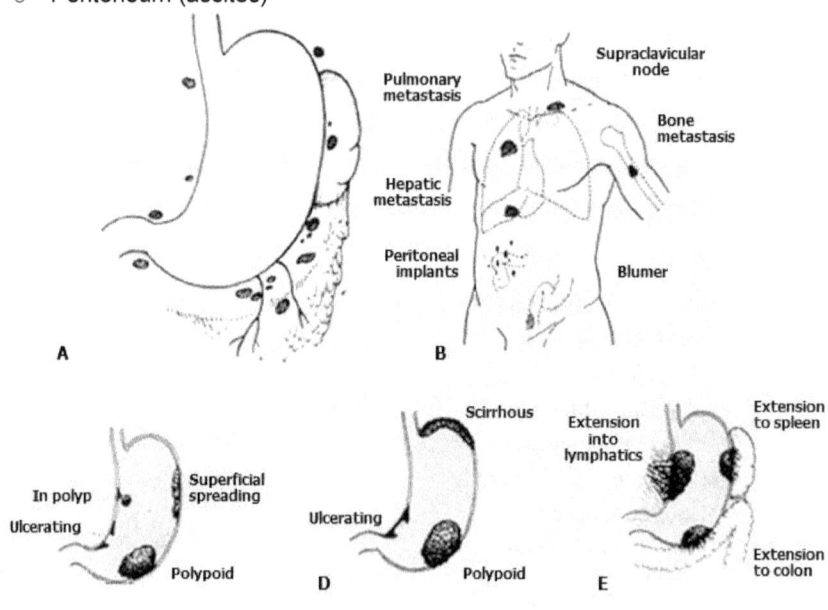

- Classification
  - Macroscopic types of gastric cancer

Please see: www.pathologyatlas.com

Types	Japanese Classification	Paris Classification
0	Superficial, flat tumors with or without minimal elevation or depression	Superficial polypoid, flat or depressed, or excavated tumors
0 – I	Protruded	Polypoid 0–Ip Protruded, pedunculated 0–Is Protruded, sessile
0 – IIa	Superficial and elevated	Non–polypoid and nonexcavated, slightly elevated 0–IIa Superficial, elevated
0 – IIb	Flat	Non–polypoid and non–excavated, completely flat 0–IIb Flat
0 – IIc	Superficial and depressed	Non–polypoid and non–excavated, slightly depressed without ulcer 0–IIc Superficial shallow, depressed
0 – III	Excavated	Non–polypoid with frank ulcer 0–III Excavated

- Causes and associations
  - Associated with the following conditions:
    - Intestinal metaplasia, type III
      - Intestinal > diffuse type of gastric cancer
    - Atrophic gastritis
    - Partial gastrectomy
    - *H. pylori* infection
    - Associated chronic gastritis (when acquired in childhood, i.e. long duration of infection)
    - Epstein Barr virus (EBV) infection
  - May be familial in some patients
  - Genetic mutations (autosomal dominant)
    - FAP
    - Seen in 10% of GCa
    - Hereditary non–polyposis cancer (HNPC)
    - E–cadherin
    - BRCA2

- Risk factors

- Name the reversible and non–reversible risk factors associated with the development of gastric adenocarcinoma.

  - Reversible – *Gastric atrophy*
    - *H. pylori* infection
    - Pernicious anemia
    - Chronic atrophic gastritis
    - Subtotal surgical resection with vagotomy for benign gastric ulcer disease
    - Diet
      - Salted, pickled or smoked foods
      - Low intake of fruits and vegetables
    - Life Style
      - Smoking (EtOH is <u>not</u> an independent risk factor)
      - Obesity
    - Esophageal — Barrett's esophagus (cancer of the cardia)

    Adapted from: Houghton, J. M. and Wang, T. C. *Sleisenger & Fordtran's Gastrointestinal and Liver Disease: Pathophysiology/ Diagnosis/ Management* 2006: page 1149.

- Non-reversible
  - Genetic
    - First degree relative with gastric cancer (hereditary diffuse gastric cancer; 2 – 3 fold ↑ risk with mutations in E–cadherin CDH1 gene)
    - Predisposition for diffuse >> intestinal–type GCa
    - Familial clustering (in 10%)
    - Twins: monozygotic HR (hazard ratio), 9.9; dizygotic HR, 6.6
  - Molecular factors
    - ↑ IL–1β → ↑ gastric myeloid–derived suppressor cells (MDSCs)
    - Polymorphisms
      - TNF–α
      - IL–10
      - TNF–α plus IL–10
  - Toll–like receptors (TLRs) have 27x ↑ risk of GCa, i.e. pattern recognition receptors, especially TLR–2
  - Syndromes
    - HNPCC >> FAP
    - Polyp — adenomatous gastric polyps (HNPCC, FAP), Peutz–Jegher syndrome (PJS), hamartomas, Ménétrier's syndrome

---

SO YOU WANT TO BE A GASTROENTEROLOGIST!

There are at least 20 genetic abnormalities occuring in GCa.

- What is the target cell upon which these gene abnormalities and expressed proteins will act?
  - It is currently thought that the target cell for the effects of genetic abnormalities to act to cause GCa is the "resident tissue stem cell", which becomes the "cancer stem cell".

Feldman, M., *et al. Sleisenger and Fordtran's Gastrointestinal and Liver Disease.* 2010. 9th Edition. *Saunders/Elsevier*, Philadelphia. page 895).

What is "the best"? The "best four clinical tests for the presence of peritonitis are: rigidity, guarding, rebound and percussion tenderness.

- ➢ Genetics
- • Give examples of common genetic abnormalities in GCa.
    - o Gene deletion or suppression
        - – TP 53
        - – Fragile histidine triad gene (FHIT)
        - – Adenomatous polyposis coli (APC) gene loss of heterogeneity
        - – Deleted in colorectal cancer (DCC)
    - o ↓ gene expression (due to epigenetic promoter hypermethylation)
        - – p16 (marker of poor differentiation)
        - – TFF_1 (human trefoil factor 1)
        - – Runt–related transcription factor 3 ($RUNX_3$)
        - – p27 (associated with poor prognosis)
        - – CDH_1
            - ▪ Encodes for E–cadherin (acts as a tumor suppressor gene)
            - ▪ Seen in hereditary diffuse gastric cancer (HDGC)
    - o ↑ gene expression (over amplification)
        - – COX–2, HGF, VEGF, c–Met, AIB–1
    - o DNA aneuploidy

Note that there are other genetic abnormalities in GCa which are less common (approximately gene frequency, 15 – 25%).

- o Mutations
    - – PIC3A that encodes for a catalytic subunit of phosphatidylinositol 3–kinase
    - – Protein–tyrosine phosphatase receptor–type (PTPRT)
- o ↑ gene expression (amplification)
    - – β–catenin
    - – EGF or EGFR (epidermal growth factor or EGF receptor)
- o ↓ gene expression (due to epigenetic promoter hypermethylation)
    - – MLH_1 and MLH_2 (MSI [microsatellite instability] phenotype)
- o Microsatellite instability

Adapted from: Abrahms, J. A. and Quante, M. *Sleisenger and Fordtran's Gastrointestinal and Liver Disease*. 9th Edition. *Saunders/Elsevier*, Philadelphia, 2016; Box 54-2, page 908, for a detailed list of genetic abnormalities in GCa.

- Name the genetic abnormalities that lead to diffuse–type GCa.
    - Gene
        - Deletion or suppression
        - ↓ expression due to hypermethylation
        - Amplification or overexpression
        - Mutations
    - DNA aneuploidy
    - Microsatellite instability

> Diagnosis
- Patients with new onset dyspepsia plus alarm symptoms ar any age, or new onset dyspepsia at age ≥ 50 – 55 years must have an EGD
- At least 6 mucosal biopsies must be taken from the edge of any gastric ulcer, or any suspicious gastric mass lesion or strictures
- Staging is performed with the following modalities:
    - CT multiplanar of chest, abdomen and pelvis
    - EUS
    - PET–CT scanning should be used in combination with EUS and CT for esophageal and for esophageal–gastric junctional tumor assessment
- Diagnosis of high grade dysplasia should be made and confirmed by "...two histopathologists, one with special interest in gastrointestinal disease"

> Diagnostic imaging
- Adenocarcinoma
    - Ulcer
        - Ulcerating mass
        - Lobulated contour of the mass
        - Irregular surface (mucosa–based lesions)
        - Nodular orifice and floor of the ulcer
        - Tissue around the ulcer is nodular
        - Tissue around the ulcer stops suddenly with an acute angle to the normal gastric tissue
        - Ulcer crater does not project beyond the expected location of the gastric wall
        - Ulcer is placed asymmetrically in the surrounding tissue

- Ulcer is wider than deep (width > depth)
    - Converging folds
        - Clubbed
        - Fused
        - Tapered
        - Amputated
        - Stop before the ulcer crater
        - Lack of mucosal markings (gastric folds) usually indicates ulceration
    - Carman meniscus sign
        - Lesser curve malignant ulcer
        - Nodular tissue around ulcer
        - Compression of both sides of the nodular surrounding tumor produces a half moon, crescent shape (pathognomonic for adenocarcinoma)
        - Usually, single
    - Infiltrative scirrhous tumor
        - Narrowing of the stomach ("leather bottle")
            - Mucosa nodular
            - Ulceration
        - Thick walls of the fundus or body
        - Contour of the stomach is irregular, scalloped
        - Stomach is not distensible
        - Long segment with intact folds
- Metastatic gastric cancer
    - Serosal contours of the gastric wall are irregular and fuzzy
    - CT shows thickened wall
    - Lymphadenopathy
        - Para–pancreatic
        - Para–aortic
        - Para–middle colic artery
    - Soft tissue masses
        - Spread to perigastric, omentum, peritoneum
    - Below renal pedicles:
        - Ovary (Krukenberg tumor)
        - Pancreas
        - Liver

- Lymphoma
  - May be localized or extensive, solitary or multiple masses
  - Masses
    - Ulcerative
    - Infiltration
    - Polypoid
    - Intraluminal fungating
  - May narrow the stomach by infiltration
  - Nodules (stomach; duodenum [crosses the pylorus])
  - Infiltration of the submucosa
  - Characteristic body of the stomach
    - Remains distended (compliant)
    - No narrowing of the lumen
  - Thickened folds

CT: lymphadenopathy of the perigastric and not below the renal pedicles

> Distinguishing diagnosis: lymphoma or adenocarcinoma
>
> | | Lymphoma | Adenocarcinoma |
> | --- | --- | --- |
> | Number | Single or multiple | Single |
> | Extent | Extensive | Localized |
> | Origin | Submucosa | Mucosa |
> | Crosses the pylorus | Yes | No |
> | Narrowed lumen | No | Yes |
> | Distensible | Yes | No |
> | Disorganized | Yes | No |

- Non–Neoplastic Gastric Filling Defects
  - Bezoar
    - Mottled, soft tissue mass (plain film)
    - Filling defect
    - Mottled, variegated appearance
    - Not attatched to the gastric wall
    - Moveable
    - Barium collects in the interstices of the concretion of ingested material

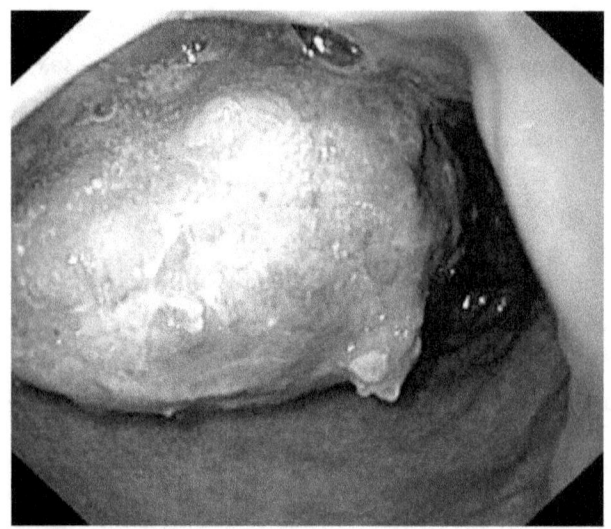

- o Ectopic pancreatic rest
    - Round submucosal filling defect
    - Central umbilication (not an ulcer)
    - Distal stomach
    - Associated with concurrent pancreatic disease
        - Pancreatitis
        - Pseudocysts
        - Adenoma
        - Carcinoma
- o Pseudotumor
    - History of surgical fundoplication
- o Gastric varices
    - Filling defects in the fundus
        - Polypoid
        - Lobulated (bunch of grapes)
        - Serpentine
    - Multiple

➤ Pathology

Patients with gastric cancer have 5–year survival rate of about 25%. In a sense, H. pylori infection may be considered a premalignant condition, and treatment of this infection is either early in life (before "point of no return") or in patients who have had EMR for early gastric cancer may reduce the risk of the development or redevelopment of GCa.

- Explain the pathological **premalignant conditions** related to GCa.
    o Chronic atrophic gastritis
        – Risk of the progression of chronic atrophic gastritis to GCa
            ▪ 1% per year
            ▪ Depends on the extend of CAG
            ▪ MAG >> corporal atrophic gastritis risk

Progression of the stages of chronic active gastritis to GCa:

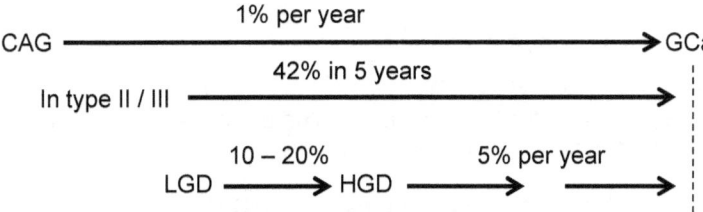

    o Production of pepsinogens (PG) from oxyntic cells
        – ↓ PG I
        – PG II, normal
        – ↓ PG I / PG II
    o Intestinal metaplasia (IM)
        – Type I
            ▪ Complete metaplasia
                – Absorptive cells with brush border membrane (BBM)
                – Paneth cells
                – Goblet cells (sialomucins)
        – Type II
            ▪ Incomplete
                – Goblet cells
        – Type III
            ▪ Intermediate
        – Risk of early GCA in type II / III IM, 42% in 5 years

- Dysplasia
    - Low grade dysplasia (LGD)
        - Regresses in 60%
        - Progresses to high grade dysplasia (HGD), 10 – 20%
    - HGD
        - Rarely progresses
        - Progresses to GCa in 5% per year
- Fundic gland polyps (FGPs) (~ 50%)
    - > 1 cm, progression to GCa is ~ 1% per year
    - FGP in FAP, dysplasia in 40%
- Adenomas (10%)
    - Progress to GCa (*in situ*), ~ 11% in 4 years
- Hyperplastic gastric polyps
    - Rare progression to GCa
- Ménétrier disease
    - Progress to GCa in ~ 15%
- Previous partial gastrectomy
    - Especially Billroth II, usually "stump cancer" begins at the anastomosis > 20 years after surgery

- What is the risk of gastric polyp progression to GCa?

Type	Progression to GCa
Adenoma	11% in 4 years
FAP	
- > 1 cm	1% per year
- In FAP	Dysplasia in 40%
Ménétrier's disease	15%
Hyperplastic hypersecretory gastropathy(HHG)	Rare

- What are the types of gastric adenoma?
    - Intestinal type
    - Pyloric gland
    - Foveolar gland type

http://www.pathologyatlas.com

- Patients with GCa have a 5-year survival rate of only about 25%
- In a sense, *H. pylori* infection may be considered premalignant, and treatment of this infection, either early in life (before "point of no return") or in patients who have had EMR for early gastric cancer, may reduce the risk of the development or redevelopment of GCa.

SO YOU WANT TO BE A GASTROENTEROLOGIST!

- *H. pylori* has been declared by the WHO to be carcinogenic, with an attributable risk of ~ 60% for gastric cancer.
- In addition to dietary and lifestyle factors, molecular factors represent a genetic basis for non–*H. pylori* GCa (cytokines [IL–1β, polymorphisms of TNF–α and IL–10), and TLRs (especially TLR–2), there are molecular factors related to *H. pylori*, which increase the risk of GCa.

- Give the **molecular factors** that increase the risk of carcinogenesis from *H. pylori*.
  - Motility
    - Proteins (Fla A, Fla B) providing spiral movement of *H. pylori*
  - Buffering of gastric acid ($\downarrow$ H^+ secretion)
    - Urease gene cluster (Ure A, Ure B)
  - Adhesion protein
    - Hop protein (outer membrane proteins)
    - Adhesion
      - Bab A (encoded by gene Bab A_2)
      - Bab A binds to blood group antigen, Lewis B
  - Cag pathogenicity island
    - Greater (or 2 – 28) risk of GCa with Cag A^+ *H. pylori*
  - Molecular needles
    - Type 4 secretion system (TFSS) enhances movement of Cag A^+ bacterial protein into gastric epithelial cells
  - Vacuolation
    - Vac A protein, a poreforming vacuolating toxin, especially in the presence of Cag A^+ *H. pylori* strains, reduce the activation of T–cells, and increase the risk of GCa

- For premalignant lesions on biopsy, what is the approximate annual risk of developing GCa from AG, IM, MMD, SD, and the recommended EGD or biopsy follow-up?

Conditions	Annual Risks	Recommended EGD or biopsy follow-up
o Atrophic gastritis (AG)	− 0.1%	None
o Intestinal metaplasia (IM)	− 0.25%	2 – 3 years
o Mild to moderate dysplasia (MMD)	− 0.6%	1 year
o Severe dysplasia (SD)	− 6.0%	Definitive therapy (EMR)

Adapted from: De Vries, A. C., et al. Gastroenterology. 2008. 134:945-52.

➢ Endoscopy

   o Sites

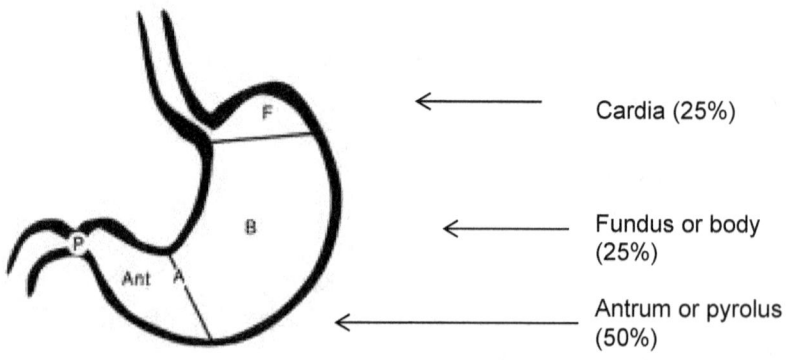

Cardia (25%)

Fundus or body (25%)

Antrum or pyrolus (50%)

   o Shape
- Polypoid or fungating mass — intestinal-type
- Infiltrating or diffuse-type ("linitis plastica") "leathery" appearance
- Not distendable with air insufflation

   o Early gastric cancers (EGC)
- Confined to the mucosa (even if lymph nodes are positive and tumor is confined)

   o Classifications have been devised, but are descriptive only, with no prognostic value

   o Intestinal-type

- Polyp
- Mass
- Ulcer
- Antrum, 50%
- Body, 25%
- Cardia 25%
  - Diffuse–type
    - Infiltrating
    - Depressed
    - Leather appearance
    - ↓ distendability (infiltration of the wall)

Clinical Tip
- EGC: localized GCa in the submucosa plus lymph nodes
- Japanese Gastroenterological Endoscopic Society (JGES) Classification
  - Endoscopic classification of GCa does not correlate well with prognosis
---

- Intestinal–type
  - Well–formed glands lined by columnar or epithelial cells with intraluminal mucin
- Diffuse–type
  - Poorly–formed nests of infiltrating cells with desmoplastic stromal response
  - Inflammatory infiltrate
  - Signet ring cells
    - Intracytoplasmic mucin displacing the nuclei to the periphery
- Mixed–type
- Medullary
  - > 50% of tumors are poorly differentiated with no fibrous stroma

- Diffuse gastric adenocarcinoma
  - Gastritis
  - Reactive endothelial cells in granulation
  - Lymphoma
- Intestinal–type may be difficult to differentiate with severe dysplasia

Features	Dysplasia	Carcinoma
Syncytial growth pattern	-	+
Back–to–back glands	-	+
Single cells throughout the lamina propria	-	+

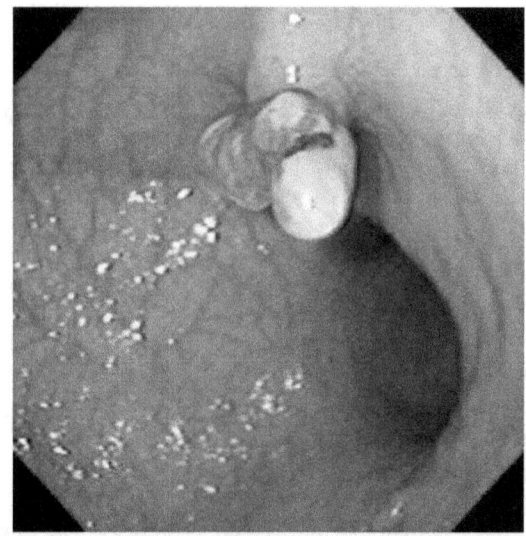

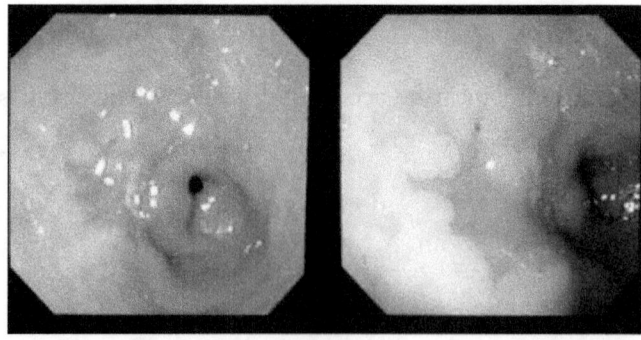

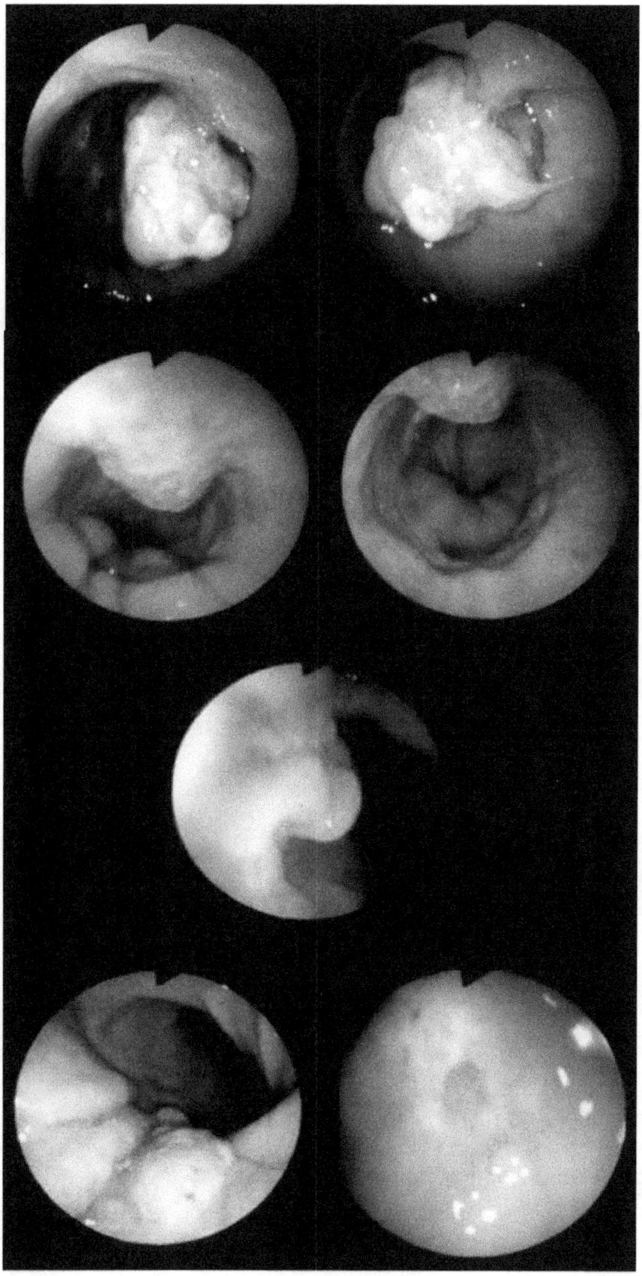

FROM COMPETENCE TO EXCELLENCE
The Stomach

© A.B.R. Thomson

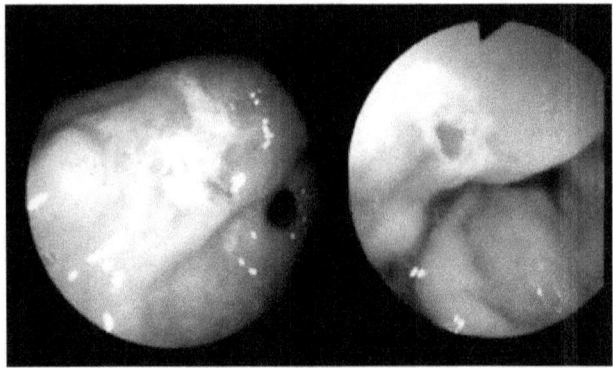

- ➤ Histopathology
  - ○ Intestinal or diffuse–type
    - – Lauren or WHO system
    - – Columnar or cuboidal epithelial cells lined with well–formed glands
    - – Intraluminal (not intracytoplasmic) mucin

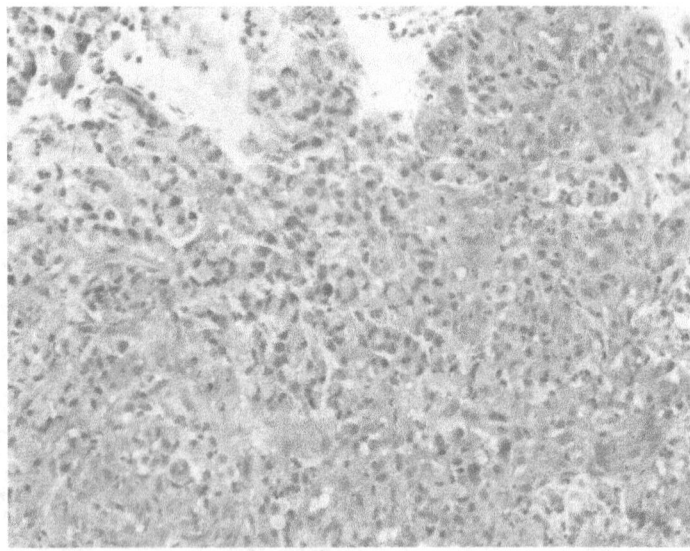

Gastric adenocarcinoma, diffuse–type

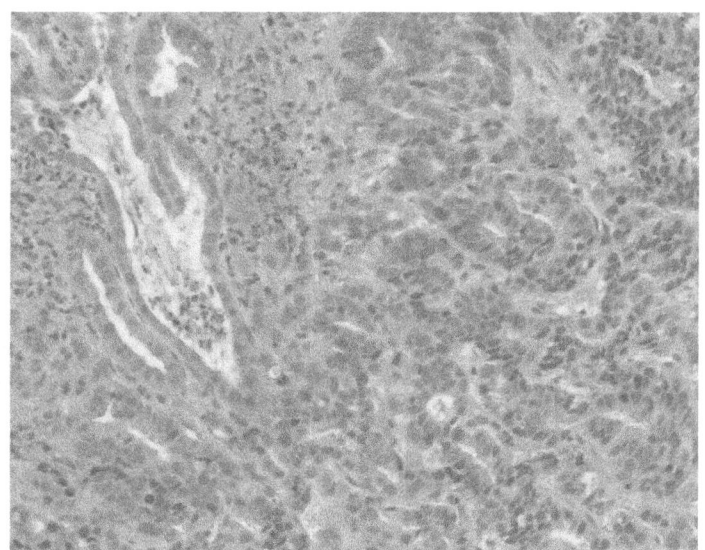

Gastric adenocarcinoma, intestinal type

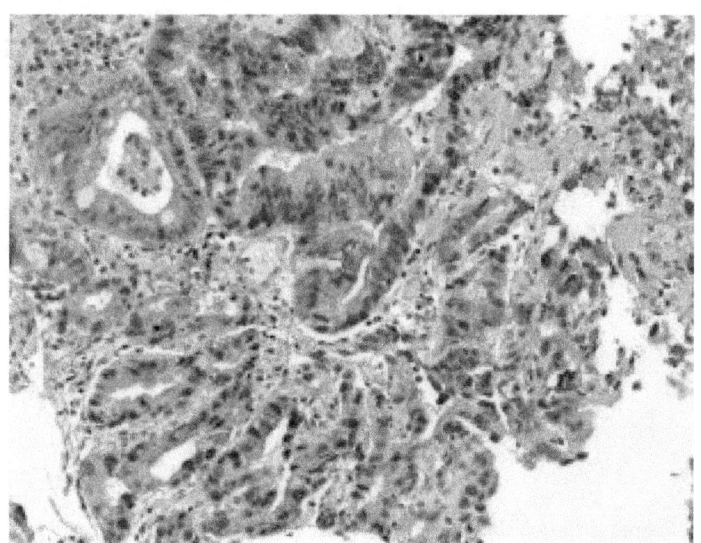

Provided kindly by Dr. Aducio Thiesen, University of Alberta

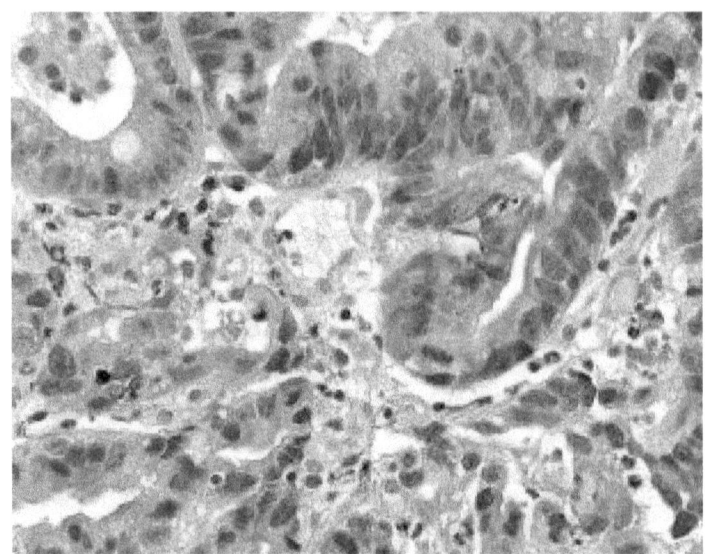

Provided kindly by Dr. Aducio Thiesen, University of Alberta

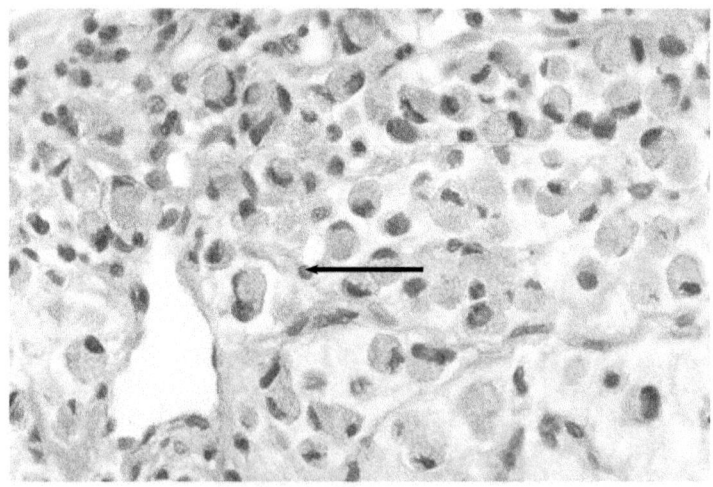

- Signet ring cell pattern of adenocarcinoma
  - Cells are filled with mucin vacuoles
  - Mucin vacuoles push the nucleus to one side (arrow)

http://library.med.utah.edu/WebPath/GIHTML/GI029.html

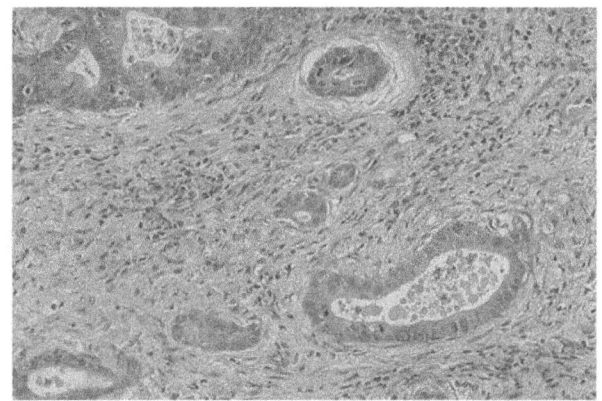

- o Neoplastic glands of GCa demonstrate the following:
  - mitoses
  - nuclear to cytoplasmic ratios (N:C ratio)
  - Hyperchromatism
- o Desmoplastic stromal reaction to the infiltrating glands

http://library.med.utah.edu/WebPath/GIHTML/GI027.html

- Differentiate pathologically intestinal– and diffuse–types of GCa (Lauren classification).

Features	Intestinal	Diffuse
o Incidence	↓	Steady
o Low risk areas	-	+
o Worse prognosis	-	+
o Risk factors: diet and environment	+	-
o Gland–like tubular structures	+	-
o Singly invasive tumor cells	-	+
o Linitis plastica	-	+

- o Another classification
  - Proximal cardia, GE junction
  - Distal fundus, body, antrum
  - Incidence
    - Proximal: ↑
    - Distal: ↓

SO YOU WANT TO BE A GI PATHOLOGIST!

- Give the Lauren and WHO classification of symptoms of GCa and its variants.

  - Lauren classification system
    - Intestinal
      - Well-formed glands
      - Columna or cuboidal cell lining
      - Single malignant cell found in the lamina propria
      - Mucin
      - Syncytial growth pattern
      - Back-to-back glands
        - ↑ in lumen of glands
        - ↓ in cells

    - Diffuse
      - Glands are not well-formed
      - Nests of malignant cells
      - Signet ring cells are common (may totally replace the gastric glands)
      - Fibrosis of stroma
      - Desmoplasia causing thick gastric wall ("linitis plastica")

  - World Health Organization (WHO) Classification system
    - Morphological subtype
      - Tubular
      - Papillary
      - Mucous
      - Signet ring cell
      - Adenosquamous
      - Undifferentiated

    - Differentiation
      - Moderate
      - Poor

    - Variants of adenocarcinoma
      - Medullary
        - > 50% of tumor is poorly differentiated
        - Lymphoepithelial appearance
        - No fibrosis
      - EBV-associated
        - Lymphoepithelial appearance
      - Hepatocellular carcinoma (HCC)-like

- Name the sites for metastatic gastric adenocarcinoma.

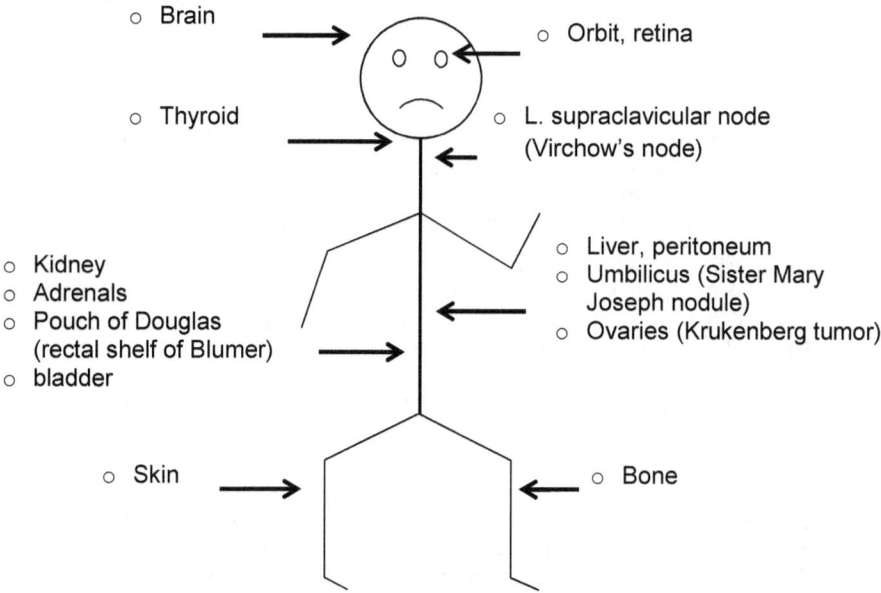

  - Brain
  - Orbit, retina
  - Thyroid
  - L. supraclavicular node (Virchow's node)
  - Kidney
  - Adrenals
  - Pouch of Douglas (rectal shelf of Blumer)
  - bladder
  - Liver, peritoneum
  - Umbilicus (Sister Mary Joseph nodule)
  - Ovaries (Krukenberg tumor)
  - Skin
  - Bone

Types	Japanese classification	Paris classification
1	Polypoid tumors that are sharply demarcated from the surrounding mucosa and are usually attached on a wide base	Polypoid carcinomas that are usually attached on a wide base
2	Ulcerated carcinomas that have sharply demarcated and raised margins	Ulcerated carcinomas that have sharply demarcated and raised margins
3	Ulcerated carcinomas that have no definite limits and infiltrate into the surrounding wall	Ulcerated, infiltrating carcinomas that have no definite limits
4	Diffusely infiltrating carcinomas in which ulceration is not usually a marked feature	Non–ulcerated, diffusely infiltrating carcinomas
5	Carcinomas that cannot be classified into any of the above types	Unclassifiable advanced carcinomas

- According to Japanese classification of GCa, in combined superficial types, the type occupying the largest area should be described first, followed by the next type (i.e. IIc + III)
- Types 0 I and 0 IIa are distinguished from each other by lesion thickness
- Type 0 I lesions have thickness more than twice the normal mucosa, and type 0 IIa lesions have thickness of up to twice the normal mucosa. Modified from data presented in Japanese classification of GCa and Paris endoscopic classification of superficial neoplastic lesions

Printed with permission: Yamamoto, H. *Nat Clin Pract Gastroenterol Hepatol* 2007. 4(9): page 513.; and Feldman, M., *et al. Sleisenger and Fordtran's Gastrointestinal and Liver Disease*. 9th Edition. *Saunders/Elsevier*, Philadelphia, 2010, Figure 54.6 II a, b, c, page 899.

- Diffuse–type ("linitis plastica") GCa tends to be more closely related to genetic factors than is the case for intestinal–type GCa, which is linked more closely to dietary and environmental factors

See: Abrahms, J. A. and Quante, M. *Sleisenger and Fordtran's Gastrointestinal and Liver Disease*. 9th Edition. *Saunders/Elsevier*, Philadelphia. 2010. Figure 54-6, page 914, for a detailed list of genetic abnormalities in GCa.

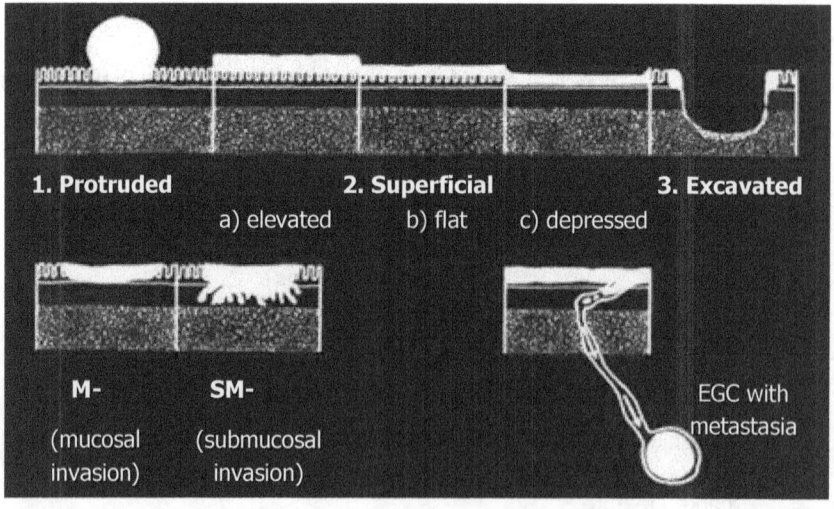

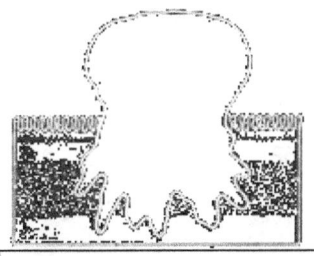
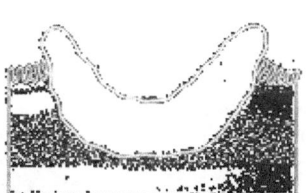

Type I: polypoid fungating | Type II: ulcerative with elevated, distinct borders

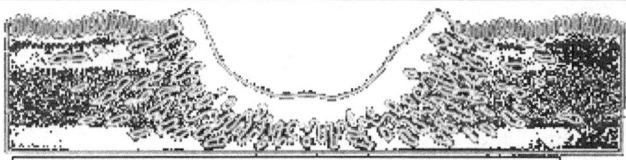

Type III: ulcerative with indistinct borders

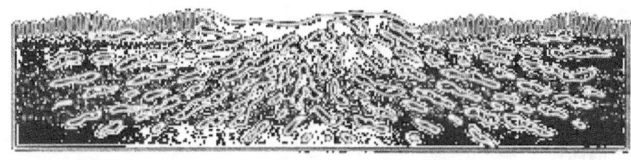

Type IV: diffuse, indistinct borders

Basic types

Type I		▬	Protruded	
			Superficial	Elevated type
	II a	▬	Elevated	
Type II	II b	—	Flat	
	II c	—⌣—	Depressed	Depressed type
Type III		⌴	Excavated	

Combined types

I + II a	▬⌣
II a + II C	⌒⌣
II C + III	⌣⌴

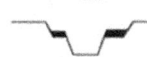

FROM COMPETENCE TO EXCELLENCE
The Stomach

© A.B.R. Thomson

Tumors found in patients with **MEN–1** and their approximate frequency (%)

Tumors	Approximate frequency (%)
o Parathyroid	78 – 97
o Pancreatic endocrine tumor	81 – 82
- Gastrinoma	54
- Insulinoma	21
- Glucagonoma	3
- VIPoma	1
o Pituitary tumors	21 – 65
- Prolactin–secreting	15 – 46
- Growth hormone secreting	6 – 20
- Cushing's syndrome	16
o Adrenal cortical adenoma	27 – 36
o Thyroid adenoma	5 – 30

- **Laurén Classification** of GCa
    - o Intestinal–type
    - o Diffuse–type
    - o Unclassified (mixed) type

		Intestinal–Type	Diffuse–Type
➢ Epidemiology	o	High risk areas	– Low risk areas
➢ Pathogenesis	o	Precursor lesions identified	
➢ Morphology	o	Cohesion	– Loss of cohesion
	o	Tubular structures	– Signet ring cells
➢ Molecular Profile	o	Depends on the studied population	– Type of alteration is partly similar

➤ **Comparison of Benign from Malignant Gastric Ulcer**

	Benign	Malignant
o Rim	- Smooth border and punched out crater	- Irregular rim with step formation to the crater
	- Soft ulcer rim or firm elastic on biopsy	- Elastic ulcer rim or firm on biopsy

o Ulcer
  - Shape
  - Crater
	- Round ulcer crater or oval
	- Edematous surroundings or later fibrotic
		- Irregular ulcer crater
		- Mucosal folds are ending abruptly away forming the rim

- Cover	- Crater covered by clean, smooth fibrinoid material	- Crater covered by "dirty" necrotic material
o Folds	- Mucosa folds radiating untill the crater and ending at the rim	- Folds in vicinity of the ulcer are broader, narrower, abruptly ending, different in color
o Surrounding mucosa	- Surrounding mucosa is evenly inflamed	- Surrounded by irregular mucosal defects or nodular elevation
o Movement	- Moving upon peristalsis, if ulcer is small	- Ulcer area is often rigid without pliability on peristalsis

- Special studies (immunostain–positive)
  - Cytokeratin
  - CEA
  - Epithelial membrane antigen (EMA)
  - CK7 (CK7$^+$ or CK20$^-$)

- Prevention of Gastric Cancer
  - Type I: Precancerous Conditions
    - *H. pylori* chronic gastritis with atrophy (RR: up to 9)
    - Autoimmune chronic gastritis with atrophy or pernicious anemia (RR: 1 – 5)
    - Post–gastrectomy stomach (RR: 1.6 BII, 1.2 BI); overall > 4% in 15 years)
    - Adenomatous gastric polyps
    - Ménétrier's–type of hypertrophic gastritis
    - Long term drug–induced a(hypo)chlorhydria a(hypo)gammaglobulinemia
  - Type II (Precancerous conditions)
    - Chronic atrophic gastritis (RR: 18)
    - Intestinal metaplasia, especially the incomplete sulphomucin secreting subtype III (high grade dysplasia develops into GCA in up to 85%)
    - Adenomatous polyp (10% focal malignancy)

- Palliation of gastric cancer
  - Obstruction
    - Resection
    - Proximal tumor (prothesis or radiotherapy)
    - Distal tumor (bypass or side–to–side antecolic gastroenterostomy)
  - Dysphagia
    - Radiotherapy
  - Bleeding
    - Radiotherapy
    - Endoscopic palliation (injection of necrotising agents, laser, etc.)
    - Best supportive care
  - Pain
    - Analgesics
    - Radiotherapy

- Treatment
  - Biopsy all gastric polyps, including the intervening non–polypoid gastric mucosa (with hyperplastic polyps, the risk of adenocarcinoma is high in the surrounding normal–appearing mucosa)

- Treat the associated *H. pylori* infection (especially if polyps are hyperplastic or adenomatous)
- Resection of polyp
  - Symptoms
  - Evidence of dysplasia on biopsy
- 1-year follow-up with EGD
  - Adenoma
  - Hyperplastic polyp

- Surgery
  - Resection of the spleen and splenic hilar nodes for proximal gastric tumors on greater curve or posterior wall
  - Gastric resection
    - Antrum
      - Subtotal gastrectomy plus distal pancreatic resection for direct immersion from the proximal stomach
    - Body
      - Total gastrectomy
    - Cardia, subcardia, EGJ
      - Transhiatal extended total gastrectomy
      - Esophagogastrectomy
    - Lymph nodes
      - D2 lymphadenectomy for gastric cancers stage II or III

- Chemoradiotherapy
  - Pre- or post-operative combination chemotherapy
  - Adjuvant chemotherapy, if neoadjuvant chemos' are not given to patient with high risk of recurrence
  - "Chemotherapy for locally advanced gastric cancer without distant metastasis can result in shrinking of tumor to the point where successful curative resection is possible
  - "Combined chemoradiation after surgical resection appears to be effective in improving progression-free and overall surgery in gastric cancer"
  - After surgical resection for the cure of GCa, if there are potential metastasis, intraperitoneal but not systemic chemotherapy may be useful

- Post-operative hyperthermic intraperitoneal chemotherapy improves the overall survival compared with surgery alone

Feldman, M., et al. *Sleisenger and Fordtran's Gastrointestinal and Liver Disease*. 9th Edition. Saunders/Elsevier, Philadelphia. 2010. page 904.

- Palliation
  - Limited resection
  - Palliative combination chemotherapy
    - Trastuzumab + cisplatin or fluoropyrimidine for HER2$^+$ tumors
    - Irinotecan for second line chemotherapy in patients with good performance characteristics

Source: Allum, et al. *Gut*. 2011; 60:1449-1472.

> Prognosis

- Give the prognostic predictors of poor outcome in GCa.

  - Patient — Older
  - Blood —
    - CEA: > 10 ng/ml
    - CA19-9: > 37 g/ml
  - Pathological stage —
    - Site
      - Proximal
    - Depth
    - Invasion of lymphatics, or venous drainage
    - Extent of involvement of the lymph node
    - Distant metastases

Early Gastric Cancer (EGC)

➢ Definition
  o Gastric cancer which is T1 and N (EGC is gastric cancer which invades no more deeply into the submucosal, regardless of the involvement of lymph nodes)

➢ Pathology
  o Synchronous and metachronous EGC

	Synchronous EGC (2nd EGC within 1 year)	Metachronous EGC
- EMR	9.2%	8.2%
- Partial gastrectomy	-	2 – 8%

  o EGC with lymph node involvement
    - Mucosal EGC   2 – 3%
    - Submucosal EGC   20 – 30%

SO YOU WANT TO BE A GI ONCOLOGIST!

- Give the primary tumors commonly metastasize to the stomach.

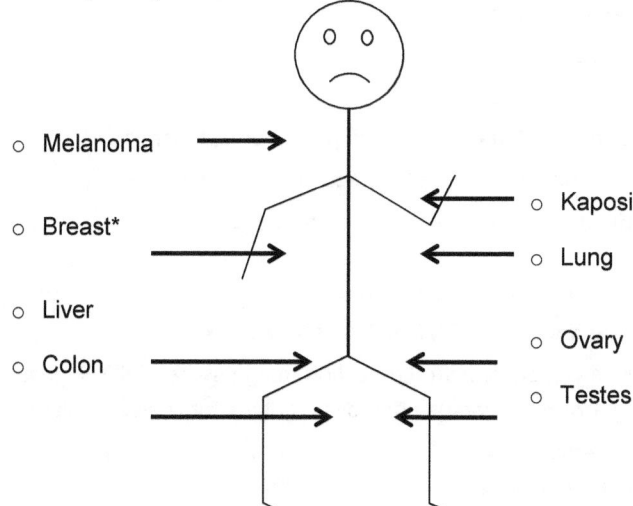

  o Melanoma
  o Breast*
  o Liver
  o Colon
  o Kaposi
  o Lung
  o Ovary
  o Testes

*Breast cancer is the most common primary tumor metastasizing to the stomach.

- What are the effects of the number of perigastric lymph nodes in the long term survival from early gastric cancer mortality from EGC?

# of nodes	Long term survival
0	92 – 95%
1 – 3	82 – 88%
4 – 6	73%
> 6	27%

> Treatment

- ❖ Endoscopic mucosal resection (EMR)
    - Successful EMR is ~ 85%
    - Lower success rates with EGCa > 2 cm
    - Ulcerated
    - Undifferentiated
    - 5–year survival rates ~ 86%
    - For incomplete resections, do the following:
        - Repeat EMR
        - Laser irradiation
        - Heater probe cautery
        - Surgical resection
    - If positive lateral margins and negative vertical margins
        - No submucosal or lymphovascular invasion
    - Piecemeal resection ↑ risk of recurrence (28%)

- ❖ Endoscopic submucosal dissection (ESD)
    - Complete resection > EMR (83% vs 24%)
    - If positive vertical or lateral resection margins after ESD → gastrectomy
        - Laparoscopic versus open distal gastrectomy give similar outcomes
    - Operative morbidity   22%
        - Operative mortality   0%
        - 5–year survival   96%
        - Disease–specific survival 98%

- ❖ Other treatment options for EGCa
    - o Photodynamic therapy (PDT)
        - – Photofrin II plus argon laser
        - – Tissue–destroying – cannot examine tissue to determine if margins are clear
    - o General indications for **gastrectomy,** with removal of perigastric lymph nodes
        - – Low probability of *en bloc* resection with EMR or ESD (i.e. endoscopic resection would be piecemeal)
        - – Diffuse rather than intestinal–type adenocarcinoma
        - – Submucosal tumor size greater than 30 mm, or tumors with ulceration
        - – Evidence of lymphovascular (lymphatic or venous) invasion in the primary tumor, or known or suspected regional lymph node metastases
        - – Gastrectomy with resection of the perigastric regional nodes
            - ▪ EGCa with positive lateral or vertical margins
        - – Laparoscopic lymph node dissection not yet ready for "prime time"
        - – 5–year survival rate for EGCa treated with gastrectomy ~ 98%

From: D. Mogan. Up To Date, "Early gastric cancer: Treatment, natural history and prognosis".

- What is the role of multidetector row CT (MDCT) in staging GCa?
    - o MDCT "…appears to have comparable accuracy to EUS in terms of T and N staging of Gca" (Feldman, M., et al. *Sleisenger and Fordtran's Gastrointestinal and Liver Disease.* 9th Edition. Saunders/Elsevier, Philadelphia. 2010. page 901).
    - o Test–and–treat for associated *H. pylori* infection
        - – Biopsies may be false negative because *H. pylori* load falls with the development of EGC
        - – Treat for *H. pylori* infection based on positive serology
        - – Treating *H. pylori* infection in EGC managed by EMR ↓ tumor recurrence in 3 years (or 0.35)
    - o Adjuvant therapy for EGC with positive nodes and observation for TlN0
    - o EMR or ESR

- Give the standard guidelines for endoscopic therapy (EMR and ESR) for intestinal–type of EGC.
    - High probability of *en bloc* resection
    - Tumor history
        - Intestinal–type adenocarcinoma
        - Tumor confined in the mucosa
        - Absence of venous or lymphatic invasion
    - Tumor size and morphology
        - < 20 mm in diameter without ulceration
        - < 10 mm in diameter of Paris classification IIb or IIc
- ➤ Expanded Criteria
    - Endoscopic resection of intestinal–type EGC
        - Mucosal tumor of any size without ulceration
        - Mucosal tumor < 30 mm with ulceration
        - Submucosal tumors < 30 mm confined to the upper 0.5 mm of the submucosal without lymphovascular invasion
        - Successful EMR ~ 85% (lower success rates with eGC > 2 cm, ulcerated, 1 cm, or undifferentiated)
        - 5–year survival rates ~ 86%
        - For incomplete resections
            - Repeat EMR
            - Laser irradiation
            - Heater probe cautery
                - Surgical resection
        - If positive lateral margins and negative vertical margins
            - no submucosal or lymphovascular invasion
        - Piecemeal resection has ↑ risk of recurrence (28%)
            - ESD
    - ESD complete resection > EMR (83% vs 24%)
        - If positive vertical or lateral resection of margins after ESD → gastrectomy

> SO YOU WANT TO BE A GASTROENTEROLOGIST!
>
> - What are the four generally accepted criteria for EMR in EGC?
>
>   According to Feldman, M., et al. Sleisenger and Fordtran's Gastrointestinal and Liver Disease. 9th Edition. Saunders/Elsevier, Philadelphia. 2010. page 902-903.
>
>   - "(gastric) cancer is located in the mucosa and lymph nodes are not included, as indicated by EUS"
>   - no ulcer scar and the maximum size of the tumor is:
>   - Type IIa less than 2 cm when the lesion is slightly elevated
>   - Type IIb or IIc, less < 1 cm when the tumor is flat (b) or slightly depressed (c)
>   - no evidence of the following:
>   - Multiple gastric cancers
>   - Simultaneous abdominal cancers
>   - "The cancer is of the intestinal–type" (i.e. not the diffuse–type)

- What are the standard guidelines for endoscopic therapy (EMR or ESR) for EGC?
  - Photodynamic therapy (PDT)
    - Photofrin II plus argon laser
    - Tissue–destroying
  - Problem: Cannot examine specific to determine if margins are clear
  - Surgical

From: Morgan, D. Up To Date. "Early gastric cancer: Treatment, natural history and prognosis".

- Surgical resection

- What are the indications for gastrectomy and perigastric regional lymph node resection for EGC?
  - Gastrectomy with resection of perigastric regional nodes
    - EGC with positive lateral or vertical margins
    - Laparoscopic lymph node dissection not yet ready for "prime time"
    - 5 year survival rate for EGC treated with gastrectomy ~ 98%

- If criteria for EMR are not met → gastrectomy and removal of perigastric lymph nodes to ↓ risk of lymph node metastases
- Type of surgery is determined by site of EGC
  - Upper 1/3 total gastrectomy
  - Lower 2/3 subtotal gastrectomy
- General indications for gastrectomy with removal of perigastric lymph nodes
  - Low probability of *en bloc* resection with EMR or ESD (i.e. endoscopic resection would be piecemeal)
  - Diffuse– rather than intestinal–type adenocarcinoma
  - Submucosal tumor size > 30 mm, or tumors with ulceration
  - Evidence of lymphovascular (lymphatic or venous) invasion in the primary tumor, or known or suspected regional lymph node metastases
  - Laparoscopic versus open distal gastrectomy give similar outcomes
    - Operative morbidity   22%
    - Operative mortality   0%
    - 5–year survival   96%
    - Disease–specific survival   98%

➢ Chemotherapy or chemoradiation
  - "Chemotherapy for locally advanced gastric cancer without distant metastasis can result in shrinking of the tumor to the point at which successful curative resection is possible."
  - "Combined chemoradiation after surgical resection appears to be effective in improving progression–free and overall surgical in gastric cancer."
  - After surgical resection for cure of GCa, if these are potential metastasis, intraperitoneal but not systemic chemotherapy may be useful.
  - Post–operative hyperthermic intraperitoneal chemotherapy improves overall survival, as compared with just surgery.

Feldman, M., et al. *Sleisenger and Fordtran's Gastrointestinal and Liver Disease*. 2010. 9th Edition. *Saunders/Elsevier*, Philadelphia. page 904.

Gastric Lymphoma

➢ Types
- o Most commont MALT
- o Diffuse B–cell
- o Marginal zone B–cell, or MALT

➢ Clinical features
- o Lymphoepithelial lesions
- o Centrocytic–like cell (low – high grade)

➢ Causes and associations

Both lymphocytic gastritis and MALT lymphoma are associated with *H.pylori* infection of the stomach.

- What is the distinction between the 2 complications of *H. pylori*?
    - o Lymphocytic gastritis
        - \> 25 lymphocytes / 100 epithelial cells
        - CD8–positive T lymphocytes
        - Reactive lymphoid follicles
        - Lymphoepithelial lesion of the glands
        - Associated with celiac disease
    - o MALT
        - Diffuse population of B–cells in lamina propria

➢ Differential diagnosis of primary gastric lymphoma
- o Secondary gastric localization other lymphomas (nodal NHL, mantel cell lymphoma)
- o Gastritis or peptic ulcer
- o Gastric carcinoma
- o Ménétrier's disease
- o Syphilis
- o Gastric metastases (lobular–type breast cancer)

➤ Endoscopy

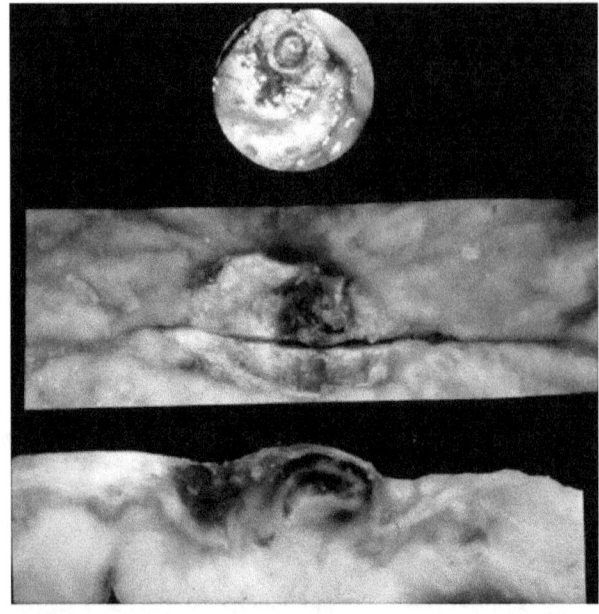

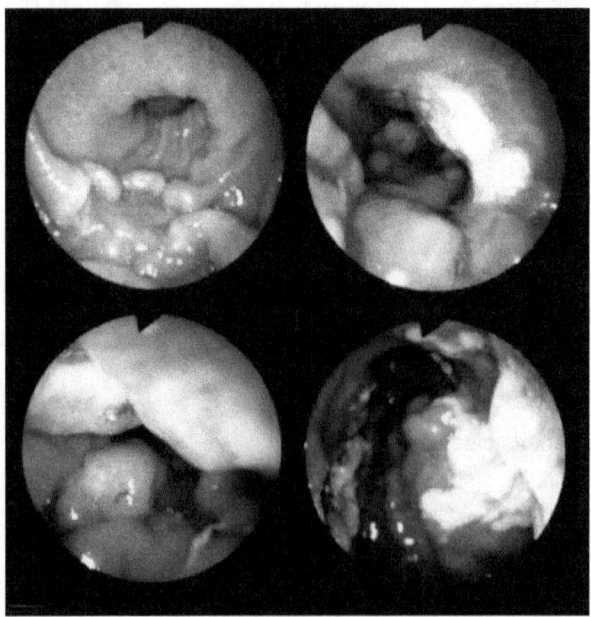

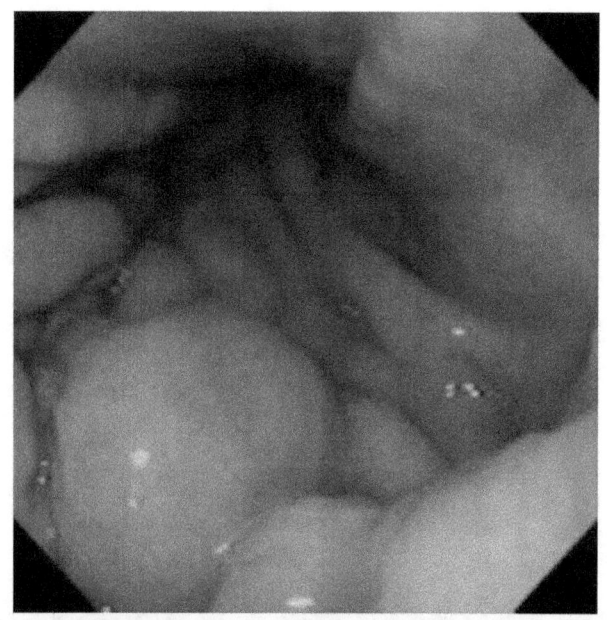

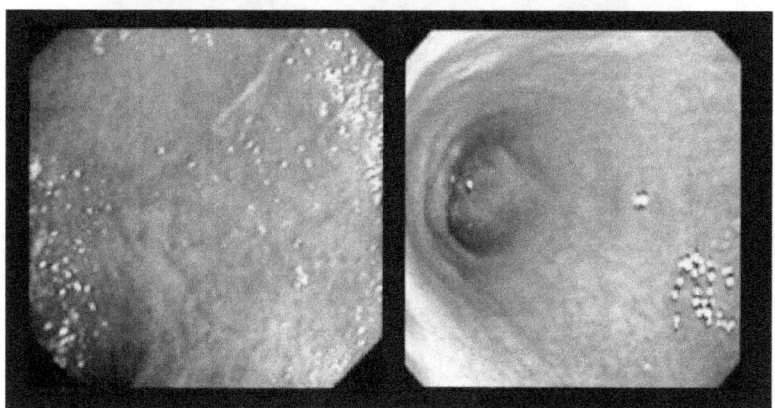

- Histopathology
  - Malignant lymphoma
  - Lymphoepithelial lesions

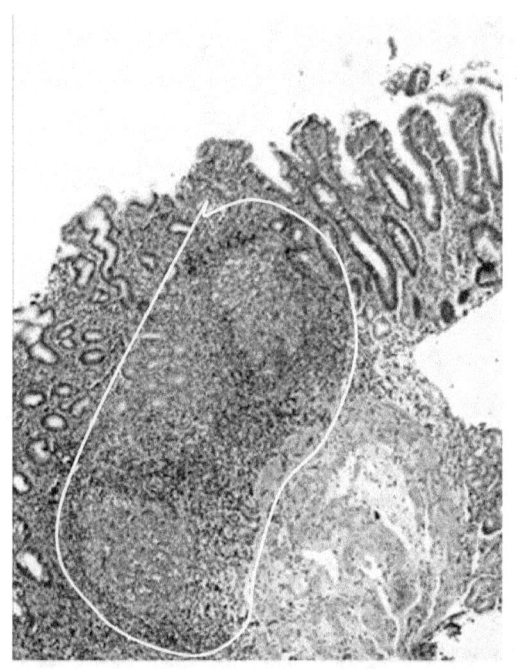
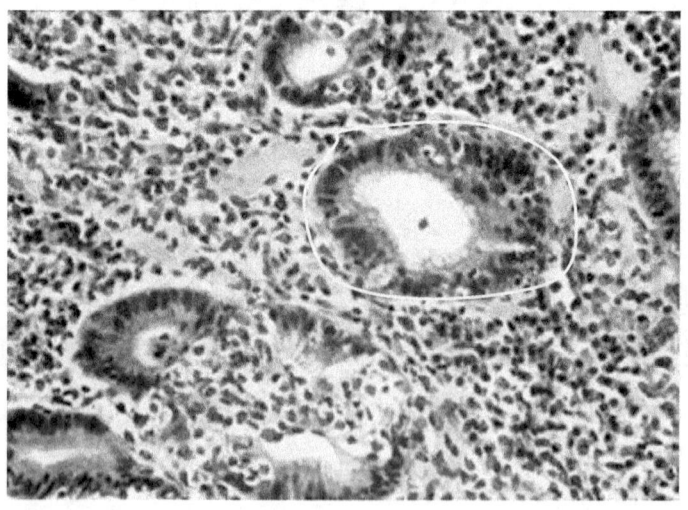

FROM COMPETENCE TO EXCELLENCE
The Stomach

Gastric MALT Lymphoma

- ➢ Definition
  - o Low grade extranodal marginal zone B–cell lymphoma arising from the MALT (Mudali, S., et al. 2012. Chapter 21, Gastrointestinal and Liver Pathology, 2nd edition. page 679)
  - o Note
    - In addition to CD20 and CD45 positive B–cells, some MALT lymphomas are comprised of T–cells, which are positive for CD3 and CD5

- ➢ Causes and associations
  - o MALT lymphoma
  - o *Helicobacter pylori* infection
  - o Rarely inflammatory or autoimmune disorders

- ➢ Genetics

SO YOU WANT TO BE A GI PATHOLOGIST!

There are four recurrent chromosomal translocations in MALT lymphomas.

- Give the significance of the t(11;18) translocation, as well as the trisomy of chromosomes 3, 12, and 18.

  - o T(11;18) and No t[11;18]
    - Commonly associated with *H. pylori* infection
  - o Trisomy 3, 12 and 18
    - ↑ risk of transformation into diffuse large B–cell lymphoma

---

- ➢ Differential
  - o B–cell MALT lymphoma
    - Lymphoepithelial lesions
    - Cellular atypia
    - IHC–positive for the following:
      - CD20
      - CD43
      - IgH rearrangement

- Lymphocytic gastritis
    - T-cell infiltration
    - No lymphoepithelial lesions
    - No cell atypia
    - Positive on IHC for CD3 and CD5
- Follicular lymphoma
    - IHC positive for the following:
        - CD10
        - BCL6
- Diffuse large B-cell lymphoma (DLBCL)

- Endoscopy
    - Size
        - Large, multifocal
    - Site
        - Body or antrum
    - Variable appearance
        - Ulcer
        - Nodules
        - Thick gastric fold

- Histopathology
    - Lymphoepithelial clusters of B-cell
        - Neoplastic
            - Marginal zone
        - Reactive
            - Follicles plus plasma cells
        - Destruction of the normal gastric tissue
    - Lymphoma cells
        - Large
        - Halo
        - Nuclear atypia
        - When sheets of the transformed cells called large B-cell lymphoma
    - Infiltrates in the interfollicular area
    - Transformed (DLBCL)

- o Plasma cells
  - Clonal
  - Reactive
- o Follicle
  - Center centrocytes
- o Monocytoid B–cell
  - Immunoblasts

- Special studies (immunohistochemistry)
  - o MALT lymphoma positive for CD20 and CD43

SO YOU WANT TO BE A GI PATHOLOGIST!

- What are the two cell populations in MALT lymphoma show positive on immunohistochemistry for CD20 and CD43?
  - o Both B–cells and T–cells are positive for CD20 and CD43
  - o Only ~ 50% of the gastric MALT lymphomas are positive for CD20 but not for CD43, give the names of the study that help make the diagnosis of rearrangement of MALT.
  - o PCR demonstration of IgH

Gastric Diffuse Large B–cell Lymphoma (DLBCL)

➤ Terminology
  - o Do not use the terms low grade and high grade lymphoma
  - o Recommended terms
    - MALT lymphoma
    - Diffuse large B–cell lymphoma (DLBCL)

➤ Demography

Both MALT lymphoma and DLBCL are most commonly (85%) in the stomach.

Give the similarities and differences of the two B-cell lymphomas

Features	MALT	DLBCL
Median age	> 50 years	> 60

- Pathology

Features	MALT	DLBCL
o Sheet of large cells		
– Immunoblasts	–	+
– Centroblasts	–	+
o Lymphoepithelial lesion	+	+/–
o Concurrent MALT plus DLBCL	–	+
o Follicle–center origin*	–	+
o "Halo" cell	–	+
o Mutation or loss of p53 1p16	–	+

- Treatment

Features	MALT	DLBCL
o When *H. pylori* infected, response to antibiotics	+	–
o Response to chemotherapy (rituximab + CHOP)	–	+
o Survival	> 50 – 90%	~ 50%

*Note: DLBCL may also be non–follicle center origin

Abbreviation: CHOP, cyclophosphamide, doxorubicin, vincristine and prednisone

---

SO YOU WANT TO BE A GI PATHOLOGY SUPERSTAR!

- Give the evidence showing DLBCL arrises from MALT lymphoma.

    o DLBCL plus MALT lymphoma
      – May exist together
      – Both have similar clonality
      – Genetic identity

Burkitt's Lymphoma

- Definition
    - Aggressive extranodal B–cell lymphoma affecting the GI tract in endemic, sporadic and immunodeficiency forms, characterized by bulky masses, and composed of a monomorphous infiltrate of medium–sized lymphocytes with "round nuclei, finely clumped chromatin, several small nucleoli and scant cytoplasm" (Mudali, S., et al. 2012. Gastrointestinal and Liver Pathology, 2nd Edition, Elsevier. Chapter 21. page 691).

- Demography

Features	Endemic	Sporadic	Immunodeficiency
o Where	Africa, Middle East	"developed" countries	Worldwide
o Age	M > F = 2:1	M > F = 2:1	
o EBV association	~ 95%	< 30%	25 – 50%

- Genetics
    - MYC deregulation as the result of MYC translocations

- Clinical
    - Bulky masses
        - Jaw
        - Orbit
        - Paraspinal
    - Bone marrow
    - Peripheral blood

- Endoscopy
    - GI site
        - Ileocecal (except for endemic areas, i.e. Africa)
        - Rectum
        - Stomach
    - Lymph nodes
        - Surrounded, but not directly affected by lymphoma tissue

- ➢ Histopathology
    - o Medium-sized lymphocytes
    - o Monomorphous infiltration
    - o Nuclei
        - Round
        - Chromatin clumps
        - Nucleoli
            - Small
            - Multiple
    - o Cytoplasm
        - Scant
        - Basophilic
        - Lipid vacuoles
        - Granulomatous reaction
    - o Macrophages
        - Contain apoptotic tumor cells
        - "Starry sky" appearance

- Special studies
    - o Immunohistochemistry positive for the following:
        - CD10
        - CD20
        - CD43
        - BCL6
    - o Ki-67 labeling (100%)
    - o Few CD3 T-cells

- ➢ Treatment
    - o Combination chemotherapy
    - o Surgical
        - Decompression
        - Debulking
    - o Treatment of associated HIV

Gastric Stump Carcinoma

➢ Demography

Stomach Ulcers following Gastric Resection

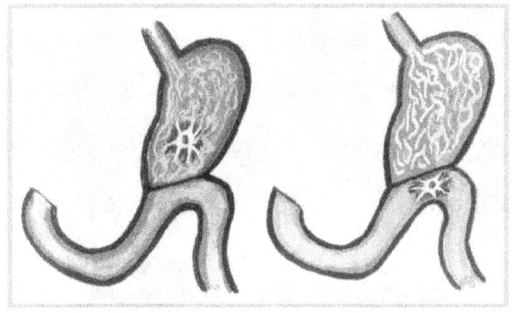

Overall incidence of cancer in gastric remnant, 3.6 –15.1%

➢ Amsterdam Survey
  o Death due to stump cancer in 9 60 years old gastrectomy patients > 3.2%
  o Cancer rate detected by prospective endoscopic screening of 535 asymptomatic gastrectomy patients (> 15 years) 4.1%

➢ Diagnostic imaging of gastric stump cancer

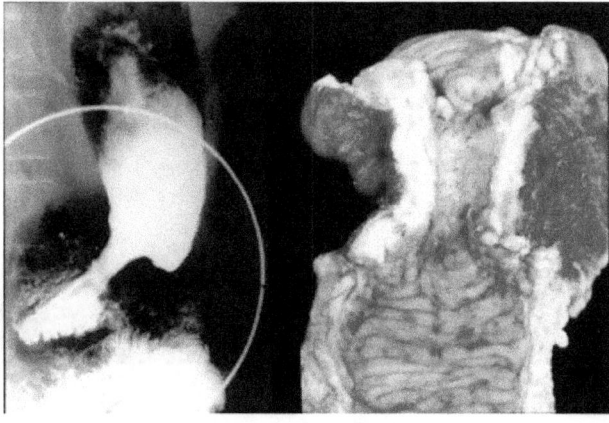

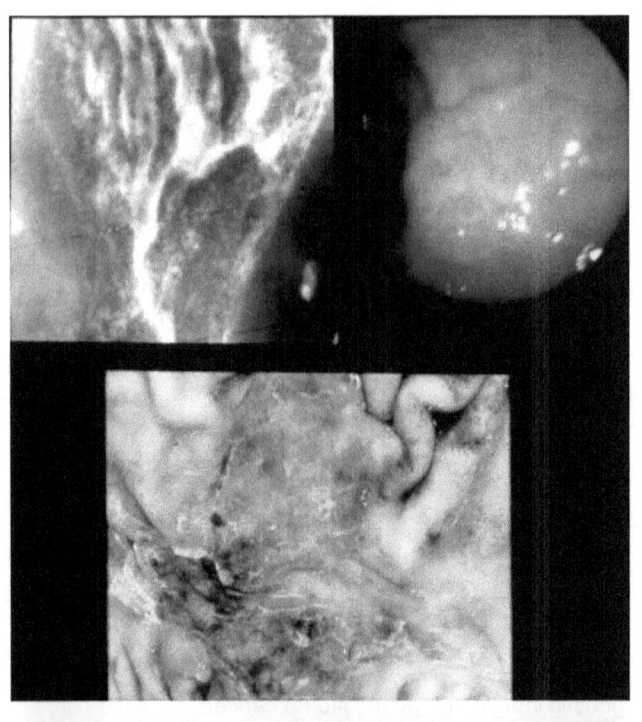
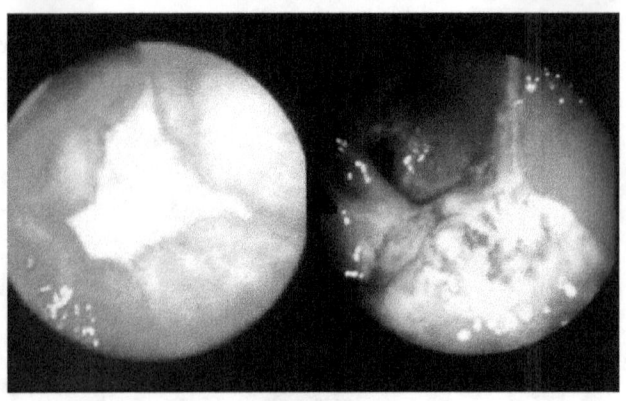

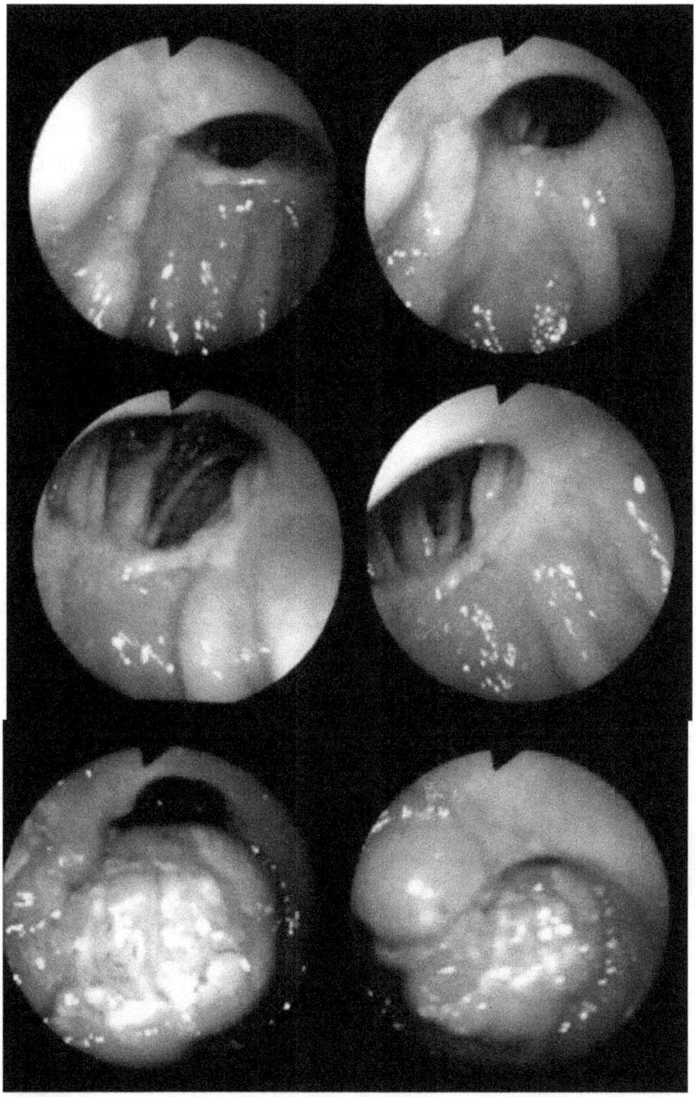

375

FROM COMPETENCE TO EXCELLENCE
The Stomach

© A.B.R. Thomson

STROMAL TUMORS AND TISSUE EOSINOPHILS

- Types
    - Inflammatory fibroid polyp
        - Spindle stroma cells mixed with blood vessels, eosinophils, stromal cells and other blood vessels
        - Stromal cells are concentrically arranged around the blood vessels
        - Loose, edematous stroma
    - Benign mesenchymal tumors
        - Leiomyoma
        - Perineuroma
        - Schwannoma
        - Solitary fibrous tumor
        - No eosinophils
        - Requires immunostains to establish the type
    - Eosinophilic gastroenteritis
        - Patchy eosinophilic infiltration
        - All layers
            - Mucosa
            - Submucosa
            - Muscularis propria
            - Serosa
    - Parasitic infection
        - Identify egg and larvae
        - Granulomatous reaction with eosinophils
- Pathology
    - Fat
        - Lipoma
            - Single
            - Pedunculated
            - Antrum
            - Prolapsed into the duodenum
            - Central ulceration
            - CT shows fat
        - Liposarcoma

- Muscle
  - Leiomyomas
    - Multiple in ~ 25%
  - Leiomyosarcomas
    - Usually exogastric
- Nerve
  - Schwannomas
- Desmoid tumors
- GIST is the most common stromal tumor in the stomach
  - Usually in the gastric fundus or small intestine
  - Endo– (into) or exogastric (away from lumen) given a dumbbell shape
  - Site
    - Stomach   ~70%
    - Small bowel   ~25%
    - Colon or rectum   5%
- Malignant potential
  - All GISTs > 10 mm

➤ Markers for GIST
  - C–kit (a stem cell factor receptor) (~ 99%)
  - CD34 (a hematopoietic cell progenitor cell antigen) (70%)
  - Smooth muscle actin (20 – 30%)
  - S 100 protein (marker of neural differentiation)

➤ Genetic mutations
  - Mutational activation of genes
    - KIT
    - PDGFRA
    - DC117

- What are the examples of CD117 negative GI spindle tumors (20%)?
    - Fat — Lipoma
    - Muscle — Leiomyomas
      - Leimyosarcoma
    - Blood vessels — Hemangiomas
    - Nerve tissues — Schawannomas

Note: Rarely the above tumors may be CD117–positive, but despite this, the non–GIST soft tissue sarcomas do not respond to imatinib.

- Endoscopic diagnosis
    - EUS plus FNA (fine needle aspiration)

Inflammatory Fibroid Polyps (IFP)

- Definition
    - Submucosal polypoid lesion composed of spindle or stellate stromal cells, mixed with stroma of inflammatory (mostly eosinophils) cells, and blood vessels in a concentric "onion skin" appearance
    - Mixture of inflammatory cells (especially eosinophils), blood vessels and a proliferation of spindle or stellate stroma cells in an edematous or myxoid stroma
    - Synonyms: Vanek's polyp, gastric submucosal granuloma with eosinophilic infiltrations, eosinophilic granuloma, fibroma, eosinophilic pseudotumor

- Demography
    - ~ 3% of gastric polyps
    - Slightly F > M
    - Mean age of 64 years

- Pathogenesis
    - Mutations in exons 12 and 18
    - Activating platelet–derived growth receptor

- ➢ Clinical
  - o Non–specific
- ➢ Endoscopy
  - o Mucosal surface
  - o Shape
  - o Size
  - o Single
  - o Site
    - Antrum (2/3); body > pylorus > incisura cardia or fundus
  - o Sessile or polypoid
  - o Average size, 1.5 cm
  - o Grey–brown color
  - o Smooth or nucleated surface
  - o Well–demarcated
- ➢ Histopathology
  - o No capsule
  - o Mucosa over the submucosal lesion is characterized by:
    - Normal
    - Reactive glandular epithelium
    - May rarely show adenoma or adenocarcinoma
  - o Muscularis mucosae
  - o Submucosa
    - ↑ spindle cells or stellate stromal cells
    - Stromal cells
      - Nuclei
      - Spindle–shaped, or oval
      - Fine granules of the chromatin
      - Small nuclei
      - Cytoplasm
        - Reddish
        - ↑ RER (EM)
        - Dense bodies (EM) within filaments in the cytoplasm
    - Myxoid
    - Nodular lymphoid aggregates

- Stromal pattern whorl "onion skin-like perivascular or periglandular
- Multinucleated giant cells

- Nodular lymphoid aggregates
- Wheel–like "onion skin" lesion caused by stromal GIST
- No marked inflammatory response, including no marked infiltration of eosinophils
- No perivascular collection of stromal cells (i.e. no "onion skin" lesion)
- Positive staining for CD117 and CKIT, as well as CD34 (both GISTs and IFPs are positive for CD34)
- Eoisinophillic gastroenteritis
  - Prominent eosinophils but they do not form a mass, as does IFP
- Parasitic infection
  - Eosinophils, granulomas, but finding schistosome egg or strongyloides larvae will give the diagnosis

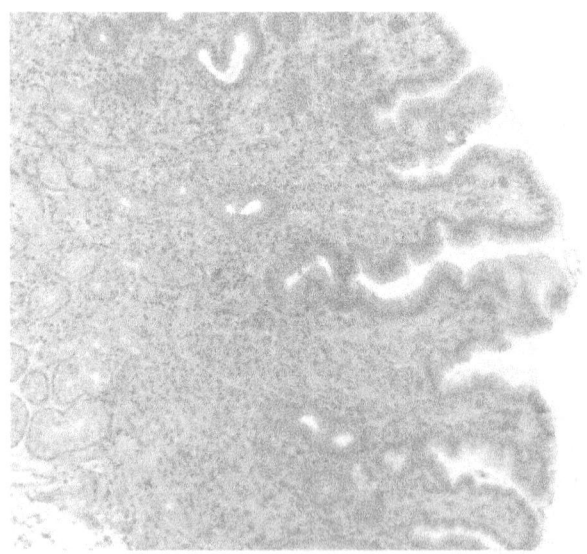

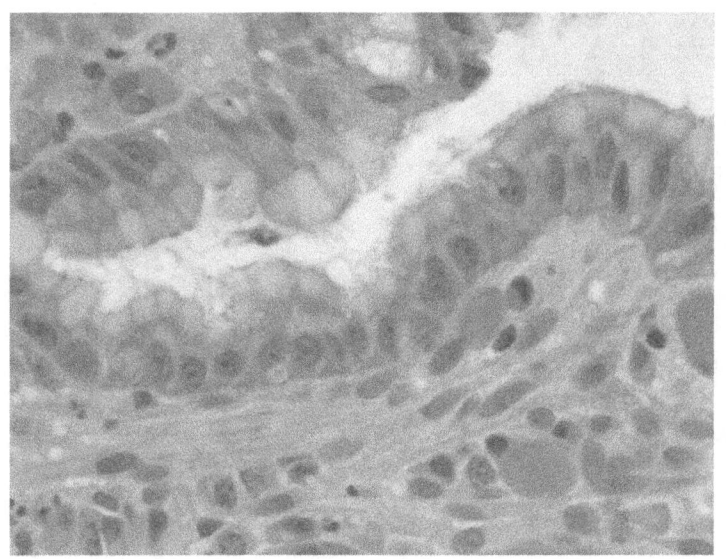

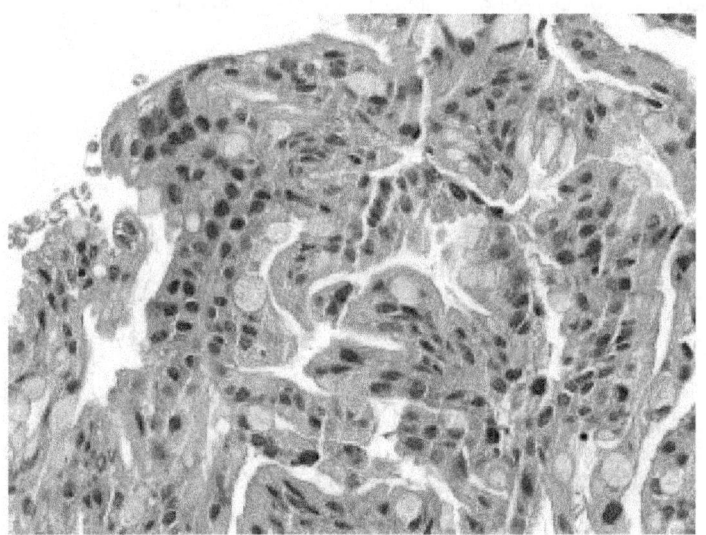

Provided kindly by Dr. Aducio Thiesen, University of Alberta

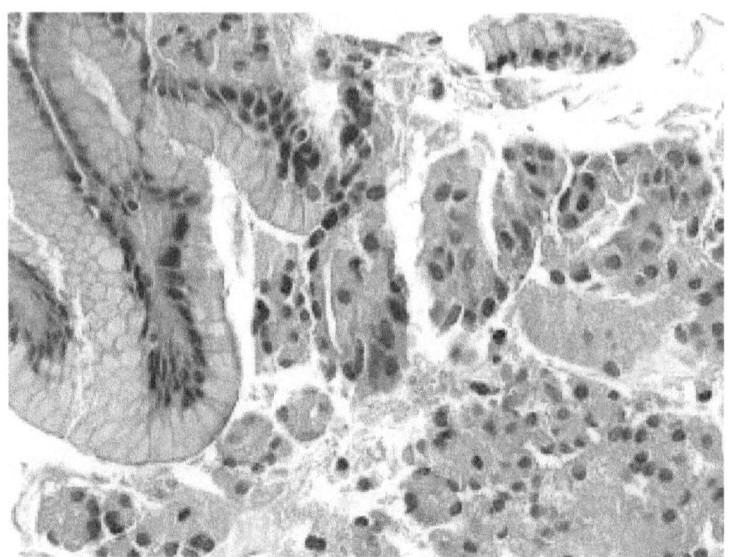

Provided kindly by Dr. Aducio Thiesen, University of Alberta

- Special studies
    - ~ 20% are positive for the following:
        - α–actin (smooth muscle)
        - Muscle specific actin (HHF–35)
        - CD68

Eosinophilic Gastritis

➤ Definition
   - Idiopathic infiltration of the stomach with large numbers of eosinophils, as part of the spectrum of involvement of other parts of the GI tract in eosinophilic gastroenteritis
   - Marked gastric mucosa infiltration with eosinophilis (> 20/hpf)

➤ Demography
   - 20% in children, 80% adults 20 – 50 years
   - M = F

- Laboratory
  - Peripheral eosinophilia in 80%
  - ↑ IgE
- Diagnostic Imaging
  - Edema and thickened gastric wall
- Clinical
  - Recurrent episodic gastrointestinal symptoms
    - Crampy abdominal pain
    - Nausea and vomiting
    - Diarrhea
    - Weight loss
  - Hypoproteinemia — edema
  - Malabsorption — steatorrhea, hypocalcemia
  - Symptoms related to anemia — fatigability, dyspnea
  - Eosinophilic ascites or pleural effusion
  - Depends on the extent and predominant layer of infiltration
    - Mucosa
      - Dyspepsia
      - Ulceration
      - Bleeding
      - Diarrhea
      - Malabsorption
      - ↓ weight
    - Muscularis propria
      - Obstruction
    - Serosa
      - Ascites
  - Associated with the following conditions:
    - Allergy
    - Food intolerance
    - Asthma
    - Drug sensitivity

- Diagnosis
    - Clinical
        - GI symptoms
        - No other causes of eosinophilia, i.e. drug reactions, parasites, Crohn's disease, lymphoma, mast cell, Langerhans cell histiocytosis, inflammatory fibroid polyp
    - Pathology
        - ↑ eosinophils (> 20/hpf) in GI tract
- Complication
    - Intestinal
        - Protein loss
        - Fat malabsorption
        - Iron deficiency
        - Vitamin B12 deficiency
        - Gastric outlet obstruction
        - Small bowel obstruction
        - Bacterial overgrowth
        - Gastrointestinal hemorrhage
    - Extra–intestinal complications
        - Mesenteric adenitis
        - Hepatosplenomegaly
        - Bone marrow eosinophilia
        - Eosinophilic pleuritis and peritonitis
        - Eosinophilic pancreatitis
        - Eosinophilic cystitis
        - Systemic reactions to food
- Differential diagnosis
    - Allergic gastroenteropathy
    - Crohn's disease
    - Carcinoma or lymphoma
    - Parasitic infestation
    - Tropical sprue, celiac sprue, Whipple's disease
    - Periarteritis nodosa
    - Amyloidosis

- Tuberculosis
- Allergic granulomatosis
- Disseminated eosinophilic collagen disease

❖ Disorders with moderate esosinophilia 1,000 – 5,000/mm^3
  - Allergic disorders
    - Asthma
    - Urticaria
    - Eczema
    - Drug allergy
  - Parasitic infections
    - Ascariasis
    - Schistosomiasis
    - Anisakiasis (Eustoma rotundatum)
    - Trichinosis
    - Tropical eosinophilia – probably due to microfilaria
    - Echinococcosis
    - Liver fluke
  - Collagen vascular diseases
    - Rheumatoid arthritis
    - Polyarteritis nodosa
  - Gastrointestinal diseases
    - Eosinophillic gastroenteritis
    - Ulcerative colitis
    - Crohn's disease
  - Neoplasia
    - Chronic myelogenous leukemia
    - Hodgkin's disease
    - Other lymphomas
    - Carcinoma (lung cancer)
    - Radiation–related eosinophilia
  - Miscellaneous
    - Pulmonary infiltrates with eosinophilia
    - Chronic peritoneal dialysis
    - Hereditary eosinophilia

- ❖ Disorders with marked eosinophilia
  - o Parasite infestations:
    - Visceral larva migrans associated with *Toxocara canis* or *T. catis* infestation
    - Tissue migration during the larval stage, including *Ascaris, Trichinella,* hookworms: *Strongyloides, Fasciola hepatica*
  - o Disseminated eosinophilic collagen disease or hypereosinophilic syndrome
  - o Eosinophilic leukemia
  - o Hodgkin disease
  - o Miscellaneous disorders, i.e. drug sensitivity and polyarteritis nodosa
- ➤ Diagnostic imaging
  - o Enlarged gastric rugal folds, i.e. antral narrowing and rigidity and irregular intraluminal mass
  - o Thickening and widening of the valvulae conniventes
  - o Regular nodular contour defects
  - o Distorted valvulae with irregular angulation and saw–toothed contour
  - o Luminal narrowing with rigid effaced folds
  - o Separation of intestinal loops
  - o "dysfunction pattern"
  - o Polypoid colonic defects
- ➤ Pathology
  - o Predominant mucosal disease
    - Fecal blood loss
    - Iron deficiency anemia
    - Intestinal protein loss with hypoproteinemia
    - Diarrhea
    - Fat malabsorption
  - o Predominant muscle layer disease
    - Pyloric narrowing and stomach outlet obstruction
    - Segmental small bowel involvement
  - o Predominant subserosal disease
    - Eosinophilic ascites

- ➢ Endoscopy
  - o May involve other parts of the GI tract
    - Eosinophilic infiltration is usually in the antrum
    - Preferentially in one layer explaining the symptoms and signs
  - o Wide range of changes, from normal reddened mucosa, nodules, erosions, ulcers
- ➢ Histopathology
  - o Marked patchy (clusters) or diffuse infiltration of the gastric antrum with eosinophils (> 20/hpf)
  - o Epithelial damage
  - o Eosinophils in mucosal epithelial cells, lamina propria, crypts (may develop crypt abscesses)
    - o Usually associated with eosinophilic gastroenteritis
    - o ↑ eosinophils (> 20/hpf)
      - Patchy or diffused
      - Found in the epithelium, lamina propria, crypts, muscularis, serosa
      - Usually is the most prominent in one layer
  - o Marked edema
  - o Epithelial damage with regeneration
  - o Antrum, eosinophilic gastritis
    - Large numbers of eosinophils infiltrate the lamina propria
    - Patchy eosinophilic infiltration of the mucosa, submucosa, muscularis propria, prominent submucosal edema
    - Characteristically, the deep mucosa is affected
    - Glands are infiltrated but not destroyed
  - o Lamina propria is expanded by edema
  - o Idiopathic eosinophilic gastritis
    - ↑ eosinophils
      - Intraepithelial
      - Crypt
      - Lamina propria
      - Patchy or diffused
    - > 20 eosinophils/hpf
    - Eosinophilic crypt abscesses

- Parasitic infection
  - ↑ eosinophils, but < 20/hpf
- Histiocytosis
  - Langerhans histiocytes (long, bean–shaped nuclei) plus eosinophils positive for CD la and S700
- Mastocytosis
  - Mast cells, positive for CD25, CD117, mast cell tryptase to distinguish them from eosinophils
- Churge–Strauss
  - Vasculitis
- Inflammatory fibroid polyp
- Miscellaneous conditions (with ↑ eosinophils)
  - Peptic ulcer disease
  - Carcinoma
  - Lymphoma
  - IBD
  - Connective tissue disease (CTD)

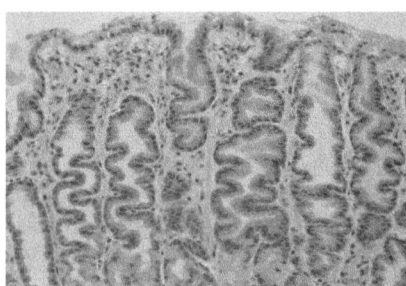

CMV inclusions

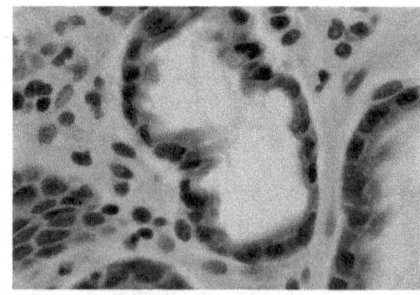

IELs in lymphocytic gastritis

- Treatment
  - Topical or systemic corticosteroids
  - Elimination diet
  - Leucokinine inhibitor

Clinical Tip
- Mucosal biopsies will not always detect eosinophils in the gastric eosinophilia, because the ↑ eosinophils per hpf may be patchy, or involve the deeper layers.
- If there is high suspicion of eosinophilic disease of the GI tract, a surgically obtained full thickness biopsy of the wall of the esophagus may be necessary.
- If mucosa biopsies are negative, then biopsies may be adequate and obtain tissues from the lamina propria.

SO YOU WANT TO BE A GASTROENTEROLOGIST!

Patients with hypereosinophilic syndrome have peripheral eosinophilia and involvement of the GI tract

- Give simple features of the hypereosinophilic syndrome (HS) distinguishing it from eosinophilic gastroenteritis (EG).

Features	EG	HS
o Peripheral eosinophilia	↑	↑↑↑ (> 1500/mm^3)
o Involvement of non–GI tissues	No	Yes
o Response to steroids	Excellent	Poor

Allergic Gastroenteropathy

- Mainly in the 1st and 2nd decades
  - Growth retardation, edema
  - ↓ albumin, ↓ globulin, protein–loosing
  - Anemia, blood eosinophilia
  - Manifestations of allergy (asthma, eczema, allergic rhinitis)
  - Small bowel eosinophilic infiltration in the mucosa and submucosa
  - Definite history of allergy to milk proteins or meat
  - Favorable response to elimination diet or corticosteroids

Disseminated Eosinophilic Collagen Disease

- Middle age, mainly male patients
- Persistent eosinophilia in the blood
- Diffuse organ infiltration by eosinophils (hepatosplenomegaly, heart disease, nervous system abnormalities, pulmonary disease)
- No other causes of eosinophilia (infectious or parasitic disease, neoplasia, etc.)
- Fever, anorexia, and weight loss, recurrent abdominal pain, persistent non–productive cough with chest pain, various neurologic abnormalities, pruritic rash, congestive heart failure, hepatosplenomegaly, lymphadenopathy
- Significant morbidity and mortality (average survival)

Hypereosinophilic Syndrome (HES)

- Middle age, mainly male patients
- Persistent hyper–eosinophilia in the blood >1500 eos/mm^3
- Diffuse organ infiltration by eosinophils (hepatosplenomegaly, heart disease, nervous system abnormalities, pulmonary disease, fever, weight loss, anemia)
- No other causes of eosinophilia (infectious or parasitic disease, neoplasia, etc.)
- Fever, anorexia, and weight loss, recurrent abdominal pain, persistent non–productive cough with chest pain, various neurologic abnormalities, pruritic rash, congestive heart failure, hepatosplenomegaly, lymphadenopathy

- Significant morbidity and mortality (average survival of 9 months) despite corticosteroids and/or antileukemic drugs
- Cardiovascular (Loeffler Fibroplastic Endocarditis), pulmonary, hematopoietic, and nervous system are most often involved, hepatic, dermatologic, gastrointestinal and renal involvement are less frequent

Gastrointestinal Stromal Tumors (GIST)

➤ Genetics

- Give the **genetics of GIST tumors** providing the rationale for the use of imatinib inr advanced (metastatic or inoperable) disease.
    - CD117
        - Positive (80%)
        - Activation mutation of KIT proto–oncogene → ↑ KIT expression
        - KIT is part of the c–kit receptor, a membrane TK
        - CD117 is part of the KIT (c–kit) receptor
        - Activation leads to tumor growth
    - CD117 mutation in the TK of GIST tumors is associated with response to imatinib
    - CD117 negative (20%), PDGFRA–positive
        - Activation mutation in another TK receptor, PDGFRA
        - Activation leads to tumor growth of ~ 66% of PDGFRA–positive GISTS are imatinib–resistant

➤ Diagnosis
    - EUS plus FNA
    - Markers for GIST on Immunohistochemical (IHC) studies

- What are the methods to distinguish GIST from leimyomas (LM) and from leimyosarcomas (LMS)?
    - C–kit (a stem cell factor receptor) (~ 99%)
        - CD34 (a hematopoietic cell progenitor cell antigen; 70%)
        - Smooth muscle actin (20 – 30%)
        - S 100 protein (marker of neural differentiation)

IHC antibody	GIST	LM or LMS
o C–kit (CD117)	+	−
o Smooth muscle actin	−	+
o Desmin	−	+

Note: EUS or FNA rather than IHC will differentiate leiomyoma from leiomyosarcoma

- Pathology
  - Fat
    - Lipoma
    - Liposarcoma
  - Muscle
    - Leiomyomas
      - Multiple in ~ 25%
    - Leiomyosarcomas
      - Usually, exogastric
  - Nerve
    - Schwannomas
  - Desmoid tumors
  - GIST is the most common stromal tumor in the stomach
    - Usually in the gastric fundus or small intestine
    - Endo– (into) or exogastric (away from lumen), given a dumbbell shape
    - Sites
      - Stomach ~ 70%
      - Small bowel ~ 25%
      - Colon or rectum 5%
    - Malignant potential
      - All GISTs > 10 mm
- Markers for GIST
  - C–kit (a stem cell factor receptor) (~ 99%)
  - CD34 (a hematopoietic cell progenitor cell antigen) (70%)

- Smooth muscle actin (20 – 30%)
- S 100 protein (marker of neural differentiation)

➢ Endoscopy

❖ Benign GIST
  - Intramural
  - Intraluminal polypoid appearance
  - Well–demarcated 90° angle between mass and normal gastric wall)
  - Smooth surface (typical of a submucosal tumor, with intact overlying mucosa)
  - Body
  - Similar appearance to the other submucosal tumors

❖ Malignant GIST
  - Larger
  - Irregular shape
  - Homogeneous
  - Intramural
  - Exophytic
  - Central necrosis
    - Fibroma
    - Neurogenic tumor
    - Vascular
    - Carcinoids

Distinguishing Diagnosis: Central Depression or Ulceration

- Malignant GIST
- Lipoma
- Ectopic pancreatic rest (umbilication; not an ulcer, since surface is covered with normal epithelium)
- Metastatic melanoma

- ❖ Metastatic Melanoma
    - o Submucosal mass
    - o Central ulceration
    - o Bull's eye ("target") lesion
    - o Multiple

> Distinguishing Diagnosis: Gastric Mass with Central Ulceration
> - o Adenocarcinoma
> - o Lymphoma
> - o GIST
> - o Metastatic melanoma
> - o Ectopic pancreatic rest

- ➢ Histopathology

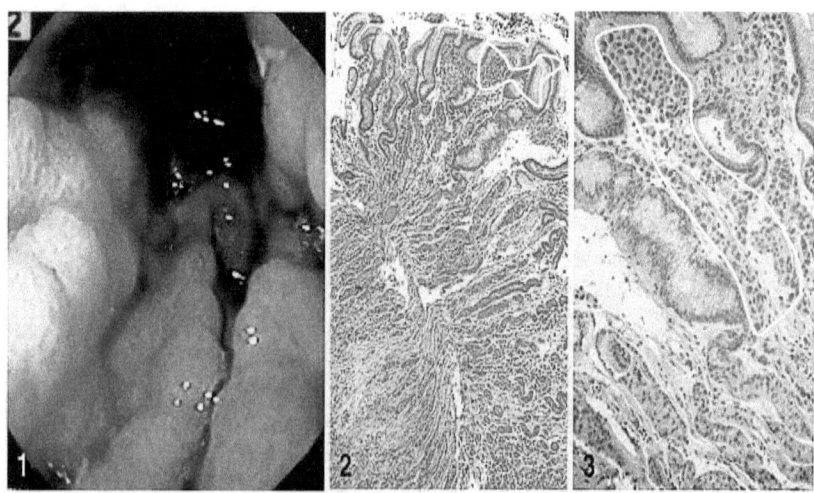

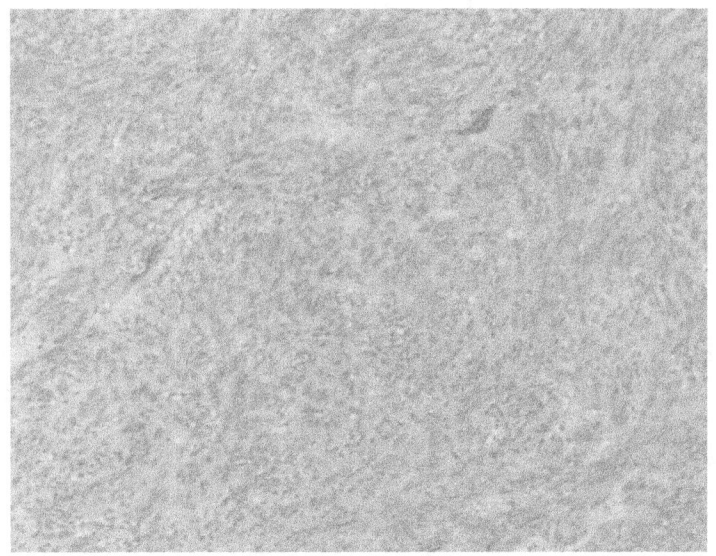

- Diffused infiltration of the elongated spindle cells

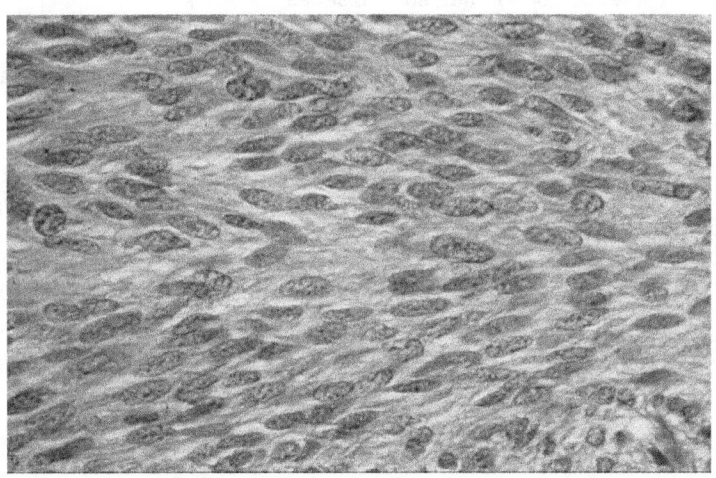

- Treatment

- Pharmacological
    - TKIs control GIST tumor growth in ~ 80%
        - Use neoadjuvant TKIs for 6 months, with imaging and reassessment for consideration, if possible, suitable for resection surgery
    - Use of tyrosine kinase inhibitors (TKIs), i.e. imatinib 400 – 800 mg/day depending on GIST mutation

Mutations	Most Common Site of GIST	Response	Dose per Day	Time (months) for Disease Progression
- Exon 11	Stomach	72%	400 mg	25
- Exon 9	Small bowel	44%	800 mg	17
- None		45%	400 mg	13

    - TKIs for GIST include imatinib and sunitinib
    - TKIs for recommended for the following:
        - Unresectable or metastatic disease
        - Adjuvant therapy and surgery
    - Stable tumor is as good as responsive tumor, i.e. response to imatinib — absence of tumor progression after 3 months of therapy
    - ↓ size of tumor in several days, but tumor may then enlarge from bleeding into the tumor or myxoid degeneration (interpretation: early ↑ size of tumor after imatinib does not necessarily mean failed therapy)
    - Difficult to determine if tumor in progressing of criteria is only tumor size, since a tumor may become cystic and appear to be stable, but new growth occurs in the cystic area ("nodule–within–a–mass") (hypodense cystic lesion becoming filled with hyperdense new tumor, used in Choi but not in RECIST criteria because of the inclusion of dense characteristics

- Surgery

- Assessment of Surgical Resectability
    - Choi Criteria for the response to imatinib assessed on contrast-enhanced CT scans depend on the size and change in tumor density on dual PET/CT scanning
        - ↓ 10% in tumor size
        - ↓ 15% in tumor density

- Choi criteria is a better predictor of tumor response than RECIST (response evaluation criteria in solid tumor)
o Segmental resection for ≥ 2 cm; leaving the tumor pseudocapsule intact
o Obtain negative tumor resection margins
o Laparoscopic resection is possible
o Neoadjuvant therapy with imatinib   GISTs ≥ 3 cm
                                        ↓ recurrence in post–op year 1
o Treatment of advanced disease, and palliation
o Surgical resection
  - For < 2 cm, resect if EUS shows the following features:
    - Irregular borders
      - Cysts
      - Ulceration
      - Echogenic foci
      - Heterogeneity (lack of homogeneity suggests area of necrosis)
    - > 2 mitoses/10 hpf
o Leiomyosarcomas
  - Adjacent structures
    - No invasion   need a nodal resection), with tumor–free margins (TFM)
    - Invasion   *en bloc* segmental resection with TFM
o Survival rates
  - 3 years   53%
  - 5 years   22%

- Tyrosine kinase inhibitors (TKIs)
  - Inhibition of receptor TKs results in ↓ growth of tumor
    - TK receptor antagonists bind to an ATP-binding site in TK receptors
    - Binding to TK receptors → ↓ phosphorylation of TK receptor
    - ↓ phosphorylation of TK receptor → ↓ activation
    - ↓ activation mutation of TK receptor → ↓ tumor growth
    - All KIT mutations are responsible to imatinib, whereas only some PDGFRA mutants are sensitive to imatinib
    - Some non-genetic inhibitory effects of TK receptor inhibitors may result from an anti-GIST immune response
  - Dose
    - Mostly small bowel GISTs require higher dose of imatinib when EXON and KIT are positive
    - Exon and KIT-positive
      - HR 0.58 for PFS for 800 mg vs 400 mg daily dose (i.e. use 800 mg imatinib)
    - Exon and KIT-negative
      - RFS 800 mg = 400 mg
      - Do not require higher dose (i.e. use 400 mg imatinib dose)

Abbreviation: RFS, recurrence-free survival

  - Trough level
    - Trough level of imatinib correlates with better clinical outcome
    - Keep trough level > 1100 ng/mL
    - Factors associated with low trough levels, and therefore a higher imatinib dose will be beneficial
      - Gastrectomy
      - ↑ serum albumin concentration
      - ↑ CCr (creatinine clearance, leading to ↓ trough concentrations of imatinib
      - Longer durations of treatment with imatinib
  - After ~ 2 years of TKI therapy, tumor develops new KIT mutations
    - Tumor may grow
    - Options
      - Continue imatinib
      - Switch from imatinib to sunitinib
      - Resection of residual disease, while continuing TKI to prolong survival

- Metastatic disease
  - Limited progression
    - Continue TKIs, plus surgery
  - Generalized progression
    - TKIs
- Liver metastases
  - Isolated
    - Hepatic resection plus TKI for non–multifocal bilobar disease (resectable disease)
  - For non–resectable (multifocal bilobar disease)
    - Hepatic arterial embolization with or without TKI (imatinib or sunitinib [a multitargeted TKI for imatinib–resistant diseases])

- Explain the **mechanism for the loss of imatinib response** in CD117–positive GIST tumors over time (> 1 year; secondary resistance).
  - Over time, there may be an increase in the renal clearance of imatinib, leading to ↓ trough levels
  - ↓ trough levels of imatinib → ↓ responsiveness of the tumor to the inhibition of TK kinases (C119 and PDGFRA)
  - Rate of tumor recurrence
    - Approximately 50% per 5 years of RFS
    - Scoring system to fine–tune the risk of recurrence
  - Although, GIST with PDGFRA EXON 18 D842V may recur, it is not sensitive to imatinib

- Explain why **PDGFRA–positive** (and therefore CD117↓negative) mutant patients with GIST may still be offered imatinib.
  - While 2/3 of PDGFRA mutants are imatinib–resistant (D842V substitution), 1/3 of PDGFRA mutants are imatinib–sensitive
  - Unless genetic testing can be done looking for the D842V substitution, PDGFRA patients still should be treated because of this 1 in 3 chance of responding to imatinib
  - Duration of treatment
    - Do not stop imatinib therapy after tumor has progressed
    - Tumor suppression with imatinib must be maintained
    - Stopping imatinib after an initial response only leads to return of progression of tumor

- Maintenance TKI must not be stopped for the fear of recurrence of GIST
- Continued (maintenance) TKI treatment for at least 3 years is necessary even after successful surgical resection of GIST
- Non-regression or local progression of GIST on imatinib is not a bad outcome as long as the tumor does not progress (i.e. stable disease is not necessarily bad) to become a generalized disease
- Generalized GIST progression while patient is on TKI has little to offer, and may be discontinued
- Sometimes, it is necessary to temporarily stop treatment with imatinib because of its AEs
- These AEs may improve even with the continuation of therapy

- What are the indications for **imatinib** neoadjuvant therapy prior to the resection of GIST?
    - Unsectable or borderline resection of locally advanced GIST
    - Potentially resectable locally advanced GIST, with extensive organ distruction
    - Source of GIST
        - Esophagus
        - Eesophagogastric junction
        - Duodenum
        - Distal rectum

- What are the **adverse effects** of imatinib?

    - Skin
        - Periorbital edema
        - Rash
    - MSK
        - Muscle cramps
    - GI
        - Nausea, vomiting, dyspepsia
        - Diarrhea
    - Hematology
        - Anemia
        - Thrombocytopenia

- Macrocytosis
- Neutropenia
  o Kidney
  - Hypophosphatemia
  o Endocrine
  - Gynecomastia
  o Heart
  - Low risk of heart failure in patients with pre-existing heart disease

---

SO YOU WANT TO BE AN ONCOLOGIST!

- What are the 4 indications for imatinib neoadjuvant therapy prior to resection of GIST?
  o Unresectable or borderline resection of locally advanced GIST
  o Potentially resectable locally advanced GIST with extensive organ destruction
  o Source of GIST
  - Esophagus
  - Esophagogastric junction
  - Duodenum
  - Distal rectum

SO YOU WANT TO BE A GASTROENTEROLOGIST!

Neoadjvant therapy for GIST with imatinib (starting TKI 6 months before surgical resection), with imaging diagnostic studies to assess response and timing of resection is a useful approach. The median time for the best response is 3.5 months, and further shrinkage is uncommon after 9 months of TKI.

- What are the findings on diagnostic imaging suggestive that GIST is responding to imatinib?
  o Optimal response to imatinib are the following:
  - Development of cystic structures
  - Change in vascularity
  o Change in tumor size is less important

Sunitinib

- Alternative to imatinib
- Switch from imatinib to sunitinib
  - Life-threatening side effects (intolerant) to imatinib
  - Imatinib-refractory condition (secondary resistance)
- Secondary resistance to imatinib may occur from the following:
  - Secondary mutations in KIT from selection of clones
  - ↑ renal clearance of imatinib → ↓ trough levels → ↓ tumor suppression
- Sunitinib blocks TK receptor vascular endothelia growth factor (VEGF)
- 50 mg *po od* for 4 out of every 6 weeks
- Response to sunitinib is higher for C119 patients with the following:
  - Primary KIT EXON 9
  - Wild-type KIT or PDGFRA mutation
  - KIT EXON 13 or 14 mutations
- Adverse effects
  - General
    - Fatigue
    - Fever
  - Skin
    - Mucositis
    - Hand-foot syndrome (acral erythema)
  - GI
    - Abdominal pain
    - ↑ lipase, amylase
    - Nausea, vomiting
    - Tumor bleeding, perforation
  - Renal
    - Renal toxicity
  - Endocrine
    - Hypothyroidism (~ 30% at 1 year)
  - CVS
    - Hypertension (47%)
    - ↓ LV ejection (28%)
    - CHF (8%)

Sorafenib

- o Use for resistance to imatinib, as well as resistance to sunitinib
- o TK inhibitor acts on:
  - KIT
  - PDGFR
  - VEGR

➢ Prognosis
- o Survival rates is 5–year 87%
- o Absolute benefit from imatinib is greatest in the high risk group
- o Standard of care for GISTs is a curable surgical resection
- o For patients who have GIST tumor which is unresectable or borderline resectable
  - Retrospective studies have shown that imatinib given initially (neoadjuvant TKI therapy), may shrink the tumor and patient's lesion may now be operable, or may allow for a more conservative local resection
  - TKI treatment is considered to be first line therapy for metastatic GIST

Gems and Pearl

- o URSO ↓ risk of gallstones by 40% after R–en–Y gastric bypass
- o Vertical banded gastroscopy (VBG) → pseudoachalasia

➢ Prognosis

Is a GIST benign or malignant?
- o Several risk stratification models (i.e. NIH, AJCC, UICC, AFIP) for discrete categories, continuous variables, or prognostic contour maps or risk of disease recurrence after complete surgical resection (i.e. tumor nomogram)
- o General concept: adverse prognostic factors and predictive of high risk for GIST recurrence, and likely benefit from TKI adjuvant therapy
  - Size ≥ 5 cm, or ≥ 10 cm

Number < 5

- Mitotic count   > 5 mitoses/hpf
- Mitotic rate   > 10/50 hpf (> 1/5 hpf)

Leiomyoma

- Histopathology

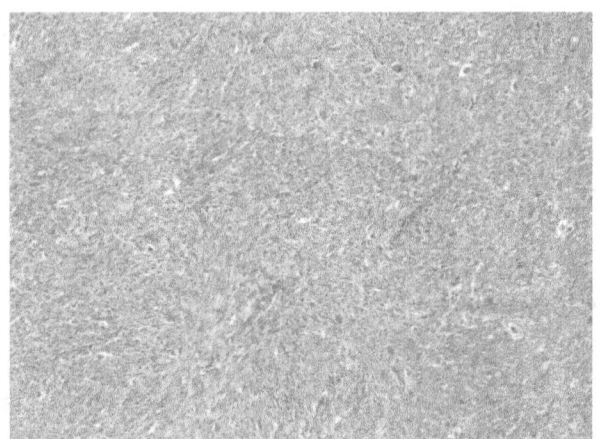

- Differential diagnosis: multiple ulcers
    - ZES — benign gastric ulcers

- Lymphoma
- Metastatic melanoma

HETEROTOPIA AND METAPLASIA

- Pancreatic heterotopia
  - Normal lobulated arrangement of acinar and ductal structures
  - Submucosal heterotopia of pancreatic acini, ducts, islet cells
  - Pancreatic acinar cells
    - Fine basophilic granules at the base of glands
    - Red granules at the apex of glands
  - No malignant cytoarchitectural features
  - No desmoplastic stromal response
  - Heterotopic components mixed in bundles of smooth muscles

- Adenocarcinoma (well-differentiated)
  - Abnormal lobulated arrangement of acini and ducts
  - Malignant cytoarchitectural features
  - Desmoplastic stromal response

- Pancreatic acinar metaplasia
  - Large, refractile red granules
  - Intestinal metaplasia
  - Associated with the following:
    - Chronic atrophic gastritis
    - Autoimmune gastritis

- Endocrine heterotopia
  - Pancreatic heterotopia involving islet cells but not the acini or ducts
  - Small microscopic nests of endocrine cells in the submucosa or muscularis
  - No desmoplastic response

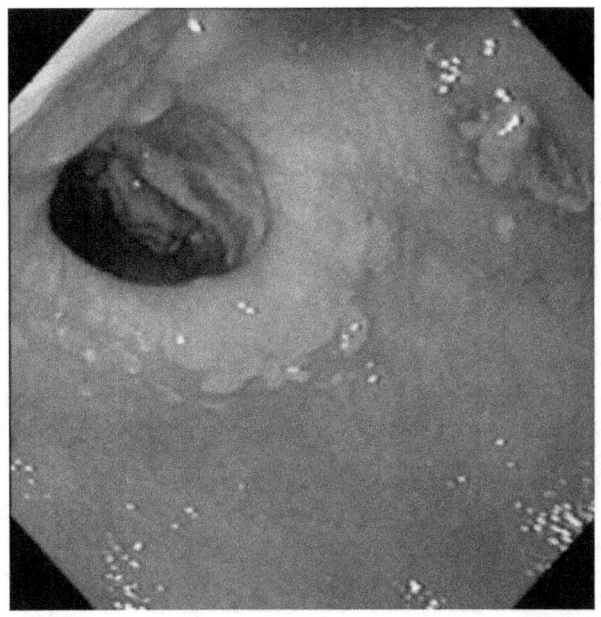

Metaplastic cancer

Pancreatic Heterotopia (pancreatic ectopia or rest)

➢ Definition
   o Pancreatic tissues found outside the pancreas forming intramural nodule
   o Pancreatic tissue not in continuity with pancreas (synonyms: pancreatic rest, ectopic pancreas)
   o Medium–power view of pancreatic heterotopia
   o This well–circumscribed submucosal nodule consists of pancreatic acinar tissue

➢ Demography
   o ~ 1% of gastric polyps
   o Slight M > F
   o Average age is 45 years

- Clinical
    - Usually asymptomatic
    - When inflamed → suggestive of pancreatiitis
    - When large → pyloric obstruction
    - May contain the following:
        - Neuroendocrine tissue
        - Adenocarcinoma
- Differentials
    - Adenocarcinoma (well–differentiated)
    - Adenomyoma (especially when only acinar cells, i.e. type III pancreatic heterotopia) mass on endoscopy (i.e. blind biopsy – why was the biopsy taken?)
        - Microscopic foci of pancreatic acini
        - Associated with inflammation, i.e. reflex esophagitis (why blind biopsies for "carditis"?)
    - Gastritis cystica profunda (occurring at the gastroenterostomy stomal sites)
    - Pancreatic acinar metaplasia: differentiated from acinar cells, i.e. exocrine type III heterotopia
        - Cardia
        - Not usually seen as a polyp
        - No ductular or islet cells

SO YOU WANT TO BE A GI PATHOLOGIST!

- What features distinguish pancreatic heterotopia from pancreatic acinar cell or Paneth cell metaplasia?

    - Pancreatic acinar cell metaplasia
        - Usually an incidental finding on mucosal biopsy of gastric cardia for suspected "carditis"
        - Inflammatory response
        - Granules

    - Paneth cell metaplasia
        - Large refractile red granules (no fine granules, and no basophilic granules at the base of the Paneth cell)
        - Associated with intestinal metaplasia in the following conditions:
            - Atrophic gastritis
            - Autoimmune gastritis

- Endoscopy
  - Well–demarcated
  - Single, small (2 – 40 mm) smooth surface
  - Submucosa
  - Hemispheric polyp (nodule, bump)
  - Central dimple erosion

  - Any part of the GI tract
    - 30% occur in the stomach
    - Rare in the following areas:
      - Gallbladder
      - Bile ducts
      - Umbilical cord
      - Mesentery
      - Mediastinum
  - Usual characteristics:
    - Single
    - Sessile
    - Well–demarcated nodule
  - Size
    - 2 – 40 mm
  - Site
    - Antrum
    - Prepylorus
  - Surface smooth
    - Central erosion or dimple (pancreatic duct)

- Histopathology
  - Endoscopic mucosal (superficial) biopsies may be normal because pancreatic heterotopia is submucosal
  - Lobulated arrangement of pancreatic tissues (ducts, acini, islet cells)
  - Often submucosal
  - Heinrich types of heterotopia

I   All cell types
    - Most common
    - No desmoplasia
    - Pleomorphism
    - Heterotopic components are mixed with bundles of smooth muscles
II Canalicular (duct)
III Exocrine (acinar cell)
IV Endocrine (islet cell)
    - Very rare
    - No stromal response
    o Note
        - Very rare that adenocarcinoma develops into duct cells

- Special studies
    o Immunostains for acinar and islet cells

Paneth Cell Metaplasia

➢ Histopathology

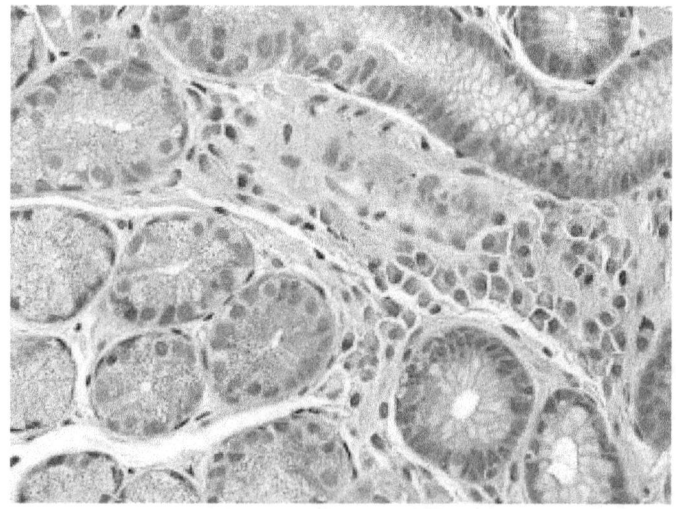

Provided by Dr. Aducio Thiesen, University of Alberta

THICKENED BASEMENT MEMBRANE

Apparent Fibrosis of Lamina Propria

- ➢ Amyloid
  - o Deposit
    - Extracellular
    - Dense
    - Homogenous
    - Acellular
    - Eosinophilic
  - o Location
    - Lamina propria
    - Submucosa
    - Muscularis propria
    - Vessels
    - Nerves

- ➢ Atherosclerosis
  - o Hyalinization of the artery may look like amyloid

Stains	Amyloid	Atherosclerosis
o Congo red	+	-
o Masson trichrome (blue;collagen)	-	+

- ➢ Systemic sclerosis
- ➢ Ischemic gastritis
  - o Fibrosis of the submucosa and muscularis
  - o Masson trichrome positive, Congo red–negative
  - o Lamina propria
  - o Ischemic injury
    - Erosions
    - Exudates
    - Microcryptitis
  - o No eosinophilic, dense, globular extracellular (amyloid) deposits

Gastric Amyloid

- ➢ Definition
  - o Extracellular, eosinopphilic, dense sheets of non-branching 7.5 – 10 nm diameter fibrils of β–pleated protein in the gastric lamina propria, submucosa, muscularis propria, vessel walls or nerve trunk of most persons with systemic amyloidosis

- ➢ Demography
  - o Present in most patients with systemic amyloidosis

- ➢ Diagnostic imaging
  - o Gastric wall
    - ↑ thickness
    - ↓ distention
  - o Erosion
  - o Ulcers
  - o Mass
  - o Serum amyloid P component scan
    - Amyloid deposits in other tissues, i.e.
      - Kidney
      - Liver
      - Spleen

- ➢ Differentiated diagnosis (mistaken as amyloid)
  - o Arteriosclerosis
    - Hyalinization of vessels stained blue with Masson's trichrome
    - Negative Congo red stains
  - o Systemic sclerosis
    - Fibrosis (collagen) of muscularis and submucosa stained blue with Masson's trichrome stain
    - Negative Congo red stain
  - o Fibrosis of the lamina propria (i.e. ischemic gastritis)
    - No vascular amyloid deposits
    - Erosion, exudates, microcrypts

- Endoscopy
  - Thick gastric rugae and folds
  - Erosions and ulcers
  - Mass
  - "waxy" appearance of the involved area
- Histopathology
  - Site
    - Patchy or diffuse
  - Extracellular deposits
    - Reddish
    - Homogenous
  - Layer
    - Lamina propria
    - Submucosa
    - Muscularis propira
    - Nerve trunk vessels
  - Slit–like space in deposits
  - Lamina propria with amyloid
  - Submucosa or muscularis propria with amyloid
  - Patchy or diffuse
  - High diagnostic yield from biopsies of stomach or rectum
  - Amyloid deposits
    - Vessel walls → fragile, leaky, bleeding
    - Muscles, nerves → dysmotility
    - Lamina propria (AA), submucosa, and muscularis propria (AC)
    - Dense, homogeneous eosinophillic (red) deposits with Congo red
    - Polarized light shows birefringence
  - Green birefringence on Congo red stain distinguishes mucosal or submucosal deposit of amyloid
  - Also present in the blood vessel walls

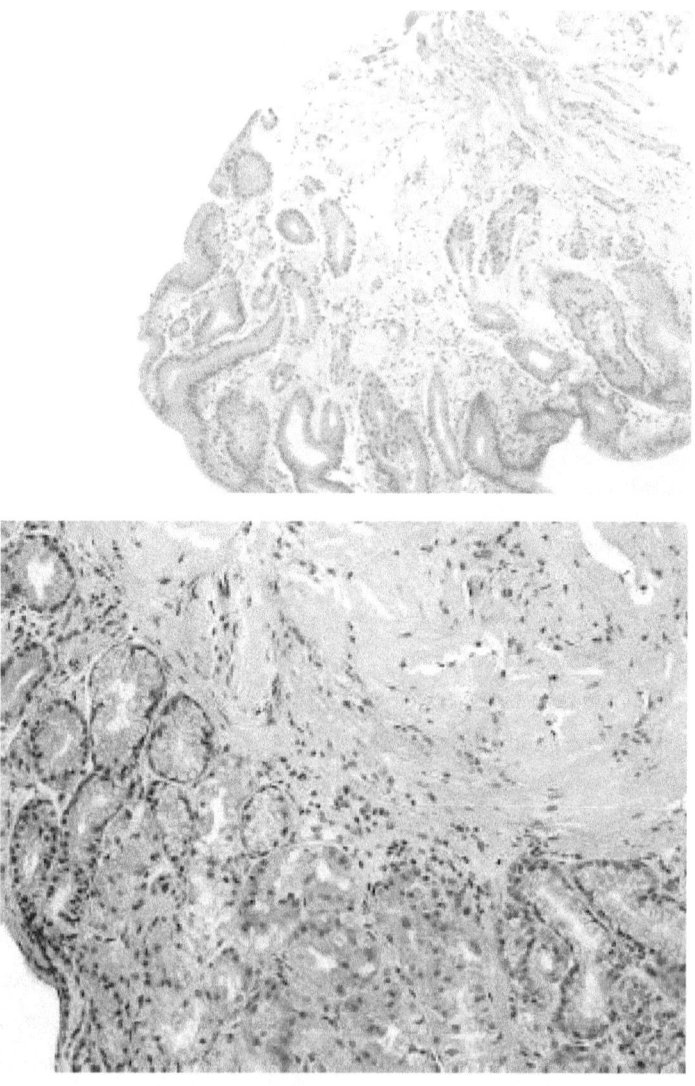

Provided kindly by Dr. Aducio Thiesen, University of Alberta

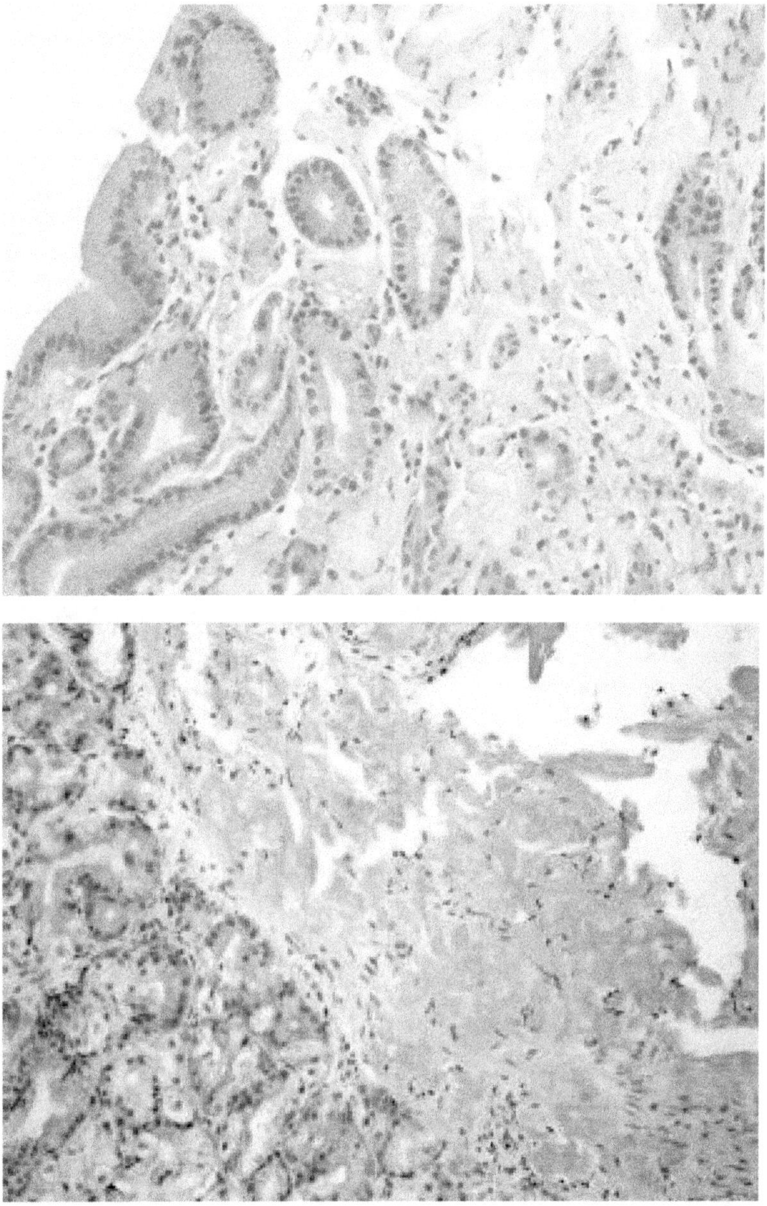

Provided kindly by Dr. Aducio Thiesen, University of Alberta

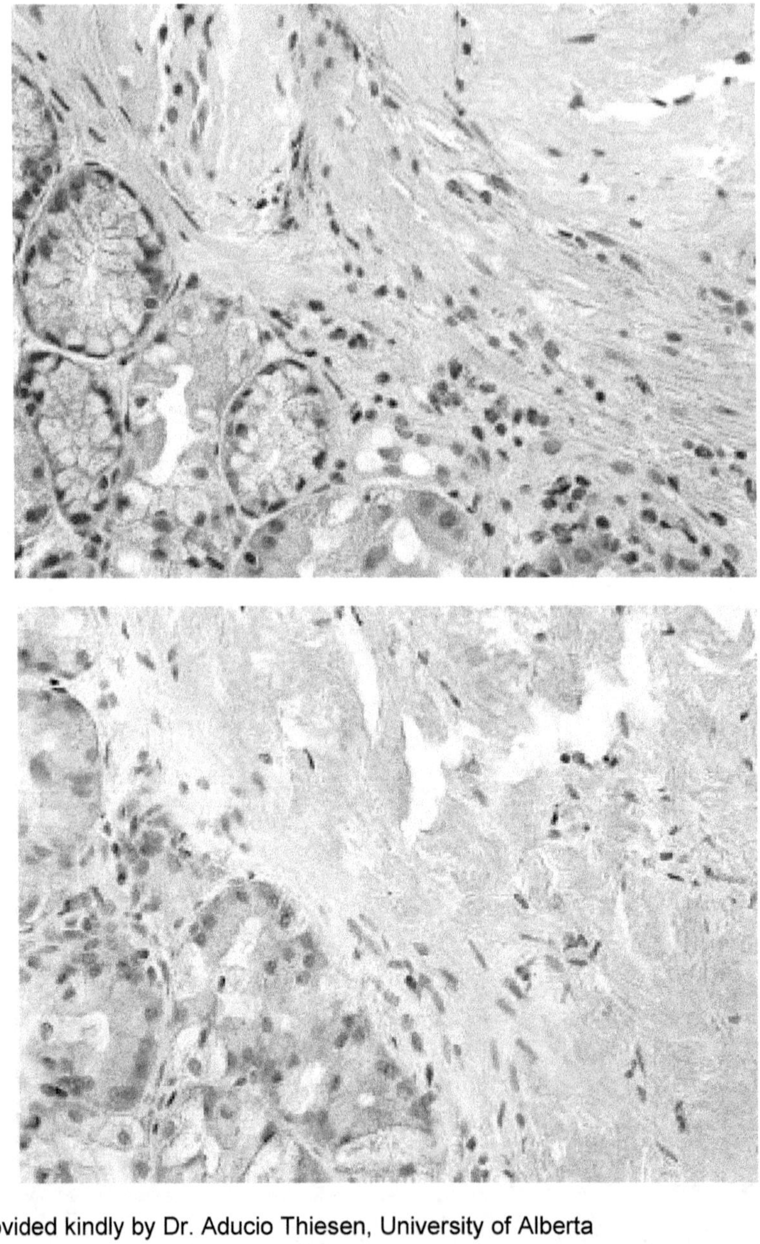

Provided kindly by Dr. Aducio Thiesen, University of Alberta

- Special studies
  - Immunostains
    - CD138, antibodies κ or λ against precursor proteins

SO YOU WANT TO BE A GASTROENTEROLOGIST!

Congo red stain makes amyloid red in white light, while polarized light turns deposits to apple–green birefringence.

- What is the role of potassium permanganate, Masson trichrome, and CD138, κ and λ antibody immunostains in the histopathological investigation of patient with suspected gastric amyloidosis?
  - Potassium permanganate

Amyloid	Pretreatment with potassium permanganate	Congo red stain (after prestain)
AL	+	+
AA	+	-

  - Thus, if the deposit is red with congo red (white light), suspicious of amyloid. Then, if the tissue is prestained with potassium permanganate and Congo red is negative, the amyloid deposit is AA.
  - Masson trichome
    - Collagen or hyaline is positive in Masson trichrome (MT) stain while Congo red (CR) is negative
    - Thus, in patient with possible atherosclerosis or scleroderma, tissue staining with MT is positive and CR is negative, helping to exclude amyloidosis

MISCELLANEOUS GASTRIC CONDITIONS

- ➢ Miscellaneous
    - o Cardia or fundus
        - Diverticulum
        - Pseudotumor
    - o Rest of stomach
        - Emphysematous gastritis
        - Partial diverticulum
        - Volvulus
    - o Barium rests
    - o Erosions
    - o Peptic ulcer
    - o Carcinoma
- ➢ Crohn's disease
    - o Thickened folds
    - o Multiple small erosions with halo (aphthous ulcers)
    - o Ulcers, confluent serpiginous
    - o Mucosal cobblestone
    - o Fibrosis
    - o Strictures
    - o Distal half of the stomach
    - o Often with associated duodenal ulcer
    - o Collagenous gastritis
    - o Amyloidosis
- ➢ Varices
    - o GE junction
    - o May be associated with esophageal varices
- ➢ Diverticulum
    - o Pouch is filled with barium
    - o Posterior surface of the fundus is near the GE junction
    - o Mucosal folds in the pouch
    - o May change the size and shape

- Partial gastric diverticum
  - Definition: "protrusion of the [gastric] mucosa into the muscular wall of the stomach without disturbing the serosa"
  - Intramural collection of barium
  - Greater curve
  - Narrow neck
  - Barium–filled pouch changes the size or shape
  - May be associated with ectopic pancreatic tissue
- Emphysematous gastritis
  - Intramural gastric air
  - Causes
    - Infection
      - *E. coli*
      - *Clostridium perfringens*
    - Ischemia
    - Ingestion of corrosive materials
    - Obstruction of the stomach
    - Gastric volvulus
- Tortion
  - Organoaxial tortion
    - 180^0 torsion along the longitudinal axis
    - Greater curvature is superior to the lesser curve
    - Gastric body is superior to the fundus ("upside–down" stomach)
  - Mesenteroaxial tortion
    - 180^0 torsion above the gastric mesentery
    - Pylorus and antrum folded anteriorly and superiorly
- Duodenal tumors
  - Benign
    - Lipoma
    - (GIST
    - Brunner's gland hyperplasia
    - Heterotropic gastric mucosa
    - Pseudopolyp (redundant mucosa at the junction of D1 or D2)
  - Malignant
    - Adenocarcinoma
    - Lymphoma
    - GIST
    - Metastases

Foamy Macrophages

- ➤ Gastric xanthomas (xanthelasmas)
  - o Lamina propria
    - Foamy macrophage filled with fat, with central nucleus in the lamina propria

- ➤ Clear cell carcinoid tumor
  - o Chemical gastropathy changes in the surrounding mucosa
  - o Histopathologically similar to gastric xanthomas or xanthelasmas

- ➤ Signet ring cell carcinoma
  - o Cytoplasm
    - Mucin vacuoles in the cytoplasm of the epithelial cells displacing the nucleus
  - o Nuclei
    - Hyperchromasia
    - Mitosis

- ➤ Whipple's disease
  - o Foamy macrophage, PAS–positive, diastase–resistant
  - o Positive immunostain for Tropheryma whipplei

- ➤ MAI infection
  - o Acid fast *Bacilli* in foamy macrophages

Gastric Xanthomas

- ➤ Definition
  - o Clusters of lipid–filled macrophages in the lamina propria
  - o Collections of macrophages filled with lipid in the gastric lamina propria
  - o Synonyms include gastric xanthelasma or lipidosis

- ➤ Demography
  - o M > F = 3:1
  - o > 60 years
  - o Present in ~ 1% of EGDs

- Causes and associations
  - Cholestasis
  - *H. pylori*
  - Chronic atrophic gastritis with intestinal metaplasia
  - Partial gastric resections
  - Gastric ulcers
  - Gastric adenocarcinoma
  - Chemical gastropathy
- Clinical usually an incidental finding

SO YOU WANT TO BE A GASTROENTEROLOGIST!

- Give the prevalence of gastric xanthomas with skin xanthelasmas.
  - There is surprisingly no association.

- Differentialdiagnosis (mistaken as fat deposits or foamy macrophages)
  - Signet ring cell carcinoma
    - Mucin vacuoles
    - Positive mucin stains
    - PAS and cytokeratin–positive
  - Granular cell tissue
    - Clusters of cells with eosinophillic granular cytoplasm
    - Positive for S–100 and CD68
  - Clear cell carcinoid
    - Positive for chromogranin and synaptophysin
  - MAI infection
    - Immunosuppressed patients
    - *Bacilli* are acid fast
  - Malakoplakia
    - Gram negative infection (i.e. *E. coli*) causing xanthogranulomatous appearance

- Whipple's disease
  - Foamy macrophage, PAS-positive and diastase-resistant
  - Immunostaining positive for *Trophyrema whipplei*
- Lepromatous leprosy
  - Foamy macrophages
  - Acid fast *Bacilli*

Gastric xanthomas stain positive for CD68, and negative for PAS, cytokeratins, S-100, mucin and chromogranin, synaptophysin and for calcium. The selection of the negative stains hints at the differential of gastric xanthomas.

- Name the lesions confused with gastric xanthomas, and for which the above stains, name the useful negative in xanthomas.

Differential lesions	Positive stains
o Signet cell adenocarcinoma	PAS Mucin Cytokeratins
o Granular cell tumor	S-100
o Carcinoid (clear cell) tumor	Chromogranin Synaptophysin
o Calcium (Michaelis- Gutmann bodies)	Von Kossa calcium stain
o Whipple's disease	PAS

- Endoscopy
  - Small (1 – 5 mm)
  - Sessile
  - Multiple
  - Yellow or white
  - Nodule or plaques
  - Single or multiple
  - Small (1 – 5 mm)
  - Sessile
  - Pale yellow nodules or plaques
  - Mostly along the lesser curve, prepyloric antrum, or at the gastric stoma
- Histopathology

- Macrophages filled with lipid forming a foamy cytoplasm
- Central bland nuclei
- Normal mitosis
- Not associated with skin xanthelasmas or hyperlipidemia
- Associated with the following conditions:
  - Cholestasis
  - Reactive (chemical) gastropathy
  - Chronic atrophic gastritis with intestinal metaplasia
  - *H. pylori* (48%)
  - Gastric ulcer, cancer, post surgical bile gastritis
- Clusters of "foamy" macrophages, from the ↑ lipid in the cytoplasm usually in lamina propria
- Surrounding mucosa
  - *H. pylori*–associated chronic gastritis
  - Chemical or bile gastropathy

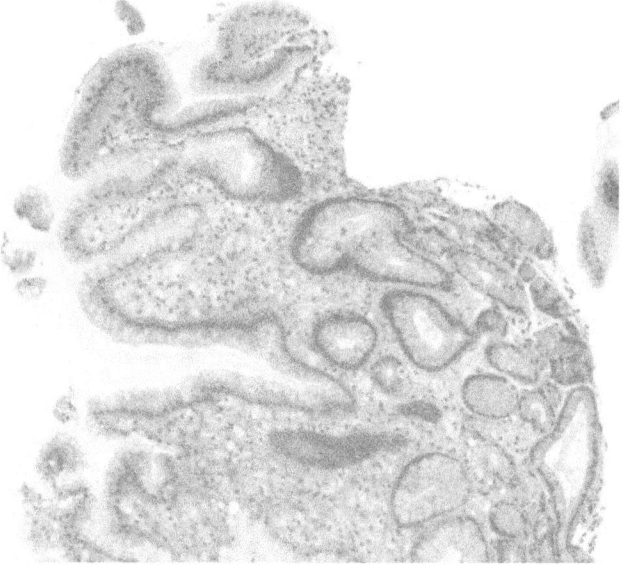

Provided kindly by Dr. Aducio Thiesen, University of Alberta

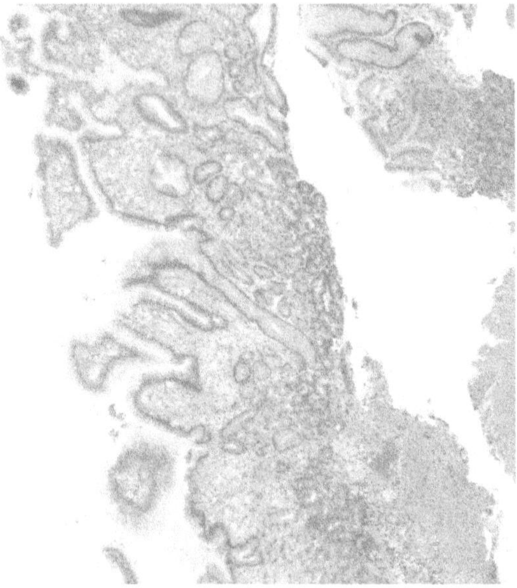

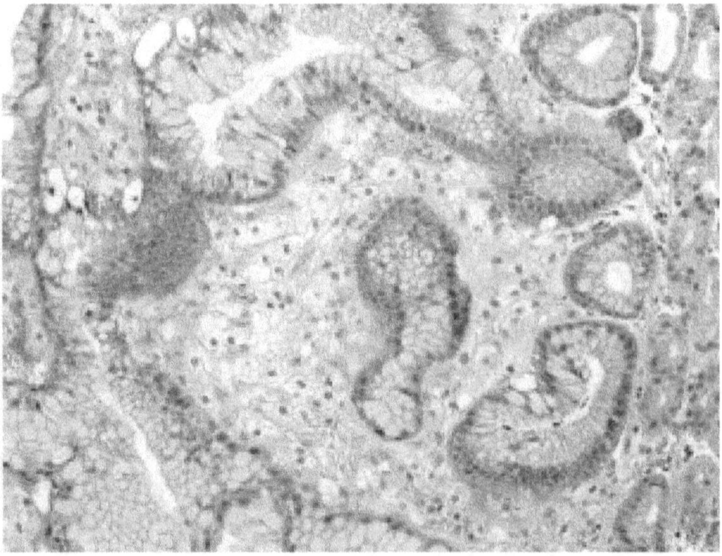

Provided kindly by Dr. Aducio Thiesen, University of Alberta

FROM COMPETENCE TO EXCELLENCE
The Stomach

© A.B.R. Thomson

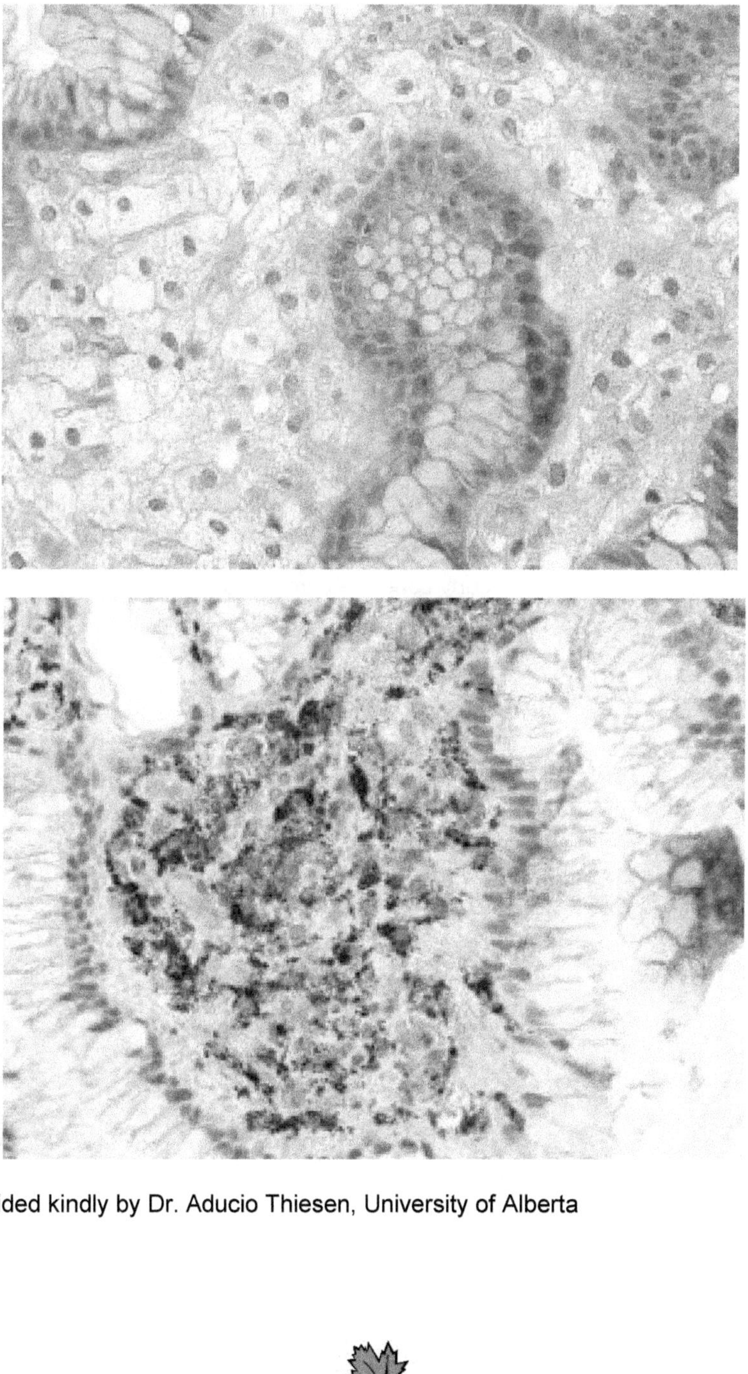

Provided kindly by Dr. Aducio Thiesen, University of Alberta

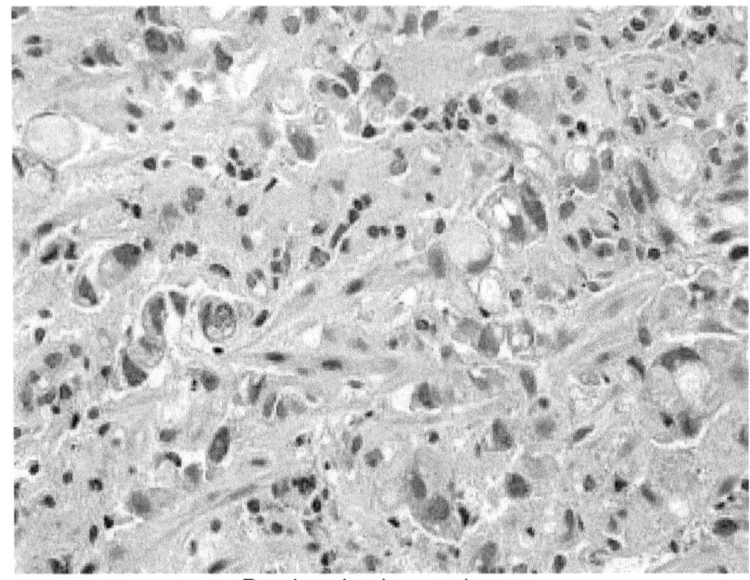
Poorly cohesive carcinoma

Provided kindly by Dr. Aducio Thiesen, University of Alberta

- Special studies
    - Fat stains (cholesterol, triglyceride)
        - Positive
            - Sudan black
            - Oil red O

Signet–Ring Cell Carcinoma

- Histopathology
    - Tumor cells with voluminous cytoplasm are scattered in the lamina propria
    - Nuclei are large and eccentric

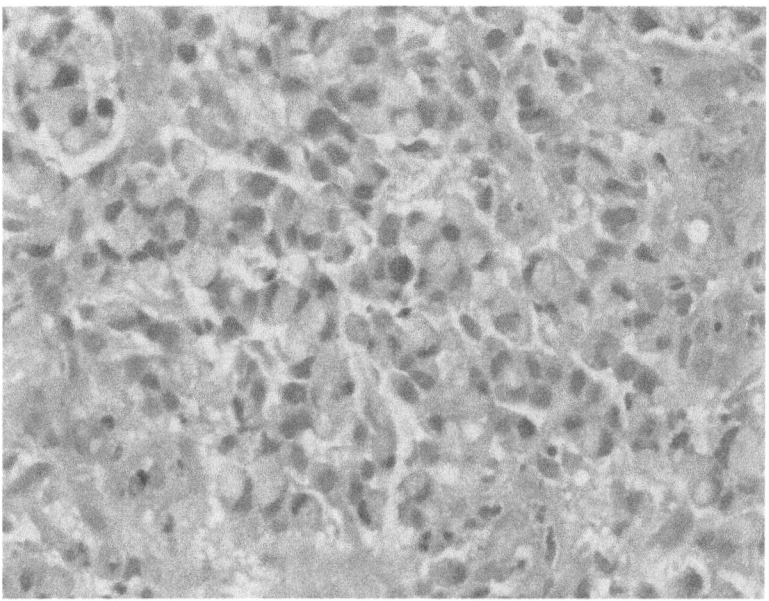

    - Tumor cells with varying degrees of cytoplasmic vacuolization fill of the lamina
    - Some have a central density giving a bull's eye appearance
    - Diffuse infiltration of signet ring cells

ABBREVIATIONS

5–HT$_3$	5–hydroxytryptamine
AA	Amino acids
ABC	Airway breathing circulation
Ach	Acetylcholine
AG	Atrophic gastritis
AMAG	Autoimmune metaplastic atrophic gastritis
ANG	Acute necrotizing gastritis
ANS	Autonomic nervous system
AP	Action potential
ASA	Acetylsalicylic acid
ASA	American Society of Anesthesiologist
BOM	Bacterial overgrowth syndrome
BOS	Bacterial overgrowth syndrome
BPD	Biliopancreatic diversion
Cag PAI	Cag pathogenicity island
CE	Capsule endoscopy
CNS	Central nervous system
COPD	Chronic obstructive pulmonary disease
COX-2	Cyclooxygenase–2
COXIBs	COX–2 inhibitors
CMV	*Cytomegalovirus*
CNS	Central nervous system
CT	Concomitant therapy
CTE	CT enterography
CV	Cardiovascular
CVA	Cerebrovascular accident
DBE	Double–balloon enteroscopy
DCAG	Diffuse corporal atrophic gastritis
DMN	Dorsal motor nucleus
DU	Duodenal ulcer
ECa	Esophageal cancer
ECL	Enterochromaffin–like

EGC	Early gastric cancer
EGD	Esophagogastroduodenoscopy
EGFR	Epidermal growth factor receptor
EHT	Endoscopic hemostatic therapy
EMAG	Environmental multifocal atrophic gastritis
EMR	Endoscopic mucosal resection
ENS	Enteric nervous system
EPS	Epigastric pain syndrome
ET	Endoscopic hemostatic therapy
ET	Eradication therapy
EUS	Endoscopic ultrasound
EVB	Esophageal variceal bleed
FAP	Familial adenomatous polyposis
FNA	Fine needle aspiration
GABA	Gamma–aminobutyric acid
GAVE	Gastric antral vascular ectasia
GCa	Gastric cancer
GCP	Gastritis cystica profunda
GERD	Gastroesophageal reflux disease
GET	Gastric emptying test
GI	Gastrointestinal
GIST	Gastrointestinal stromal tumor
GRP	Gastrin related peptide
GU	Gastric ulcer
GVB	Gastric variceal bleed
GVE	Gastric vascular ectasia
GVHD	Graft–versus–host disease
H2RA	H2 receptor antagonist
HDGC	Hereditary diffuse gastric cancer
HGF	Hepatocyte growth factor
HHG	Hyperplastic hypersecretory gastropathy
HHT	Hereditary hemorrhagic telegangiectasia
HNPCC	Hereditary non–polyposis colon cancer

HP-NAP	*H. pylori* neutrophil–activating protein
HPG	*H. pylori* gastritis
HSV	*Herpes simplex* virus
IBS	Irritable bowel syndrome
ICC	Interstitial cells of Cajal
IFN-γ	Interferon–gamma
IM	Intestinal metaplasia
IML	Intermediolateral columns
IMMC	Interdigestive migrating motor complex
IPPN	Isolated pyloric pressure waves "pylorospams"
ITP	Idiopathic thrombocytopenic purpura
LAGB	Laparoscopic adjustable gastric banding
Les	Liver enzymes
LES	Lower esophageal sphincter
LFTs	Liver function tests
LGD	Low grade dysplasia
LPS	Lipopolysaccharide
MAG	Multifocal atrophic gastritis
MALT	Mucosa-associated lymphoid tissue
MDCT	Multi-detector row CT
MDSCs	Myeloid-derived suppressor cells
MEN	Multiple endocrine neoplasia
MHC	Major histocompatibility
MMD	Mild to moderate dysplasia
mToR	Mammalian target of rapamycin
MU	Marginal ulcer
n	Nerve
NA	Nucleus ambiguous
NERD	Non–erosive reflux disease
NFAT	Nuclear translocation of a transcription factor
NNT	Number needed to treat
NO	Nitric oxide
NOD_1	Nucleotide-binding oligomerization domain-1

NPV	Negative predictive value
NPY	Neuropeptide Y
NSAIDs	Non–steroidal anti–inflammatory drugs
NUD	Non–ulcer dyspepsia
NVUGIB	Non-variceal upper GI bleeding
OGIB	Obscure GI bleeding
OTC	Over–the–counter
PACAP	Pituitary adenylate cyclase-activating polypeptide
PAMPS	Pathogen-associated molecular receptors
PDT	Photodynamic therapy
PE	Push enteroscopy
PG	Phlegmonas gastritis
PHG	Portal hypertensive gastropathy
PI3K	Phosphatidylinositol 3–kinase
PLR	Positive likelihood ratio
PNS	Parasympathetic nervous system
PONV	Post–operative nausea and vomiting
PP	Plateau potential
PPD	Post–prandial distress
PPIs	Proton pump inhibitors
PPV	Positive predictive value
PR	Pulse rate
PRBC	Packed red blood cells
PTPRT	Protein–tyrosine phosphatase receptor–type
PUD	Peptic ulcer disease
PYY	Peptide YY
RFA	Radiofrequency ablation
RMP	Resting membrane potential
RR	Relative risk
RUNX$_3$	Runt–related transcription factor 3
SBE	Single balloon enteroscopy
RYGB	Roux–en–Y gastric bypass
SBP	Systolic blood pressure

SCF	Stem cell factor
SD	Severe dysplasia
SE	Sleeve gastrectomy
SHR	Endoscopic stigamata of recent hemorrhage.
SIBO	Small intestinal bacterial overgrowth
SIDS	Sudden infant death syndrome
SK	Substance K
SNS	Sympathetic nervous system
SOD	Sphincter of Oddi
SP	Substance P
SSRI	Selective serotonin reuptake inhibitors
SST	Somatostatin
T & T	Test and treat
TB	Tuberculosis
TFF_1	Trefoil protein
TFM	Tumor–free margins
TGF-α	Transforming growth factor–alpha
TIPS	Transjugular intrahepatic portosystemic shunt
TK	Tyrosine kinase
TLRs	Toll–like receptors
TNF-α	Tumor necrosis factor–alpha
Treg	Regulatory T–cells
TS	Tractus solitaries
UBT	Urea breath test
UCDA	Ursodeoxycholic acid
UGIB	Upper GI bleeding
VBG	Vertical banded gastroplasty
VEGF	Vascular endothelial growth factor
VIP	Vasoactive intestinal peptides
ZES	Zollinger–Ellison syndrome

433

© A.B.R. Thomson

SUGGESTED READINGS

Atrophy

Systemic Reviews and Meta-analysis

Neumann, W. L., et al. Autoimmune atrophic gastritis--pathogenesis, pathology and management. Nat Rev Gastroenterol Hepatol. 2013. 10(9):529-541.

Bariatric Surgery

Papers and Reviews

Kumar, N. and Thompson, C. C. Endoscopic management of complications after gastrointestinal weight loss surgery. Clin Gastroenterol Hepatol. 2013. 11(4):343-353.

Miras, A. D. and Le–Roux, C. W. Mechanisms underlying weight loss after bariatric surgery. Nat Rev Gastroenterol Hepatol. 2013. 10(10):575-584.

Strohmayer, E., et al. Metabolic management following bariatric surgery. Mt Sinai J Med. 2010. 77(5):431-445.

Systemic Reviews and Meta-analysis

Eisendrath and Deviere, J. Major complications of bariatric surgery: endoscopy as first-line treatment. Nat Rev Gastroenterol Hepatol. 2015. 12(12):701-710.

Guidelines and Consensus

American Society for Gastrointestinal Endoscopy Standards of Practice Committee, et al. The role of endoscopy in the bariatric surgery patient. Gastrointest Endosc. 2015. 81(5):1063-1072.

Mechanick, J. I., et al. American Association of Clinical Endocrinologists, The Obesity Society, and American Society for Metabolic & Bariatric Surgery medical guidelines for clinical practice for the perioperative nutritional, metabolic, and nonsurgical support of the bariatric surgery patient. Obesity (Silver Spring). 2009. 17 Suppl 1:S1-70.

Cancer

Papers and Reviews

Abnet, C. C., et al. Diet and upper gastrointestinal malignancies. Gastroenterology. 2015. 148(6):1234-1243.

Tan, P. and Yeoh, K. G. Genetics and Molecular Pathogenesis of Gastric Adenocarcinoma. Gastroenterology. 2015. 149(5):1153-1162.

Veitch, A. M., et al. *Optimizing early upper gastrointestinal cancer detection at endoscopy. Nat Rev Gastroenterol Hepatol.* 2015.12(11):660-667.

Guidelines and Consensus

Allum, W. H., et al. *Guidelines for the management of oesophageal and gastric cancer. Gut.* 2011. 60(11):1449-1472.

Dyspepsia

Papers and Reviews

Camilleri, M. and Stanghellini, V. *Current management strategies and emerging treatments for functional dyspepsia. Nat Rev Gastroenterol Hepatol.* 2013. 10(3):187-194.

Feldman, M. J. Edward Berk. *Distinguished [corrected] lecture: Gastric acid secretion: still relevant? Am J Gastroenterol.* 2013. 108(3):347-352.

Graham, D.Y. and Rugge, M. *Clinical practice: diagnosis and evaluation of dyspepsia. J Clin Gastroenterol.* 2010. 44(3):167-172.

Lacy, B.E., et al. *Review article: current treatment options and management of functional dyspepsia. Aliment Pharmacol Ther.* 2012. 36(1):3-15.

Guidelines and Consensus

Yang, Y. X., et al. *American Gastroenterological Association Institute Guideline on the Role of Upper Gastrointestinal Biopsy to Evaluate Dyspepsia in the Adult Patient in the Absence of Visible Mucosal Lesions. Gastroenterology.* 2015. 149(4):1082-1087.

Gastric Cancer

Systemic Reviews and Meta-analysis

McLean, M. H. and El-Omar, E.M. *Genetics of gastric cancer. Nat Rev Gastroenterol Hepatol.* 2014. 11(11):664-674.

Endoscopy

Guidelines and Consensus

ASGE Standards of Practice Committee, et al. *The role of endoscopy in the management of premalignant and malignant conditions of the stomach. Gastrointest Endosc.* 2015;82(1):1-8.

Gastroparesis

Papers and Reviews

ASGE Standards of Practice Committee, *et al.* The role of endoscopy in gastroduodenal obstruction and gastroparesis. Gastrointest Endosc. 2011. 74(1):13-21.

Camilleri, M., *et al. Clinical guideline: management of gastroparesis. Am J Gastroenterol.* 2013. 108(1):18-37.

Gastritis

Papers and Reviews

Neumann, W. L., *et al.* Autoimmune atrophic gastritis--pathogenesis, pathology and management. *Nat Rev Gastroenterol Hepatol.* 2013. 10(9):529-541.

Peptic Ulcer Disease (PUD)

Papers and Reviews

Feldman, M., *et al.* J. Edward Berk Distinguished [corrected] lecture: Gastric acid secretion: still relevant? *Am J Gastroenterol.* 2013. 108(3):347-352.

H. pylori Infection (HP)

Papers and Reviews

Graham, D. Y. *Helicobacter pylori* update: gastric cancer, reliable therapy, and possible benefits. Gastroenterology. 2015. 148(4):719-731.

McColl, K. E. Clinical practice. *Helicobacter pylori* infection. *N Engl J Med.* 2010. 362(17):1597-604.

Non-Variceal Upper Gastrointestinal Bleeding (NVUGIB)

Papers and Reviews

Hayes, S. M., *et al.* Barriers to the implementation of practice guidelines in managing patients with nonvariceal upper gastrointestinal bleeding: A qualitative approach. *Can J Gastroenterol.* 2010. 24(5):289-296.

Laine, L. and Jensen, D. M. Management of patients with ulcer bleeding. *Am J Gastroenterol.* 2012. 107(3):345-360.

Lau, J. Y., *et al.* Omeprazole before endoscopy in patients with gastrointestinal bleeding. *N Engl J Med.* 2007. 356(16):1631-1640.

Sreedharan, A., *et al.* Proton pump inhibitor treatment initiated prior to endoscopic diagnosis in upper gastrointestinal bleeding (Review). The Cochrane Library. 2012. 3: http://www.thecochraanelibrary.com

Tsoi, K. K., et al. Second-look endoscopy with thermal coagulation or injections for peptic ulcer bleeding: a meta-analysis. *J Gastroenterol Hepatol*. 2010. 25(1):8-13.

Villanueva, C., et al. Transfusion strategies for acute upper gastrointestinal bleeding. *N Engl J Med*. 2013. 368(1):11-21.

Systemic Reviews and Meta-analysis

Fletcher, E. H., et al. Systematic review: Helicobacter pylori and the risk of upper gastrointestinal bleeding risk in patients taking aspirin. *Aliment Pharmacol Ther*. 2010. 32(7):831-839.

Laine, L. and McQuaid, K. R. Endoscopic therapy for bleeding ulcers: an evidence-based approach based on meta-analyses of randomized controlled trials. *Clin Gastroenterol Hepatol*. 2009. 7(1):33-47.

Wang, C. H., et al. High-dose vs non-high-dose proton pump inhibitors after endoscopic treatment in patients with bleeding peptic ulcer: a systematic review and meta-analysis of randomized controlled trials. *Arch Intern Med*. 2010. 170(9):751-758.

Guidelines and Consensus

American Society for Gastrointestinal Endoscopy. The role of endoscopy in the management of acute non-variceal upper GI bleeding. Gastrointestinal Endoscopy. 2012. 75(6): 1132-1138.

ASGE Standards of Practice Committee, et al. The role of endoscopy in the management of patients with peptic ulcer disease. *Gastrointest Endosc*. 2010. 1(4):663-668.

Bitar, K. N., et al. Tissue engineering in the gut: developments in neuromusculature. Gastroenterology. 2014. 146(7):1614-1624.

Upper Gastrointestinal Bleeding (UGIB)

Papers and Reviews

Laine, L. and Jensen, D. M. Management of patients with ulcer bleeding. *Am J Gastroenterol*. 2012. 107(3):345-360.

Kim, J. J., et al. Causes of bleeding and outcomes in patients hospitalized with upper gastrointestinal bleeding. *J Clin Gastroenterol*. 2014. 48(2):113-118.

Systemic Reviews and Meta-analysis

Chavez-Tapia, N. C., et al. Meta-analysis: antibiotic prophylaxis for cirrhotic patients with upper gastrointestinal bleeding - an updated Cochrane review. *Aliment Pharmacol Ther*. 2011. 34(5):509-518.

Guidelines and Consensus

Barkun, A. N., *et al*. International consensus recommendations on the management of patients with nonvariceal upper gastrointestinal bleeding. *Ann Intern Med*. 2010. 152(2):101-113.

Dworzynski, K., *et al*. Management of acute upper gastrointestinal bleeding: summary of NICE guidance. *BMJ*. 2012. 344.

Scottish Intercollegiate Guidelines Network. Management of acute upper and lower gastrointestinal bleeding: A national clinical guideline. http://www.sign.ac.uk/pdf/sign105.pdf.September 2008. Accessed March 10, 2015.

Gastrointestinal Bleeding (GIB)

Systemic Reviews and Meta-analysis

Raju, G. S., *et al*. American Gastroenterological Association (AGA) Institute technical review on obscure gastrointestinal bleeding. *Gastroenterology*. 2007. 133(5):1697-1717.

NSAID

Guidelines and Consensus

Lanza, F. L., *et al*. Guidelines for prevention of NSAID-related ulcer complications. *Am J Gastroenterol*. 2009. 104(3):728-738.

Rostom, A., *et al*. Canadian consensus guidelines on long-term nonsteroidal anti-inflammatory drug therapy and the need for gastroprotection: benefits versus risks. *Aliment Pharmacol Ther*. 2009. 29(5):481-496.

Gastric Antral Vascular Ectasia (GAVE)

Guidelines and Consensus

Swanson, E., *et al*. Medical and endoscopic therapies for angiodysplasia and gastric antral vascular ectasia: a systematic review. *Clin Gastroenterol Hepatol*. 2014. 12(4):571-582.

Stress-related Mucosal Disease

Papers and Reviews

Bardou, M., *et al*. Stress-related mucosal disease in the critically ill patient. *Nat Rev Gastroenterol Hepatol*. 2015. 12(2):98-107.

Polyps

Papers and Reviews

Goddard, A. F., *et al*. The management of gastric polyps. *Gut*. 2010. 59(9):1270-1276.

Shaib, Y. H., *et al*. Management of gastric polyps: an endoscopy-based approach. *Clin Gastroenterol Hepatol*. 2013. 11(11):1374-1384.

Tumors

Papers and Reviews

Crosby, D. A., *et al*. Gastric neuroendocrine tumours. *Dig Surg*. 2012. 29(4):331-348.

Shaib, Y. H., *et al*. Management of gastric polyps: an endoscopy-based approach. *Clin Gastroenterol Hepatol*. 2013. 11(11):1374-1384.

INDEX

Note: Page number followed by f and t indicates figure and table respectively.

A
Acetylcholine (Ach), 15–16, 16f
Ach. *See* Acetylcholine
Acid rebound, 33
Acupuncture, 163
Acute erosive gastritis (AEG)
   causes, 227
   vs. CG, 230t
   clinical, 227
   definition, 227
   endoscopy, 227
   histopathology, 227–228, 228f–229f
   treatment, 230, 230t
Adenocarcinomas, 406
   diagnostic imaging, 333–334
   vs. lymphoma, 335t
AEG. *See* Acute erosive gastritis
AIG. *See* Autoimmune gastritis
Allergic gastroenteropathy, 224, 390
Aluminocalcinosis. *See* Gastric mucosal calcinosis
AMAG. *See* Autoimmune metaplastic atrophic gastritis
Amyloid, 411
   definition, 412
   demography, 412
   diagnostic imaging of, 412
   differentiated diagnosis of, 412
   endoscopy, 413
   histopathology, 413, 414f–416f
   special studies, 417
ANS. *See* Autonomic nervous system
Antiemetics
   drug interactions of, 179t
   other drugs on effect of, 180t
   for treatment of nausea and vomiting, 179t–180t
Antral filling and pyloric pump
   body contractions, 165
   emptying, 166–169
   food–related factors, 164–165
   gastric narrowing, 169
   gastric scarring, causes of, 169
   physiological function, 164

Antral gastritis
  active, 225
  diffuse, 226, 226f
Antrum, 8–9, 9f
APS. See Autoimmune polyglandular syndrome
Atherosclerosis, 411, 411t
Autoimmune gastritis (AIG)
  vs. APS, 248t
  clinical, 246
  definition, 246
  demography, 246
  differential diagnosis, 247–248, 247t, 248t
  vs. EMAG, 247t
  endoscopy, 248, 248f
  histopathology, 249–250, 249f–250f
  laboratory, 246–247
  pathogenesis of, 246
Autoimmune metaplastic atrophic gastritis (AMAG), 203
Autoimmune polyglandular syndrome (APS), 248t
Autonomic nervous system (ANS), 146

B
BAO. See Basal acid output
Bariatric surgery
  benefits of, 124
  complications, 126–128
    biliopancreatic diversion, 128
    CNS, 126
    gastric banding, 128
    gastric bypass, 127
    gastroplasty, 127
    GI, 127
    lung, 126
    metabolic, 127
    surgical, 127
  diagnostic imaging
    afferent loop syndrome, 131
    bile reflux gastritis, 131
    jejunogastric intussusceptions, 131
    post-gastric surgery, 131
    stomal cancer, 131
    stomal (marginal) ulcer, 131
    thicknened folds, 132
  indications of, 124
  pathophysiology, 128–130

post-operative stomach, 128–136
  diarrhea, 129–130
  gastric stump cancer, 129
  iron deficiency, 128–129
  metabolic bone disease, 129
  non-nutritional complications of, 128
  peptic ulceration, 130, 130f
 treatment, 132–139
  anti-depressants for, 139
  antiepileptics for, 139
  cannabinoid–1 receptor antagonist for, 139
  diabetes-treating drugs, 139
  dietary supplements for, 139
  diethylpropion, 139
  disorders, lookout for, 133–134
  endoscopic, 134–136
  medications, 133
  nutrition, 132
  for obesity, 136–139, 137f
  Orlistat®, 138–139
  pharmaceuticals, 137
  phentermine, 139
  serotonin agonist, 138–139
  for weight loss, 137
 types of
  malabsorption–producing procedures, 124
  mixed procedures, 124–125
  restriction procedures, 124
  for weight loss, 125f
Basal acid output (BAO), 25, 38–39, 42
B-cell MALT lymphoma, 367
Benign gastric ulcer, 291–292
 causes, 292
 endoscopic findings, 295f–297f
 types, characteristics and pathological features, 292t–294t
Benign mesenchymal tumors, 376
Bupropion, 139
Burkitt's lymphoma
 clinical, 371
 definition, 371
 demography, 371
 endoscopy, 371
 genetics of, 371
 histopathology, 372
 special studies, 372
 treatment, 372

C

Calcitonin gene related peptide (CGRP), 15
Candidiasis
  definition, 252
  demography, 252
  differentials, 252
  endoscopy, 253, 253f
  histopathology, 254, 254f
Capsule endoscopy (CE), 109–110
Cardiac glands, 3
Carditis
  causes and associations, 220–221
  definition, 220
CE. *See* Capsule endoscopy
CG. *See* Chemical gastropathy
CGRP. *See* Calcitonin gene related peptide
Chemical gastropathy (CG), 230t
Chief (peptic) cells, 10t
Chronic atrophic gastritis of body, 233–234, 233f, 234f
Clear cell carcinoid tumor, 420
Clinical syndromes, 71t–72t
Collagenous gastritis
  clinical, 211
  definition, 210
  demography, 210
  diagnosis, 211
  differential, 210–211
  differential diagnosis, 212t
  endoscopy, 212
  histopathology, 213–215, 214f
  treatment, 215
Congestive gastropathies, 277
Crohn's disease, 262
Cytomegalovirus (CMV)
  clinical, 255
  definition, 255
  demography, 255
  differential diagnosis, 255, 256t
  endoscopy, 256
  histopathology, 256, 257f–258f
  vs. HSV, 256t

D

DBE. *See* Double balloon enteroscopy
DCAG. *See* Diffuse corporal atrophic gastritis
Diabetes, gastroparesis and
  abnormalities, 171
  demography, 170
  pathophysiological processes, 170–171
Diarrhea, 129–130
Diethylpropion, 139
Diffuse corporal atrophic gastritis (DCAG), 203, 234f
Diffuse large B-cell lymphoma (DLBCL), 368
  demography, 369, 370t
  vs. MALT, 370t
  pathology of, 370t
  terminology, 369
  treatment, 370t
Disseminated eosinophilic collagen disease, 390
Distention, 24
DLBCL. *See* Diffuse large B-cell lymphoma
DMN. *See* Dorsal motor nucleus
Dorsal motor nucleus (DMN), 15
Double balloon enteroscopy (DBE), 109
Dyspepsia
  clinical, 43–45
  definition, 43
  demography, 43
  diagnosis, 46t–47t, 47
  gastric radiological features in, 201
  NSAIDs and, 112
  and pregnancy
    demography, 50
    diagnosis, 50–51
    endoscopy in, 51
    treatment, 51
  treatment
    for acid inhibition with PPIs, 49–50
    empiric therapy, 48
    for gastric folds, 49
    test and investigate, 48–49
    test–and–treat (for H. pylori), 48
  types, 43

E

Early gastric cancer (EGC)

chemotherapy/chemoradiation for, 362
definition, 357
expanded criteria for treatment, 360–362
pathology of, 357–358, 357t, 358t
treatment, 358–360
EGC. *See* Early gastric cancer
EHT. *See* Endoscopic hemostatic therapy
EMAG. *See* Environmental multifocal atrophic gastritis
Endocrine cells, 10t
Endocrine heterotopia, 406
Endoscopic hemostatic therapy (EHT)
  for bleeding peptic ulcer, 98
ENS. *See* Enteric nervous system
Enteric nervous system (ENS), 145, 146
Enterochromaffin cells (EC), 4t
Enterochromaffin-like (ECL) cells, 4t
Enterogastric reflux gastritis
  diagnosis of, 235, 235f
  endoscopy, 236f–238f
  pathophysiology, 235
Enterogastrones, 28–29
Environmental multifocal atrophic gastritis (EMAG), 203
  vs. AMAG, 247t
Eosinophilic collagen disease
  clinical, 225
  demography, 224
  histopathology, 224
  prognosis, 225
Eosinophilic gastritis
  clinical, 383
  complication of, 384
  definition, 382
  demography, 382
  diagnosis of, 384
  diagnostic imaging of, 383, 386
  differential diagnosis, 384–386
  endoscopy, 387
  histopathology, 387–388, 388f
  laboratory, 383
  pathology of, 386
  treatment, 389
Eosinophilic gastroenteritis (EG), 376
  vs. hypereosinophilic syndrome (HES), 389t

F

Fasting basal gastric acid secretion, 24–25
Fluoxetine, 139
Follicular lymphoma, 368
Forrest endoscopic classification of bleeding gastroduodenal ulcers, 86–87
Foveolar cell cytoplasm, 8
Fundic gland polyp
  associations with, 299
  clinical, 298
  definition, 298
  demography, 298
  differential diagnosis, 300
  dysplasia and cancer, progression to, 300
  endoscopy, 300, 301f
  histopathology, 302–304, 303f–304f
  pathogenesis of non-FAP, 298
  special studies, 305
  types of, 299, 299t

G

Gastric acid secretion, 14–42
  AA in stomach, 24
  acetylcholine, 15–16, 16f
  acid rebound, 33
  acute pathways, 17
  cephalic and gastric phases of, 27t
  chronic pathways, 18
  direct, 29
  distention, 24
  enterogastrones, 28–29
  fasting basal, 24–25
  gastric inhibitory peptide, 28
  gastrin, 16–17
  GI peptides, 24
  histamine, 19
  hormonal ("indirect") pathway, 18–19, 18f
  hormones, 14
  indirect, 29
  intestinal phase of, 28
  parietal cells, 14
  pharmaceutical control of, 33–35
  prostaglandin E2 (PGE2), 28
  prostaglandins, 23
  secretin, 28

secretory cells, 14
somatostatin, 20–22, 20f
stimulated, 26
  calcium, 26
  HCl secretion, 26
  hormonal (indirect) pathway, 26
  neurocrine (direct) pathway, 26, 26f
  paracrine pathway, 26
Gastric adenocarcinoma
  Benign vs. malignant gastric ulcer, 353t
  causes and associations, 330
  classification, 329, 329t
  clinical, 327–328, 328f
  demography, 326
  diagnosis of, 333
  diagnostic imaging
    adenocarcinoma, 333–334
    lymphoma, 335
    metastatic gastric cancer, 334
    non-neoplastic gastric filling defects, 335–336, 336f
  endoscopy, 340–342, 340f, 342f–344f, 342t
  genetics, 332–333
  histopathology, 344, 344f–347f, 346–352, 347t, 350f–351f, 352t
  intestinal– vs. diffuse–type of gastric cancer, 327t
  Laurén classification of, 348, 352, 352t
  metastasis of gastric cancer, sites for, 328, 328f
  pathological conditions with gastric cancer, 327
  pathological types (Lauren classification), 326t, 327t
  pathology of, 337–340, 338t, 340t
  prevention of gastric cancer, 354
  prognosis of, 356
  risk factors of
    non-reversible, 331
    reversible, 330
  risk of gastric polyp progression to, 338t
  sites for metastatic, 349f
  special studies, 353
  treatment of, 354–356
  World Health Organization (WHO) classification system, 348
Gastric adenomas
  definition, 313
  demography, 313
  differential diagnosis, 314
  endoscopy, 314, 315f–316f
  histopathology, 316, 316t
  pathogenesis, 314

types, 314, 338–339
Gastric amyloid, 411
  definition, 412
  demography, 412
  diagnostic imaging of, 412
  differentiated diagnosis of, 412
  endoscopy, 413
  histopathology, 413, 414f–416f
  special studies, 417
Gastric anatomy, 3
  diagnostic imaging, 4, 4f
  endoscopy, 5, 5t
  enterochromaffin cells vs. enterochromaffin–like cells, 4t
  gastric glands
    cardiac glands, 3
    parietal glands (oxyntic/fundic) glands, 3
    pyloric (antral) glands, 4
  general comments, 6–7
  goblet cells, 7–11
  histopathology, 6, 6f
Gastric antral vascular ectasia (GAVE), 110, 111t
  clinical, 192
  definition, 191
  demography, 191
  endoscopy, 193, 193f
  histopathology, 193–194, 194f
  liver transplantation for, 183
  vs. PHG, 192t
Gastric conditions
  Crohn's disease, 418
  diverticulum, 418
  duodenal tumors, 419
  emphysematous gastritis, 419
  miscellaneous, 418
  partial gastric diverticum, 419
  tortion, 419
  varices, 418
Gastric dieulafoy lesion
  definition, 190
  demography, 190
  endoscopy, 190, 191f
  treatment, 191
Gastric electrical therapy, 163
Gastric emptying
  background, 140
  causes and associations, 156–157

clinical, 157–158
definition, 140
diagnosis, 159
factors alternating rate of
  body mass index, 169
  CCK and ileal break, 168
  food, 167
  gastric narrowing, 169
  glucagon–like polypeptide–1 (GLP–1), 168
  hormones, 167, 168
  motility–related factors, 167, 168
of food and fluids, 150–151
modulation of rate of, 152–154, 153f, 166–167
pathophysiology of, 143–156
  autonomic nervous system, 146
  enteric nervous system, 145–146
  GI peptides, 149
  ICC (pacemaker cells), 146–147
  migrating myoelectrical complex, 147–148
  parasympathetic nervous system, 145
  peristaltic reflex, 145–146
  smooth muscle cells, 143–144, 144t
  sympathetic nervous system, 145, 146–147
process of, 141–143, 143f
treatment for, 159–163
Gastric epithelial dysplasia (GED)
  architecture, 223t
  cells, 223t
  definition, 221
  demography, 221
  differential diagnosis, 223
  endoscopy, 222
  histopathology, 222, 223t
  risk factors of, 221
Gastric foveolar adenoma
  differentials, 324
  endoscopy, 325
  histopathology, 325, 325f
Gastric function, 11
Gastric inhibitory peptide (GIP), 28
Gastric lymphoma
  causes and associations of, 363
  clinical features of, 363
  differential diagnosis, 363
  endoscopy, 364f–365f
  histopathology, 365, 366f

types, 363
Gastric MALT lymphoma
  causes and associations, 367
  chromosomal translocations in, 367
  definition, 367
  differential, 367–368
  endoscopy, 368
  genetics, 367
  histopathology, 368–369
  special studies, 369
  two cell populations in, 369
Gastric mucosal calcinosis (GMC), 280
Gastric pathology, immunohistochemistry (immunostains) for diagnosis of, 11–13
  immunostaining of gastric tumors, 13t
  stains, 12–13
Gastric polyps
  causes and associations, 284
  classification, 281–282
  clinical, 284
  demography, 281
  diagnostic imaging of gastric cancer, 285–288, 285f–286f
    Carman meniscus sign, 287
    converging folds, 287
    infiltrative scirrhous tumor, 287
    lymphoma, 288, 289f
    metastatic gastric cancer, 288
    ulcer, 287
  differential diagnosis, 289–290, 290f
  filling defects, 291
  HFoP, 283
  HFuP, 283
  pathology
    benign gastric ulcer, 291–297
    fundic gland polyp, 298–305
    gastric neuroendocrine tumors, 305–313
  tumor–like lesion, 283
Gastric stump cancer, 129
Gastric varices (GV)
  endoscopy, 184–185, 184f–185f
  to glue/band, 182
  primary prophylaxis, 183–184, 183t
  SARIN classification of, 182
Gastric vascular ectasia (GVE), 183
  liver transplantation for, 183
Gastric xanthomas (xanthelasmas), 420

Gastrin, 16–17
Gastritis
  acute erosive/hemorrhagic, 227–230
  allergic gastroenteropathy, 224
  AMAG, 203
  antral
    active, 225
    diffuse, 226, 226f
  autoimmune, 246–250
  Candidiasis, 252–254
  carditis and
    causes and associations, 220–221
    definition, 220
  causes of, 196–197
  chronic
    endoscopy, 231f
    histopathology, 231–232, 231f–232f
  chronic atrophic gastritis of body, 233–234, 233f, 233f–234f
  CMV, 252, 255–258
  collagenous gastritis
    clinical, 211
    definition, 210
    demography, 210
    diagnosis, 211
    differential, 210–211
    differential diagnosis, 212t
    endoscopy, 212
    histopathology, 213–215, 214f
    treatment, 215
  cystica polyposa, 251
  DCAG, 203
  diagnostic imaging, 201
  EMAG, 203
  enterogastric reflux gastritis, 235–238
  eosinophilic collagen disease, 224–225
  and gastropathies, 215
    diagnostic imaging, 215–216
    endoscopy, 216, 216f
  GCP, 215
  GED, 221–223
  granulomatous, 260–263
  Helicobacter pylori–associated, 239–245
  HSV, 252
  hypereosinophilic syndrome, 225
  infections, causes of, 252
  lymphocytic, 210, 264–268

lymphoid hyperplasia, chronic antral gastritis with, 225
mycobacterial, 259, 259t
NSAIDs and, 113, 114
  endoscopy, 217, 217f–218f
  histopathology, 218, 219f
  pathophysiology, 217
pathological types
  H. pylori gastritis, 198, 198f
  patterns of gastritis, 199t–200t
pathology, 201f–202f
phlegmonous gastritis, 204
  clinical, 204
  endoscopy, 204f–208f
  histopathology, 208, 209f
suppurative (phlegmonous), 259
terminology, 195
type A, 203
types of, 195t, 196
Gastritis cystica glandular (GCG), 324
Gastritis cystica polyposa, 251
Gastritis cystica profunda (GCP), 215
Gastritis cytica polyposa
  clinical features, 319
  definition, 319
  demography, 319
  diagnostic imaging of, 319
  endoscopy, 319
  histopathology, 319–320
Gastroenteropathy, 224
Gastroesophageal varices (GEV)
  SARIN classification of, 182
Gastrointestinal stromal tumors (GIST)
  diagnosis of, 391, 392t
  endoscopy, 393–394
  genetics of, 391
  histopathology, 394f–395f
  vs. leimyomas (LM) *vs.* leimyosarcomas (LMS), 391, 392t
  markers for, 392–393
  pathology, 392
  prognosis of, 403, 404t
  treatment
    imatinib, 400–401
    imatinib response in CD117-positive GIST tumors, 399
    PDGFRA-positive, 399–400
    pharmacological, 396, 396t
    sorafenib, 403

sunitinib, 402
surgery, 396–397
tyrosine kinase inhibitors, 398–399
Gastroparesis
  background, 140
  causes and associations, 156–157
  clinical, 157–158
  definition, 140
  diabetes and
    abnormalities, 171
    demography, 170
    pathophysiological processes, 170–171
  pathophysiological defects and pharmaceutical approach in diabetic, 156t
  pathophysiology of, 143–156
    autonomic nervous system, 146
    enteric nervous system, 145–146
    GI peptides, 149
    ICC (pacemaker cells), 146–147
    migrating myoelectrical complex, 147–148
    parasympathetic nervous system, 145
    peristaltic reflex, 145–146
    smooth muscle cells, 143–144, 144t
    sympathetic nervous system, 145
  prokinetic drugs for, 161–162
  treatment for, 159–163
  with type I diabetes, 155
Gastropathies, 215
  congestive, 277
  diagnostic imaging, 215–216
  endoscopy, 216, 216f
  gastric folds and, 269–270
    diagnostic imaging, 270, 270f
    differentials, 270
    histopathology, 271, 271f
    Ménétrier's disease, 271–276
  hypertrophic, 277–279
GAVE. *See* Gastric antral vascular ectasia
GCG. *See* Gastritis cystica glandular
GCP. *See* Gastritis cystica profunda
GED. *See* Gastric epithelial dysplasia
GEV. *See* Gastroesophageal varices
GIP. *See* Gastric inhibitory peptide
GIST. *See* Gastrointestinal stromal tumors
GMC. *See* Gastric mucosal calcinosis
Granulomatous gastritis
  antrum, 262, 262f–263f

causes, 260
Crohn's disease and, 262
definition, 260
endoscopy, 261
histopathology, 261–262
Gut endocrine tumors, clinical syndromes of, 71t–72t
GV. *See* Gastric varices
GVE. *See* Gastric vascular ectasia

H

Helicobacter heilmannii, 241
Helicobacter pylori gastritis (HPG), 198, 198f
  clinical, 239–240
  complications of, 240
  definition, 239
  demography, 239
  differential diagnosis, 241
  endoscopy, 242
  histopathology, 242–243, 244f–245f
  lymphoid hyperplasia *vs.* gastric MALT lymphoma, 240t
  pathogenesis of, 239
  tests for, 241t–242t
Helicobacter pylori infection, 7
  carcinogenesis from, 339
  and negative peptic ulcer disease
    clinical, 67, 67t
    demography, 67
    diagnosis, 68
  and peptic ulcer disease
    causes and associations, 58–59
    demography, 51–53
    diagnosis, 61
      performance characteristics of tests for, 62f, 62t
      tests for, 61
    gastric acid secretion and, 54
    histopathology, 63, 63f
    laboratory, 59–61
    pathophysiology, 54–58
    risk of carcinogenesis from, 58
    treatment, 63–67
  and positive peptic ulcer disease
    differential diagnoses for, 69–70
    pathophysiology, 68–69
    treatment, 70–71
HES. *See* Hypereosinophilic syndrome

HFoP. *See* Hyperplastic foveolar polyp
HFuP. *See* Hyperplastic fundic polyp
HHG. *See* Hyperplastic hypersecretory gastropathy
Histamine, 19
HP. *See* Hyperplastic polyps
HPG. *See Helicobacter pylori* gastritis
Hypereosinophilic syndrome (HES), 225, 390–391
  vs. eosinophilic gastroenteritis (EG), 389t
Hypergastrinemia, 35–39
  diagnostic imaging, 37–39
  endoscopy, 37
  laboratory tests, 36
  overview, 35–36
Hyperplastic foveolar polyp (HFoP), 283
Hyperplastic fundic polyp (HFuP), 283
Hyperplastic hypersecretory gastropathy (HHG), 269
Hyperplastic polyps (HP), 269–270
  clinical, 320–321
  definition, 320
  demography, 320
  differential diagnosis, 321
  endoscopy, 321
  histopathology, 322, 323f
  pathophysiology of, 320
  special studies, 324
  treatment, 324
Hypertrophic gastropathies
  clinical, 277
  definition, 277
  demography, 277
  diagnostic imaging, 278
  endoscopy, 278, 278f
  histopathology, 278–279
  laboratory, 278

I
IFP. *See* Inflammatory fibroid polyps
IGV. *See* Isolated gastric varices
Inflammatory fibroid polyps (IFP), 376
  clinical, 379
  definition, 378
  demography, 378
  endoscopy, 379
  histopathology, 379–380, 380f–382f
  pathogenesis of, 378

special studies, 382
Ischemic gastritis, 411
Isolated gastric varices (IGV), SARIN classification of, 182

J
Jejunogastric intussusceptions, 131

L
Leiomyoma, 404–405
  differential diagnosis, 404–405
  histopathology, 404f
Lorcaserin, 138–139
Lymphocytic gastritis, 210, 215, 240, 363, 368
  clinical, 264
  definition, 264
  demography, 264
  diagnostic imaging, 264
  differentials, 264
  endoscopic and histological changes in, 268
  endoscopy, 265
  histopathology, 265, 266f–267f
  strains, 268t
Lymphoid hyperplasia, chronic antral gastritis with, 225
Lymphoma
  vs. adenocarcinoma, 335t
  diagnostic imaging, 335
  gastric
    causes and associations of, 363
    clinical features of, 363
    differential diagnosis, 363
    endoscopy, 364f–365f
    histopathology, 365, 366f
    types, 363
  gastric MALT
    causes and associations, 367
    chromosomal translocations in, 367
    definition, 367
    differential, 367–368
    endoscopy, 368
    genetics, 367
    histopathology, 368–369
    special studies, 369
    two cell populations in, 369

M

MAI infection, 420
MALT. *See* Mucosa associated lymphoid tumors
MAO. *See* Maximal acid output
Maximal acid output (MAO), 25, 38–39, 42
MD. *See* Ménétrier's disease
Meckel scan, 110
MEN-1. *See* Multiple endocrine neoplasia-type I
Ménétrier's disease (MD), 220, 269
  causes and associations, 271
  clinical, 272
  definition, 271
  demography, 271
  diagnostic imaging, 274
  differential diagnosis, 273–274, 274t
  endoscopy, 275, 275f
  histopathology, 276, 276f
  laboratory, 272
  pathophysiology, 272
  risk factors, 272
Metabolic bone disease, 129
Metaplastic cancer, 407f
Metformin, 139
Migrating myoelectrical complex (MMC), 147–148
MMC. *See* Migrating myoelectrical complex
Mucosa associated lymphoid tumors (MALT), 68
  gastric lymphoma
    causes and associations, 367
    chromosomal translocations in, 367
    definition, 367
    differential, 367–368
    endoscopy, 368
    genetics, 367
    histopathology, 368–369
    special studies, 369
    two cell populations in, 369
  lymphoma with *H. pylori*, 240
Mucous neck cells, 8, 10t
Mucus, 25
Multifocal atrophic gastritis, 234f
Multiple endocrine neoplasia-type I (MEN-1)
  biochemical screening program for, 76
  end genetics of, 277
  gastrinomas *vs.* sporadic gastrinomas, 77t

tumors in patients with, 76t
Mycobacterial gastritis, 259, 259t

N
Nausea and vomiting
  causes of, 172
  definition, 172
  in newborn, differential diagnosis, 174
  pathophysiology, 172
  post–operative
    mechanisms, 173
    methods to reduce risk of, 174
    risk factors for, 173
  treatment, 175–180
    antiemetics for, 179, 179t–180t
    during breastfeeding, 180–181, 181t
    causes and classes of medication, 175t–176t
    drugs, 176–177
    during pregnancy, 177–178, 178t, 180–181, 181t
    prolong QTc and/or PR interval, 179
NET. *See* Neuroendocrine tumors
Neuroendocrine tumors (NET)
  classification, 306–307
  clinical, 307
  definition, 305
  demography, 305, 305t–306t
  differential diagnosis, 307, 308t
  endoscopy, 308, 309f
  vs. glomus tumor, 308t
  histopathology, 309–310, 310f–311f
  immunostains to diagnose benign mesenchymal tumors, 312t
  prognosis, 313t
  special studies, 311
  synthetic somatostatin and octreotide in human GI tract, 312–313
  WHO types of, 308t
Non–steroidal anti–inflammatory drugs (NSAIDs)
  antiplatelet drugs and, 121
  dyspepsia and, 112
  effects of, 112t–113t
  endoscopy, 123f
  gastritis, 113, 114
  and gastroprotection, 114–116
  GI toxicity, 113
  pathophysiology of, 112
  prevention, 121, 122t, 123

risk stratification, 116–119
    COXIBs, 119
    H. pylori, 119–120
    of high dose, 119t
    ulcer, 116t–117t
    with upper gastrointestinal clinical events, 117t, 118
  scoring system for, 113
  summary, 120–121
  upper GI tract and, 113–114
Non-variceal upper GI bleeding (NVUGIB). *See also* Upper GI bleeding (UGIB)
  causes and associations, 81f, 82
  clinical, 80–81, 86
  demography, 80
  diagnosis of, 83t
  diagnostic imaging, 87f–89f
  Forrest endoscopic classification of bleeding gastroduodenal ulcers, 86–87
  hypotension and prognosis, 85t
  pathology, 89, 90f–95f
  persistent/recurrent, risk of
    clinical, 100–102
    treatment, 102–103, 103t
  prognosis
    predictors of poor outcome, 98
    Rockall Risk Score Scheme, 99t–100t
    variables, 99
  risk
    initial bleeding, stratification of, 83t, 84t
    for ulcers and bleeding, 84t
  treatment
    chronic liver disease, 96
    endoscopic hemostatic therapy, 96t, 97, 97t, 98
  volume depletion estimation, clinical methods to, 85t
NSAIDs. *See* Non-steroidal anti-inflammatory drugs
NVUGIB. *See* Non-variceal upper GI bleeding

O

Obesity, 136, 137f
Obscure GI bleeding
  angiography, 110
  capsule endoscopy, 109–110
  CT enterography, 110
  demography, 107
  diagnostic imaging, 107–108
  EGD/colonoscopy, 109

findings and treatments, 111t
Meckel scan, 110
RBC scan, 110
small bowel endoscopy, 109
Orlistat®, 138–139

P
Pancreatic acinar cell metaplasia, 408
Pancreatic acinar metaplasia, 406
Pancreatic heterotopia, 406
  clinical, 408
  definition, 407
  demography of, 407
  differentials, 408
  endoscopy, 409
  histopathology, 409–410
  special studies, 410
Paneth cell metaplasia, 408, 410f
Parasitic infection, 376
Parasympathetic nervous system (PNS), 145
Parietal cells
  cellular acid secretion, 30–32, 31f
  gastric acid secretion, 14
  gastric hydrochloric acid secretion, 29–32
    components of, 30t
    requirements of system, 30
Parietal glands (oxyntic/fundic) glands, 3
Parietal (oxyntic) cells, 10t
Pepsin
  autoactivation of, 40–41
  BAO / MAO vs., 42
  biochemistry, 39
  physiology, 39–40
  secretion of, 41–42
Pepsinogen
  autoactivation of, 40–41
  biochemistry, 39
  physiology, 39–40
  secretion of, 41–42
Peptic ulcer
  clinical, 86
  endoscopy, 86
  laboratory, 86
Peristaltic reflex, 145–146
Peutz-Jeghers polyps, 324

PRACTICE REVIEW
GASTROENTEROLOGY

© *A.B.R. Thomson*

Pharmaceutical control, of acid secretion, 33–35
Phentermine, 139
PHG. *See* Portal hypertensive gastropathy
Phlegmonous gastritis, 204
  clinical, 204
  endoscopy, 204f–208f
  histopathology, 208, 209f
PNS. *See* Parasympathetic nervous system
Polyposis syndromes, 318, 318f
PONV. *See* Post-operative nausea and vomiting
Portal hypertensive gastropathy (PHG), 110, 111t
  definition, 185
  endoscopy, 185, 186f–187f
  vs. GAVE, 192t
  histopathology, 188–189, 188f–189f
  liver transplantation for, 183
  pathogenesis of, 185
  treatment, 190
Post-operative nausea and vomiting (PONV)
  mechanisms, 173
  methods to reduce risk of, 174
  risk factors for, 173
PPIs. *See* Proton pump inhibitors
Pregnancy
  and dyspepsia
    demography, 50
    diagnosis, 50–51
    endoscopy in, 51
    treatment, 51
  nausea and vomiting during, 177–178, 178t, 180–181, 181t
Prostaglandin E2 (PGE2), 28
Prostaglandins, 23
Proton pump inhibitors (PPIs), 33–35, 34f
Pyloric (antral) glands, 4
Pyloric gland adenomas
  definition, 317
  demography, 317
  differential diagnosis, 317
  endoscopy, 317
  histopathology, 317–318
  pathogenesis of, 317
  special studies, 318
Pyloric pump and antral filling
  body contractions, 165
  emptying, 166–169
  food–related factors, 164–165

gastric narrowing, 169
gastric scarring, causes of, 169
physiological function, 164

R
Roux-en-Y stasis syndrome, 126, 171

S
SBE. *See* Single balloon enteroscopy
Secretin, 28
Serotonin agonist, 138–139
Signet ring cells, 7
  carcinoma, 420, 427, 427f
Single balloon enteroscopy (SBE), 109
Smooth muscle cells, 143–144
  electrophysiology of, 144t
SNS. *See* Sympathetic nervous system
Somatostatin (SST), 15, 20–22, 20f
Sorafenib, 403–404, 404t
Sporadic *vs.* familial fundic gland polyposis, 299t
SST. *See* Somatostatin
Stomach
  AA in, 24
  cells and functions of, 10t
  gastric
    acid secretion, 14–42
    anatomy, 3–11
    function, 11
    pathology, immunohistochemistry (immunostains) for diagnosis of, 11–13
  primary tumors to, 357f
  trefoil factors, physiological effects of, 11
Stromal tumors and tissue eosinophils
  allergic gastroenteropathy, 390
  disseminated eosinophilic collagen disease, 390
  endoscopic diagnosis, 378
  eosinophilic gastritis, 382–389
  gastrointestinal stromal tumors, 391–401
  genetic mutations, 377–378
  GIST, markers for, 377
  hypereosinophilic syndrome, 390–391
  inflammatory fibroid polyps, 378–382
  leiomyoma, 404–405
  pathology of, 376–377

sorafenib, 403–404
sunitinib, 402
types, 376
Sunitinib, 402
Superficial epithelial cells, 10t
Suppurative (phlegmonous) gastritis, 259
Sympathetic nervous system (SNS), 145
Systemic sclerosis, 411

T
Trefoil factors, physiological effects of, 11
Type A gastritis, 203
Type1 diabetics, 171

U
UGIB. See Upper GI bleeding
Upper GI bleeding (UGIB), 104–106

V
Vascular lesions
  gastric antral vascular ectasia (GAVE), 191–194
  gastric dieulafoy lesion, 190–191
  gastric varices (GV), 182–185
  portal hypertension gastropathy (PHG), 185–190
Vasoactive intestinal peptide (VIP), 15
VIP. See Vasoactive intestinal peptide
Vomiting and nausea
  causes of, 172
  definition, 172
  in newborn, differential diagnosis, 174
  pathophysiology, 172
  post–operative
    mechanisms, 173
    methods to reduce risk of, 174
    risk factors for, 173
  treatment, 175–180
    antiemetics for, 179, 179t–180t
    during breastfeeding, 180–181, 181t
    causes and classes of medication, 175t–176t
    drugs, 176–177
    during pregnancy, 177–178, 178t, 180–181, 181t
    prolong QTc and/or PR interval, 179

W
Weight loss, 137
Wharton, 7
Whipple's disease, 420

X
Xanthomas
  causes and associations, 421
  clinical, 421
  definition, 420
  demography, 420
  differential diagnosis, 421–422, 422t
  endoscopy, 422
  histopathology, 422–423, 423f–426f
  special studies, 426

Z
ZES. *See* Zollinger-Ellison syndrome
Zollinger-Ellison syndrome (ZES), 25, 132, 269
  clinical features of, 72–73
  diagnostic imaging, 75
  endoscopy, 74
  gastric hypersecretion and, 78
  gastrin triangle, 73, 73f
  laboratory tests, 74
  malabsorption in, 75–76
  pathology of, 76t–77t
  provocative tests, 74
  secretin-stimulated gastrin test in, 79
  treatment, 77–79
Zymogens, 39

www.ingramcontent.com/pod-product-compliance
Lightning Source LLC
Chambersburg PA
CBHW071409180526
45170CB00001B/23